# ❖ Primary Care of Women and Children with HIV Infection

# Jones and Bartlett Books on Oncology and HIV-Related Illnesses

# ❖ Primary Care of Women and Children with HIV Infection
## A Multidisciplinary Approach

*Edited by*

Patricia Kelly

Susan Holman

Rosalie Rothenberg

Stephen Paul Holzemer

**Jones and Bartlett Publishers**
**Boston**            **London**

*Editorial, Sales, and Customer Service Offices*
Jones and Bartlett Publishers
One Exeter Plaza
Boston, MA 02116
1-800-832-0034
617-859-3900

Jones and Bartlett Publishers International
7 Melrose Terrace
London W6 7RL
England

**Library of Congress Cataloging-in-Publication Data**
Primary care of women and children with HIV infection : a
   multidisciplinary approach / edited by Patricia Kelly . . . [et al.].
      p.   cm. -- (Jones and Bartlett series in oncology and HIV-
related illnessess)
   Includes bibliographical references and index.
   ISBN  0-86720-709-4
   1. AIDS (Disease)  2. Women--Diseases.  3. AIDS (Disease) in
children.  4. HIV infections.  5. Primary care (Medicine)
I. Kelly, Patricia. MS.  II. Series
   [DNLM:  1.  HIV infections--prevention & control.  2.  HIV
Infections--in infancy & childhood.  3.  Primary Health Care.
4. Women's Health Services.     WD 308 P9518 1995]
RA644.A25P757   1995
362. 1 ' 969792 ' 0082--dc20
DNLM/DLC
for Library of Congress                    94-34337
                                    CIP

Printed in the United States of America
98  97  96  95        10  9  8  7  6  5  4  3  2

*This book is dedicated to*

*the families affected by HIV with whom
we have had the privilege to work*

*and to*

*Henry Paquin.*

# ❖ Contents

# ❖ Foreword

No longer members of an "invisible epidemic" (Corea, 1992), women today are becoming infected with the human immunodeficiency virus (HIV) in unprecedented numbers. Worldwide, developing countries have as many infected women as men, industrialized countries are quickly catching up, and the epidemic in children is paralleling that of women.

In the United States, it has taken us until the second decade of the epidemic to recognize women's vulnerability to HIV and to acknowledge its unique disease manifestations. Our main educators have been women living with HIV, their advocates, and a few clinicians. They have provided us with the information, demanded the service programs, and collaborated with the research. Their efforts have increased our understanding of the interrelationships between the manifestations of HIV disease, women's lives and their coping and healing strategies. Their efforts have moved us away from viewing women as merely the "vectors" of HIV infection to men and unborn children. Finally, their efforts have reminded us of women's intrinsic worth and the indispensable role they play as caretakers of children and other family members, even when they themselves are critically ill.

Care of HIV-infected people has spread beyond the venue of infectious disease specialists. It is now firmly established in the primary care practices of all communities. As a result, primary care clinicians throughout the United States have a special need and responsibility to become competent in the prevention and management of HIV disease among women and children. These clinicians are uniquely able to provide a broad range of health care services for patients, not just HIV-related medical care. They already recognize that to work effectively with any community of patients they must offer care that is accessible and close to the community; comprehensive, spanning prevention and early diagnosis to rehabilitation; continuous, offering stable relationships with patients and providers; coordinated, ensuring families the best use of their time and resources; and accountable, so that patients can demand and professionals can ensure high-quality services. Quality HIV care depends on an open dialogue with colleagues from all health care disciplines and with patients and activists.

The contributors to this book are not only experienced providers and researchers, but also advocates who have listened and learned throughout the epidemic. From the women and children living with HIV, they learned of their needs, hopes, fears, and concerns. In each chapter, the authors share special knowledge of HIV disease, keeping us centered on the needs of women and children. The book's framework integrates practice, politics, and caring, which clinicians, advocates, and policymakers can utilize in their day-to-day work.

We must confront crucial issues in this next decade of the HIV epidemic. The complexity of women's social roles has shaped their choices in self-care, reproductive health, and relationships to partners, all of which are essential to preventing the epidemic's spread. HIV-specific education and early intervention programs for both sexes must focus on modifying the behaviors of substance abuse, sexuality, and violence. However, truly effective prevention will require the improvement of the social and economic status of women and children. The spread of HIV has been facilitated by poverty and by women's powerlessness in negotiating sexual relations. Women are learning that empowerment that excludes economic, political, cultural, and social advancement leaves them with few tangible resources. If our society is to succeed in halting the HIV epidemic, real steps must simultaneously be taken toward achieving women's true equality.

Helen Rodriguez-Trias, MD, MPH, FAAP

## Reference

Corea, G. (1992). *The invisible epidemic: The story of women and AIDS.* New York: Harper Collins.

# ❖ Introduction

Women and children represent a rapidly growing population of persons with HIV infection. AIDS is already one of the leading causes of death among young women in the United States. Based on identified trends, HIV disease in women and children is expected to emerge as a significant health problem in many new areas of the United States over the next decade. Because primary care settings provide most of the health care for both women and children, primary care professionals will play an increasingly critical role in HIV-related care for these families. As the HIV epidemic spreads throughout the United States, there is a need for a comprehensive reference that addresses the questions and knowledge needs of providers in primary care settings throughout the United States. This book is intended to offer the benefits of the experience and expertise of health professionals who have been caring for women and children in high-prevalence areas.

This book seeks to fill the void in the literature by addressing the comprehensive health care needs of both women and children with HIV infection, and it does so from a multidisciplinary perspective. Using a care focus that spans early to late disease, each chapter discusses a topic found to be most relevant to women and children. The contributors were selected from a wide range of disciplines, including medicine, nursing, social work, anthropology, and epidemiology. They have been active in the care and research of families with HIV disease since early in the epidemic. This book is directed to all health care practitioners who provide care to women and children with HIV infection—physicians, nurses, midwives, social workers, counselors, and chaplains. We also hope that administrators and program planners will find this a valuable resource. This book can be used by health care providers who are currently working in their respective fields as well as by students of these disciplines.

Chapter 1, "The Voices of Women with HIV Infection," written by anthropologist Patricia Antoniello, reveals intimate facets of the lives of women with HIV infection. Important emerging themes for these women are the discovery of HIV-positive status, pregnancy and the importance of children, interactions with the health care system, living with HIV, and empowerment.

In chapter 2, "HIV Disease in the Primary Care Setting," Mardge Cohen and Patricia Kelly delineate the philosophy and essential features of programs of comprehensive health services in the primary care setting for women and children infected with HIV. Together, chapters 1 and 2 define the client-centered, multidisciplinary framework on which HIV services are ideally based.

Three chapters focus specifically on HIV disease in women. First, the epidemiology and natural history of HIV in women is discussed in chapter 3 by Sheldon Landesman and Susan Holman. In chapter 4, "Care of Women with HIV Disease," by Catherine Lyons and Jack DeHovitz, current approaches to the primary health care of women with HIV, including gynecologic and medical management, are described. Ann Kurth and Howard Minkoff then address the reproductive issues of women with HIV infection, including pregnancy, contraception, and reproductive decision making in chapter 5.

The epidemiology, natural history, and state-of-the-art care of children and adolescents with HIV infection are presented in the next three chapters. In chapter 6, "Epidemiology and Natural History of HIV Infection in Children," Robert Simonds and Margaret Oxtoby outline the major issues of the HIV epidemic in children. In chapter 7, "Care of Children with HIV Infection," Mary Jo O'Hara discusses the comprehensive pediatric care of HIV-exposed and HIV-infected children. Unique adaptations of care for adolescents are examined in chapter 8, "Adolescents and HIV," by Judy Cohn and Donna Futterman.

The psychosocial, supportive counseling, and educational aspects of health care are of great importance to the lives of women and children with HIV infection. Chapter 9, "HIV Counseling and Testing for Women," by Susan Holman and Ann Kurth, provides readers with a comprehensive discussion of the essential components of HIV counseling and testing.

The major stages of adaptation and related psychosocial issues faced by families throughout the HIV disease spectrum are discussed by Judy Weaver Mason, Joyce Preisinger, and Sister Mary Donohue in chapter 10.

The economic and cultural gap between providers and most of the women and children affected by HIV cannot be ignored if primary care providers are to offer appropriate care and treatment. In chapter 11, "Cultural Sensitivity," Joanne Bradley describes the impact of these cultural factors on families with HIV and suggests strategies for bridging the gap.

In chapter 12, "Continuity of Care," Stephen Paul Holzemer, Rosalie Rothenberg, and Carolyn Fish discuss the variety of settings available for the delivery of care to families with HIV infection and their changing nature through the illness continuum. They explore strategies for facilitating the transition of care, accessing supports and resources for home care, and identifying alternative sources of care.

Belief in the mind-body connection and use of a variety of alternative health care practices sustain many patients with HIV disease. In chapter 13, "Complementary Therapies," Ana Oliveira and Rae Crowe outline the therapies used most often by women with HIV infection.

Substance abuse, including alcoholism, affects many families dealing with HIV infection. Ann Williams and Patrick O'Connor highlight many of the issues raised by substance abuse in chapter 14. These include the effect on families, special concerns for women, and the impact on primary health care.

Michele Russell discusses HIV disease among lesbians in chapter 15, a topic that has been largely overlooked in the professional literature. Her contribution outlines how primary care providers can demonstrate greater sensitivity to lesbians and bisexual women and discusses issues of concern for this group of women, including HIV transmission risks and safer sex strategies.

In chapter 16, "Ethical, Legal, and Policy Considerations," Elizabeth Cooper and Kathleen Powderly present a broad perspective on many of the legal and ethical issues that affect the lives of families with HIV infection. This chapter discusses mandatory testing, contact tracing, and access to health services and clinical trials. Lauren Shapiro provides readers with an extensive practical guide to the legal concerns and needs of women and families with HIV infection in chapter 17, "Legal Concerns of Women with HIV Infection." The issues discussed include advance directives, long-term planning, and custody.

Because providers play an important role in the primary and secondary prevention of HIV transmission, the theoretical basis and design of patient and community education programs is presented in chapter 18, "Prevention and Education," by Kathleen Nokes and Marilyn Auerbach.

Finally, the personal concerns of primary care providers who see women and children with HIV infection on a daily basis as well as the concerns of providers who work with this patient group infrequently are discussed by Janice Bell Meisenhelder in chapter 19, "Caring for the Caregiver."

HIV disease is the most poignant health challenge of the last half of this century. The problem of HIV in women and children is growing and will continue to stretch resources that are already thin. Primary care professionals will be called on to provide comprehensive care to seriously ill multiproblem families that are experiencing a continuum of physical, emotional, and legal stresses. It is our hope that the contributors to this book can provide the helping hand of experience to fellow professionals undertaking this important task.

Patricia Kelly
Susan Holman
Rosalie Rothenberg
Stephen Paul Holzemer

# ❖ Contributors

PATRICIA ANTONIELLO, PHD, Assistant Professor, Department of Health and Nutrition Sciences, Brooklyn College, City University of New York

MARILYN I. AUERBACH, DRPH, Assistant Professor of Community Health Education, Hunter College, City University of New York

JOANNE BRADLEY, EDD, Vice Provost for Nursing and Allied Health, State University of New York Health Science Center at Brooklyn

MARDGE H. COHEN, MD, Director, Women's and Children's HIV Program, Cook County Hospital, Chicago, Illinois

JUDY COHN, RPA-C, Physician Assistant, Special Treatment and Research Program, State University of New York Health Science Center at Brooklyn

ELIZABETH B. COOPER, JD, Gibbons Fellow in Public Interest and Constitutional Law; Grummy, Del Deo, Dolan, Griffinger & Vecchione, Newark, New Jersey

RAE L. CROWE, PHD, RN, Assistant Professor, College of Nursing, State University of New York Health Science Center at Brooklyn

JACK A. DEHOVITZ, MD, MPH, Associate Professor of Preventive Medicine and Community Health and of Medicine, State University of New York Health Science Center at Brooklyn

SISTER MARY DONOHUE, MS, MA, Chaplain, University Hospital of Brooklyn, New York

CAROLYN A. FISH, MPH, RN, Professor of Nursing, Westbrook College, Portland, Maine

DONNA FUTTERMAN, MD, Medical Director and Acting Director, Adolescent AIDS Program, Montefiore Medical Center, Bronx, New York

SUSAN HOLMAN, RNC, MS, Project Director, Women's Interagency HIV Study, State University of New York Health Science Center at Brooklyn

STEPHEN PAUL HOLZEMER, PHD, RN, Dean of the School of Nursing, Long Island College Hospital, Brooklyn, New York

PATRICIA KELLY, MS, MPH, FNP, Practitioner-Teacher, Rush University College of Nursing, Chicago, Illinois

ANN KURTH, MPH, MSN, CNM, Director of Clinical Data and Research, Indiana State Department of Health, Indianapolis

SHELDON H. LANDESMAN, MD, Professor of Medicine, State University of New York Health Science Center at Brooklyn

CATHERINE LYONS, MS, MPH, Nurse Practitioner, Outpatient AIDS Clinic, San Francisco General Hospital

JUDY WEAVER MASON, CSW, MSW, Social Work Supervisor–Obstetrics and Gynecology, Mount Sinai Medical Center, New York

JANICE BELL MEISENHELDER, DNSC, Director, Center for Nursing Research, New England Deaconness Hospital, Boston, Massachusetts

HOWARD L. MINKOFF, MD, Professor of Obstetrics and Gynecology and Director of Maternal-Fetal Medicine, State University of New York Health Science Center at Brooklyn

KATHLEEN M. NOKES, PHD, RN, FAAN, Associate Professor and Project Director, Nursing of Persons with HIV/AIDS Program, Hunter College–Bellevue School of Nursing, City University of New York

PATRICK G. O'CONNOR, MD, MPH, Director of the Primary Care Center, Yale University School of Medicine, New Haven, Connecticut

MARY JO O'HARA, RN, MSN, CPNP, Clinical Educator, National Pediatric HIV Resource Center, Newark, New Jersey

ANA L. OLIVEIRA, MA, LAc, Director of Program Services, Osborn Association, New York

MARGARET J. OXTOBY, MD, Chief, Pediatric and Family Studies Section, Division of HIV/AIDS, Centers for Disease Control and Prevention, Atlanta, Georgia

KATHLEEN POWDERLY, MSN, CNM, MPHIL, Associate Director, Division of Humanities in Medicine, State University of New York Health Science Center at Brooklyn

JOYCE E. PREISINGER, CSW, MS, Clinical Social Worker, Mount Sinai Medical Center, New York

HELEN RODRIGUEZ-TRIAS, MD, MPH, FAAP, Immediate Past President of the American Public Health Association and Consultant in Health Programming, Brookdale, California

ROSALIE ROTHENBERG, RN, EdD, Acting Dean, College of Nursing, State University of New York Health Science Center at Brooklyn

MICHELE RUSSELL, CSW, MSW, Clinical Social Worker, New York Hospital–Cornell Medical Center

ROBERT J. SIMONDS, MD, Pediatric and Family Studies Section, Division of HIV/AIDS, Centers for Disease Control and Prevention, Atlanta, Georgia

LAUREN SHAPIRO, JD, HIV Project Director, Brooklyn Legal Services Corp. B, New York

ANN B. WILLIAMS, RNC, EdD, FAAN, Associate Professor, Yale University School of Nursing, New Haven, Connecticut

# ❖ Chapter 1

# The Voices of Women with HIV Infection

Patricia Antoniello

*My physician spends time with me. She does. I trust her, I really do. I trust her. She told me different things about HIV. She told me about some problems. She told me to eat right. My doctor told me that some people live a long time.*

---

*I can talk to the people in the clinic about my complications and my sickness.... They are not rushing. They spend time, and they sit down. I can say nothing negative about them.*

---

*The doctor basically just diagnosed me, gave me my medication, sent me home. I didn't know nothing from nothing.*

Although HIV infection in women has been analyzed by panels, seminars, papers, and books, missing from most of these discussions are the voices of the women affected by the epidemic. This chapter attempts to provide some of the words, thoughts, and beliefs of women whose lives have been profoundly influenced by HIV infection, in the hope that primary care practitioners can listen and integrate these concerns into the clinical care they provide to families.

Interviews were conducted with women at two New York City hospitals that provide clinical services to women and at Life Force, a community-based organization that provides training and education for women affected by or infected with HIV. Responses were gathered using open-ended questions based on specific themes identified through focus groups and clinical experiences. This chapter offers a snapshot of women's views throughout HIV infection because perceptions change as women learn more about their disease and as they experience the reality of its impact on their lives. The comments are recorded here with only minor changes for clarity and flow.

## ❖ Discovery

Women were eager to discuss events surrounding the discovery of their HIV status. The following vignettes represent those who have experienced different stages of the HIV epidemic. Women who were diagnosed in the 1980s tend to have some relationship to intravenous drugs, either as users themselves or as partners of drug users. In contrast, women who learned of their HIV status in the 1990s more commonly identify heterosexual transmission as the source of their infection.

Lillian G. is a 40-year-old African-American woman who was born in New York City. She has a history of intravenous drug use and has been aware of her HIV status for 6 years:

> I am a recovering addict, but I had been clean since 1984. Even when you are a recovering addict, you know, when you hear that you are infected, it's no different than a woman that is in a heterosexual relationship. I was very upset. I was tested at the Board of Health and I was by myself. I had no one with me, and I was crying and real upset. The counselor there told me, and she was real sensitive and everything.... I was down the stairs, bouncing up against the wall I was so upset, but then I kind of got it together, and I called my church and I called a friend. She prayed with me over the phone, we talked. She was a recovering addict for about 10 years and I think she was the only person I could talk to.

Nadia S. is a 53-year-old woman from Guyana who has no history of drug use and has been employed as a nurse's aide in a nursing home for more than 10 years:

> I was living with the man since 1984. I had known him for almost 20 years. He died in Guyana. When they told me it was AIDS related, I was in shock. I thought I would die. I never knew he was with other women. He kept it a secret. I wish I would have known all these things. You know men, you never know what they do. He was so nice, but then, you don't know....
>
> My daughter is a lab technician and said I should have the test. I found out in February [two months ago]. I was so devastated. I cried and cried, I thought I could never stop crying. I said, I have no hopes now. I was trying to quit everything and stop work. The counselor that they gave me here, she builds me up and gives me the hope to carry on. The doctor, too, she gives me hope. I asked her a lot of questions, and she gave me that hope. And now, I continue working.

Ruth M. is a 37-year-old Haitian woman who is at a complete loss to understand the source of her newly discovered HIV positivity:

> I have been in New York for 10 years. I don't use drugs. I was always working. I don't drink. I don't even smoke cigarettes. I don't know how I could have gotten this. She [the counselor] asked me, do you have a boyfriend? I said, yes, I had one guy, I don't know if he carried that disease. He went back to Haiti. He died at his mother's house 3 or 4 years ago. I don't know if it was AIDS. And about 3 or 4 years after that, I started getting sick.

Carmen T. is a 32-year-old Puerto Rican with a history of intravenous drug use. She has been seropositive for more than 5 years. She moved to the United States at age 7:

*In 1987, the doctor recommended that I get an AIDS test. That's when I found out I was positive. I forgot everything. I wished I could forget my name. I wanted to die. That day I came out of that place, I just wanted to die. I walked like a zombie. I was just crying. I almost got hit by a bus. From there, I didn't want to live. Who the hell would want to live? Since then, I'm not the same person I used to be.*

The remarks of these women have implications for those providing HIV counseling and testing services (chapter 9). Adequate time must be allowed for the initial expression of pain and grief when test results are given. Equally important to the women are nurturing behaviors, such as touch and supportive silence. Always schedule at least one additional visit; most patients, even those expecting positive results, require at least two visits to begin to absorb the information about their HIV status. Those who give positive HIV results in a supportive manner provide an important bridge to this new reality.

## ❖ Pregnancy and Children

Many women discover that they are infected with HIV during pregnancy because a health professional has recommended "routine" antepartum HIV testing. Although issues surrounding pregnancy were a real concern of the women in this sample, their actual knowledge about pregnancy outcomes and the effect of pregnancy on their health status reflected considerable misinformation.

Marie B. is a 30-year-old Haitian woman who had two abortions in Haiti before giving birth to a daughter 10 years ago. Since learning of her HIV status, Marie had two more pregnancies, one of which she terminated by abortion before she delivered a son who is now 1 year old. The HIV status of the baby is still unclear, although he has been symptom free:

*I didn't have it. I was afraid to have a baby. If you have a baby, it's going to be sick. I don't want to cause any pain. I know that I am HIV and that the baby is going to be sick. The first time I went and got the abortion. The second time I told my husband that I was pregnant, he wouldn't give me money to have an abortion. He said, if you are really for me, you have to keep it. What are the chances that I would have some problem with it? The doctor said that I could be sick or the baby could be sick and die. But after I talk to the nurse, I thought that I could take a chance and just pray. Only God can know.*

Wilma L. is a 38-year-old white woman who has a history of intravenous drug use and found out that she was HIV positive during her pregnancy 2 years ago:

*I was pregnant at the time, and I asked her [the provider], can I keep the baby? She just shook her head. She looked at me with real sympathy and said I cannot keep it. She took that choice away from me. I got rid of the baby.*

Sharon W. is a 34-year-old African-American from North Carolina who recently learned that she is HIV positive:

*I'm having a hard time dealing with the fact that I may not be able to have children. If I do decide to have children and I choose to get pregnant, I am endangering the life of my own child. It hurts. I think that part of the whole deal stinks.*

Although pregnancy decisions were difficult, children provided a life focus for all of the women interviewed. Children gave them the best and the most painful moments of their newly aware life.

*Carmen T.: If I didn't have my kids, I wouldn't care what happened. When I am with them, I can forget about myself, about HIV. That's the future. Their needs are now. I live for my kids. Otherwise, I'd commit suicide.*

---

*Marie B.: I have my son to take care of, to cook and clean for. To take care of him makes me feel really good. You can think about him every night and every day. No, I don't have to think all the time that I will die. I want to live to see what he will be like when he grows.*

---

*Lillian G.: The worst time, even worse than when I got my diagnosis, was finding out that the baby for sure had it. When he got sick, I couldn't leave the hospital. I stayed by his side for 2 weeks.*

---

*Ruth M.: I am getting sicker now. I know I am. Their father is already dead. I have no family. Who is going to raise my children?*

Counseling patients about reproductive issues and HIV disease raises difficult issues for providers, who often have conflicting feelings (chapter 16). Do women with HIV infection have the same reproductive rights as women without infection? What about the future of both infected children and uninfected children who might become orphans? Providers should be aware of their own feelings and should express them fully with peers, not with patients. Women with HIV infection have burden enough in making decisions about pregnancy and children without adding the negative opinions and judgments of providers (chapter 5).

The statements of these women also indicate their need for both ongoing support and education. The facts about vertical transmission of HIV infection are difficult to comprehend, and pregnancy always raises complex emotional issues that must be explored. When a patient is anxious or depressed, she may be unable to comprehend or integrate much of the information presented to her. Questions about contraceptive practices, pregnancy, and future plans for the woman's children must be brought up on a regular basis, it is hoped with further exploration possible each time. The facts about HIV transmission must be reiterated until the patient is able to explain them in her own words.

## ❖ Living with HIV

This section describes ways in which women cope with their HIV infection. Their solutions to specific problems vary but generally represent resolutions based on limited resources.

*Nadia S.: I'm still working at a nursing home. I love work because it keeps my mind [busy]. I don't want to be sitting around and doing nothing and worrying about this. I want to just get up in the mornings, be well, and go on to work. [Laughing] Probably in my last dying breath I will be working. I think.*

---

*Carmen T.: There was a while when I was taking care of myself real good for about 8 months. But now I've been very depressed. So about two or three times I got high. To tell you the truth, it makes me relax. It's not like I want to do it. It's just that I want to get away from my problems, my depression, from the stress.*

---

*Marcia D.: Women should get a mind-set of "I have to take care of myself." Because in the beginning, it was all about my husband and my daughter getting through college.*

---

*Diane H.: I think I'm healthier. [Laughing] I mean I'm infected. That's sort of strange. Before, I'd eat all sorts of things. Now I'm more cautious about how I take care of myself. I think I care about people more, too. I spend more time with people. I have compassion for people, and I think I'm wiser.*

Support groups have provided a mechanism for women and families with HIV disease to share experiences and learn how others have coped with HIV infection, physical and emotional difficulties, and other problems. Groups also allow patients to develop emotional bonds with one another. Although many women are initially reluctant to attend such groups, encouragement to sit in on at least one session has often proved worthwhile.

## ❖ Medical Care

In response to questions about their medical care, many of the women focused on the patient-provider relationship as their chief concern.

*Amanda P.: There is another thing I want to add. I think some of these doctors need to be trained or retrained or updated about HIV. Because when I first went to the doctors, they told me no more sex and to get rid of my animals.*

---

*Audrey N.: I need a doctor to be a little more sensitive and just listen. I had an incident with a female doctor. She asked me about HIV and how I got the virus. When I told her that I had shot drugs, her attitude changed towards me. And I picked up on it right away. It was very unprofessional. [I thought,] I don't trust you, I don't want you to touch my body because you might misdi-agnose me because of your attitude.*

---

*Tracy A.: Last week I had a headache all week long, and I'm scared. The doctor said, don't worry, everything is going to be okay. I really want somebody to sit and talk to me and explain something....*

*Another thing I think the doctors could do better is to treat the patient as a whole and not just treat the symptoms. You know, I think with this virus, people get stressed and they get sick.*

---

*Sandra V.: The only thing about it is the inconvenience of getting a prescrip-tion, going to another building to wait on an extremely long line in order to get your medicine. Sometimes, they may have run out of the medication or the doctor might have made a mistake on the prescription, and you have to go outside, travel all the way back [to the clinic], and then you have to wait in order for that doctor to come out. And you have to say, please rewrite my prescription. And that takes all day long, and if you are sick, you can forget it. You're going to end up being even sicker.*

It is clear that primary care providers play an important role in the lives of women with HIV disease. However, the ability to respect and to care about the patient is as important as knowing the specifics about initiation of antiretroviral therapy. Allow time to understand a woman's medical situation and her social situation. Answers to women's questions are not always necessary; affirmation that she has been heard and silent support are also strong indications of caring. Encouraging self-care and health-promotion activities maximizes the patient's psychological and immunologic resources. The HIV primary care encounter may be the first time that these concepts have been introduced to many women, and they are strong self-esteem and ego boosters for them.

Access to health care service is an ongoing problem for poor women; those with HIV infection are caught in the middle of a system that is already inadequate to meet the needs of women and children. Long waiting times, physical distances, services not available to those with Medicaid or limited insurance coverage, and negative caretaker attitudes make the receipt of needed health care services unpleasant at best and truly burdensome and to be avoided at worst. Physicians, nurses, social workers, and counselors can all work to be advocates for families, both at their individual sites and in the larger community.

### ❖ Empowerment

*Empowerment* has been defined as enabling individuals and groups to participate in action and decision making (Mason, Backer, & Georges, 1991). It is a process that involves individuals in a group effort to assess their problems with an understanding of their place in current society. It is important in the care of women with HIV disease, many of whom have been alienated from the support of their own families and communities. Women cannot be given empowerment but must themselves work through the process that identifies their individual goals and the needs and values of the community (Freire, 1985). As an individual's self-esteem is built, so also is a comprehension of her place and value in society. However, women must be given the opportunity to understand and build self-esteem; it is not a birthright for those born into economic or cultural poverty. The transformation process that has occurred for many women with HIV infection is proof that empowerment is possible when the resources are provided to work with women at activities that benefit them and their communities.

The quotes that follow are from women who are members of Life Force, a New York City community-based organization that trains women to be advocates for themselves and for families affected by HIV disease. Membership in this group has been a defining experience for most of the women interviewed. They discuss the consequences of the training they have received and the importance of the organization as a support for themselves, their families, and their community.

*Miriam C.: In Life Force, we were trained to go back into the community to different sites and do HIV education. I mean hospitals, prisons, clinics, offices, schools. We really go anywhere. This helps you stay empowered, gives you more control of your life.*

*Grace J.: After I came here and got empowered, so to speak, I can now work with my doctor. I know that I don't have to take everything that's given to me. I say, let me go home and do some research on this. For me, the doctors aren't gods, especially with this virus. It's a very new disease. I think a lot of us know as much as the doctors.*

*Pam Y.: You have to believe in what you're doing. It's not like I have x amount of free time and I'm going to volunteer in Life Force because I don't have anything else to do. I think that you really need to believe.*

*Linda B.: There are different ways that you can empower yourself. Some girls help out by working in the office, answering the telephone, and listening to other people who have problems.... But the majority of us go out and educate. Not everyone is willing to go to some of my sites, like the AIDS Clinic at the [local hospital]. Sometimes girls are afraid because they see people who are sick, sometimes they can't even sit up long enough to talk, they got to lay down on the chair. There are people there with sores all over their body or wasting away. Sometimes they have diarrhea at the time that you are present. So, it's just how people handle it. [Life Force] gives you the education, but it is up to you to see how you want to internalize and use it. We have to get them to understand they are the captains of their ships.*

*Miriam C.: We have our work cut out for us. We go to homes to do safer sex parties. We'll go in and we'll educate. We go to our friends who are not in Life Force and confront them about their teenagers and the sex they are having. We say, come on, people are dying. You know, a lot of people stay in denial until someone in their family turns HIV positive. Last week, we had someone who was 18 years old. She had never used drugs.*

---

*Annette P.: I don't think that I would have empowered myself to the extent that I have today if I was not infected. I know that I would not have....*
*We have situations where we go out and hand out condoms, and they hand the condoms back. [They say,] my husband doesn't fool around and neither do I. Like my girlfriend, 55 years old and married for 27 years, who one day decided to get tested. Today she is 55 years old and HIV positive.*

## ❖ Summary

This chapter has examined the perspectives of women with HIV disease through their own voices. Through recorded interviews, the diversity of the women has been shown, and the common patterns that affect their lives have been highlighted. Although all of the women included in this chapter are residents of inner-city communities, there is a heterogeneity of background and social circumstances. These women's comments provide important insights for the delivery of health care services to families with HIV infection.

Primary care providers of women with HIV infection must initiate technical medical workups and must oversee the completion of complex applications for needed services. However, primary care involves more than these tasks. Equally important is listening. The words of women with HIV infection tell us about some of the realities of their lives and clearly remind us of the prominence of nonmedical factors. The ability of primary care providers to be responsive to these factors can assist in strengthening the patient's self-care abilities and can be an important determinant of long-term adherence to a medical treatment regime.

## ❖ References

Freire, P. (1985). *Education for critical consciousness.* New York: Continuum Press.
Mason, D. J., Backer, B. A., Georges, C. A. (1991). Toward a feminist model for the political empowerment of nurses. *Image: Journal of Nursing Scholarship,* 23, 72–77.

## ❖ Chapter 2

# HIV Disease in the Primary Care Setting

MARDGE H. COHEN

PATRICIA KELLY

## ❖ A Primary Care Orientation

Patients with AIDS and HIV were initially treated by infectious disease medical subspecialty clinics. Time and experience have shown that infection with HIV is better viewed as a chronic illness affecting virtually every aspect of the life of the patient and her family. A comprehensive model of care is now necessary to provide appropriate services. However, delivery of such services is difficult. A shortage of primary care providers, in combination with the social and financial barriers to care that exist in the United States, has forced the patient population that is most vulnerable to the HIV epidemic—poor, minority, urban, uninsured—to rely on emergency rooms and Medicaid mills when acute illness strikes. In particular, women and children with and at risk for HIV infection often receive episodic sickness care rather than true health care. It is our contention that interventions that will slow the progression of HIV disease and will have an impact on the lives of women and children can better be given within a primary health care setting that promotes and provides health, rather than sickness, care.

The natural history of HIV disease, with its long asymptomatic period, makes it well suited to a primary health care setting. Indeed, advances such as chemoprophylaxis of the common opportunistic infections has further extended the symptom-free period in which the major focus of care of patients with HIV is on health maintenance activities and psychosocial concerns. The general principles of primary health care and the biopsychosocial model provide appropriate guidelines for the implementation of services to women and children with HIV disease (Engel, 1980). Such services should be comprehensive, continuous, coordinated, and accessible (Starfield, 1992) as well as multidisciplinary, family centered, and specific to the communities in which the services are delivered (World Health Organization, 1978). Integrating these standards into existing programs and making them integral to new ones will result in high-quality services that meet the diverse health needs of women, children, and families affected by HIV.

## Comprehensive

Primary care clinics for families with HIV infection must provide health maintenance activities, general medical care, and HIV-specific care in one visit. For women, this means integrating a range of preventive and therapeutic medical, gynecologic, and psychological services into the same setting. Children with HIV need a provider who addresses issues related to growth and development, general pediatrics, HIV infection, and intercurrent illnesses. When these services are provided at a single site, especially one that also cares for uninfected children and other family members, the integrity of the family unit is maintained, and access to needed medical services is ensured. Arrangements must be made for 24-hour availability of staff by rotating beeper or telephone coverage to assist patients through acute medical events. Clinic programs should have agreements with emergency rooms to facilitate transfer of medical information and notification of program staff when patients receive services.

## Continuous

Having the same providers over time allows families to develop appropriate confidence and trust in the health care staff. Successful communication about sensitive HIV-related issues, such as sexual practices, prevention, family support, disclosure, confidentiality, drug use, and death and dying, requires a long-term patient-provider relationship. Staff who have ongoing relationships with patients can more accurately assess changes in clinical and social conditions faced by the women and children and their families as HIV disease progresses.

## Coordinated

Families affected by HIV have multiple medical and psychosocial needs. A recent study conducted in Boston demonstrated that each family with HIV must apply for services at 12 to 16 different institutions (Carr, 1990). Although it would be ideal to be able to provide all of these services in one setting, this is often impossible. Many clinics, especially newer ones or those in communities with a relatively small number of patients, have limited the services provided in one setting. The careful coordination of treatment plans, services, and referrals can assist in overcoming these limitations. Communication among staff members about a family's major problems and the agreed-upon plans prevent problems from being overlooked in a system. The organization of all care under the aegis of one primary provider, meticulous attention to documentation, and follow-up of every referral, especially those to outside agencies, will help to ensure that all problems are addressed.

## Accessible

Cultural, financial, and geographic barriers limit most women and children with HIV from obtaining services in public-sector institutions. These institutions are often poorly equipped to meet the needs of poor women and their families, and few are able to provide needed services, such as child care, transportation, or food vouchers. Also, many agencies have obstacles to access, such as long waiting periods or difficult application procedures, that serve to ration limited resources. Some agencies demonstrate insensitivity to the health beliefs, cultural concerns, or language of families from many backgrounds, which can contribute to inaccessibility for people with HIV. Others may intentionally discourage those who have used or are using drugs from participating or may adopt a punitive approach that blames women and their families for the HIV infection and the situation in which they find themselves. Many families have experienced negative interactions with health care institutions, social service agencies, drug treatment programs, and legal services. To make primary care HIV sites accessible and to engage families in ongoing care, a concerted effort must be made to acknowledge these previous experiences, to be sensitive to the causes of these negative interactions, and to create care settings that communicate an appreciation of and respect for the families and their concerns. The establishment and maintenance of such a caring and respectful environment is as important as any service provided.

## Multidisciplinary

The mental health and social service needs of those with HIV need to be addressed regardless of the clinical stage of HIV disease. Psychologists and social workers or case managers are an essential part of the multidisciplinary primary care team. They often deal with underlying psychological issues as well the particular crises that women and their children face during the course of the illness. Critical events for families span the life cycle and include the following:

- ❖ Initial diagnosis of HIV seropositivity
- ❖ Disclosure of HIV status to family members
- ❖ Pregnancy
- ❖ Childbirth
- ❖ Anticipation of a child's HIV serostatus
- ❖ Decline in T cells
- ❖ Initiation of antiretroviral therapy
- ❖ Initial hospitalization
- ❖ Advancing disease
- ❖ Terminal illness

Addressing such a wide range of issues is greatly facilitated by having a multidisciplinary staff of medical and psychosocial providers, with families relying on different providers during different stages of the illness. Even individual problems that affect families with HIV disease usually demand more than one provider and more than one discipline to develop appropriate solutions. Such continuity of care is best provided by a multidisciplinary staff. This allows patients to have their many needs met by more than one provider, and it allows providers to share with other staff the sometimes overwhelming patient care responsibilities.

## Family Centered

For women and children, HIV is a family disease. The modes of heterosexual and perinatal transmission link the life-affirming activities of love, sex, and birth with disease and the death of oneself and loved ones. Many women, at risk for HIV because of a history of injection drug use, often are also at risk because their sexual partners are injection drug users. In the 1990s, more than 90% of children with HIV contracted the infection via perinatal transmission. A healthy mother is very important to the future health of her children and other family members because most women with HIV infection serve as caretakers for their children and their partners, often to the detriment of their own health. Solutions that help mothers also help their families. It is difficult for the family to negotiate multiple visits to different medical providers and institutions. Scheduling appointments for children and mothers to have all care provided at a single visit relieves the family of the need to make visits at different times or to different sites. Family-centered care also means that the mother's needs and the child's needs are not seen as conflicting. Rather, events in the lives of one member must be viewed as family events.

## Community Specific

The structure of an HIV clinic and the range of services provided to the population of women and children with HIV infection vary by community and depend on the rates of HIV and the services that are available in the area. It is essential for providers to learn what these services are, to assess which needs are not met, and to design a clinic program that meets the needs of the specific patient population without duplicating services. The formation of a community advisory board allows staff to stay in touch with community needs and helps to set short-term and long-term goals for the services that the clinic can provide. A board can also be a vehicle for patients to express their criticisms and to communicate suggestions for improving the clinical program.

## ❖ Essential Services for Women and Children with HIV Disease

### Medical

A variety of medical, nursing, and psychosocial services are needed by women and children who have HIV infection. Limiting clinic services to monitoring CD4 cells and providing medication does not address the many related needs that affect HIV disease progression.

The medical care offered to women and children with HIV should be as comprehensive as possible, addressing appropriate screening and preventive services and treatment for most other conditions in addition to HIV-related care. HIV-specific care includes protocols for the initiation of antiretroviral and opportunistic infection therapy for adults and children, tuberculosis screening and diagnosis, and treatment and hospitalization for acute sickness. Basic gynecologic care includes breast examinations, regular pelvic examinations to screen for sexually transmitted diseases and cervical cancer, contraceptive counseling, access to barrier and hormonal contraceptives, pregnancy testing, and counseling about reproductive choices, including abortion. A mechanism must be readily available to provide pregnancy termination and prenatal and postpartum care on site or through easy referral. Health maintenance services include immunizations for adults and children, mammograms and other age-appropriate health screening for adults, well-child care, and growth and development monitoring. Age-appropriate health counseling must be provided. Common acute and chronic diseases, including respiratory and ear infections in children, hypertension, diabetes, arthritis, and depression in adults, should be managed in this primary care setting, with consultation as required.

The primary provider should monitor hospitalizations, either directly or by regular contact with both the patient and the acute care physicians. This will maintain continuity between inpatient and outpatient treatment regimens and also will assist the patient through a stressful period. Nursing and case management also will assist in coordinating an appropriate discharge plan that will meet the patient's needs and will be compatible with family and outpatient resources.

These services can all be provided by a primary care team, which might include family practitioners, pediatricians, internists, nurse practitioners, and physician assistants, each acting as a primary care provider and consulting with infectious disease specialists and gynecologist/obstetricians as necessary.

### Health Education

Clear, comprehensive, and explicit education about HIV infection for women at risk for or recently diagnosed with HIV disease is a critical component of care and a continuous process. After the initial devastation of learning of a positive HIV test result, patients and their families require ongoing education and counseling, including information about transmission, prevention, treatment options, disease progression, and life changes that may be anticipated as a result of the diagnosis. The health educator is a critical staff member. He or she may provide the original HIV pretest counseling for patients, inform them of the results, refer them to the clinical program, and be available for supportive counseling as needed. The professional bond that can be created with a patient by an educator who informs a woman of her positive status in a supportive and caring manner may lead to a special relationship if the educator is integrated into the clinical setting. The educator can teach about perinatal transmission, contraception, disease manifestations in women, and antiretroviral therapies in individual follow-up and group counseling sessions.

## Case Management

Most women with HIV and their children start out poor or become poor as a result of unemployment and the costs associated with disease progression. It is therefore imperative to have skilled staff to assist in the procurement of social service entitlements. This is the role of case managers, who serve as advocates for women and their families through the bureaucratic maze of maternal-child health benefits, Social Security disability, public assistance, transportation services, foster care agencies, housing, chemical dependency treatment programs, early intervention programs, schools, home nursing and hospice care, and funeral arrangements. In addition to sorting out the different application procedures and eligibility requirements, case managers provide ongoing assistance to families as their clinical and social service needs change. By ongoing telephone contact or home visits with families, case managers also can play a role in increasing compliance with clinic appointments and referrals.

## Psychological Health

Some women and children have previously existing psychological problems that require attention within the primary care setting. Others find that the stresses of HIV disease progression often exacerbate problems. One such problem is chemical dependency, especially in women who have a history of sexual or physical abuse or other psychological problems. Although all staff will be supportive, social workers, psychologists, and psychiatrists are essential and must be readily available to provide intervention and management at these times.

## Support Groups

Women with HIV and their families often feel isolated in their communities. Support groups can relieve some of this isolation. These groups may be either open, with a drop-in format for women attending clinic, or closed, with regularly scheduled sessions that require a greater commitment from participants. Group sessions allow women with HIV to talk to one another, express their fears and concerns, and share coping strategies about their disease. As women continue to express their feelings and frustrations, support groups become an integral part of the treatment program.

Membership in HIV support groups can be heterogeneous or homogeneous. Homogeneous groups are especially appropriate for women working on preventing substance abuse relapse, women for whom English is not their first language, or women with infected children. Groups for partners, for caregivers, or for extended family members are also helpful. The variety of support groups that can be made available depends on the number and types of patients in a specific community.

All support groups need staff facilitators (health educators, case managers, psychologists) and a pleasant private setting to encourage open participation. Child care and snacks may be helpful. A group process that allows full participation and that discourages monopolization of conversation is essential. Topics can be solicited from the group, or a schedule can be developed.

## Chemical Dependency Services

Many women with AIDS or HIV disease in the United States have had substance abuse problems, relationships with partners who abused drugs, or both. The issue of chemical dependency must be addressed to promote adherence to other aspects of HIV care, such as keeping appointments, preventing further HIV transmission, and caring for family members. Chemical dependency counselors in clinics can provide crisis intervention, relapse prevention, and continued individual and group counseling sessions. Women who are actively using drugs and wish to enter a detoxification program often encounter a waiting list for available treatment slots and may need specific hand-holding and encouragement to facilitate their entrance into treatment programs. The continued support of primary care staff is important for women in these programs. A major problem for women with children is that there are few women-centered drug treatment programs that assist with arrangements for child care. Clinic staff can be helpful in assisting women to place children with family members during these times. Weekly individual and/or group sessions are important to support women awaiting enrollment in detoxification or long-term treatment programs.

## Nutrition

A nutritionist who reviews the dietary histories of clinic patients and encourages appropriate eating habits with a culturally sensitive perspective can have a major impact on improving the health of patients. Education should be available, either individually or in groups, on such topics as wasting syndrome, vitamin supplements, healthy meals on a limited budget, and eating tips for nausea, vomiting, and diarrhea.

## Pastoral Care

Pastoral care is an important component of comprehensive care and may be of particular comfort during hospitalizations or terminal stages of illness for the patient and the family. However, beginning the relationship prior to these stages is often useful. A trusting relationship can be initiated while the patient and the family are well, when time is available to anticipate the needs of later disease stages. The skills of the pastoral care staff enhance the counseling given by other members of the multidisciplinary team throughout the disease process.

## Child Care

Providing child care is essential to delivering family-oriented HIV care. Trained, sensitive child-care staff and designated play space show respect for the entire family and allow the clinic visit to be a more pleasant and orderly event. Although art therapists or child-life experts can be utilized, the availability of secure, safe, and caring staff and space is most important. In addition, assisting the patient in making arrangements for child care in the home or with relatives or friends enhances compliance with clinic visits and appointments for diagnostic tests.

## Legal Services

Most people with HIV and their families have not had occasion to use legal services other than for crises or emergencies. HIV legal services that emphasize advance planning, such as living wills, power of attorney, advance directives, and guardianship, ensure that the patient's desires will be carried out. Legal staff can provide the thought, guidance, advocacy, and flexibility for such services and also can assist when issues of discrimination in jobs, housing, schools, or entitlements are brought to the staff's attention.

## Staffing Issues

Working in the HIV primary care setting can be one of the most rewarding of present-day health care jobs. HIV teams are, more than most medical fields, receptive to the contributions of staff from different backgrounds and areas of expertise, as well as from patients. HIV health care providers believe that they are on the cutting edge of medical science, in which research and clinical findings change almost on a daily basis. In most settings, this changing information is shared with the entire multidisciplinary staff.

Because of the continuing discrimination and isolation that they experience, women, children, and families affected by HIV often show particular gratitude and appreciation toward their providers. They are thankful for the support they feel as well as the concrete help they receive in coping with the illness. The clinical staff is often viewed as a new family, and the setting is seen as a place where patients share their intimate successes and difficult struggles.

HIV health care providers may also find inspiration in the strength that patients demonstrate in overcoming the many difficult stages of HIV illness. Staff members are often impressed by the ability of most patients to joke and to enjoy and look forward to their visits. Clinic sessions are not somber occasions; rather, they are filled with jocularity and familiarity, breaking through much of the formality of other clinical settings. Children help to make the settings feel familiar and friendly.

The composition of the clinic staff should reflect the community that it serves. At least one staff member must be able to speak the languages of the patient population. Although finding such staff may take extra time and effort, the benefits of improved communication with patients make the effort worthwhile. Staff recruitment is enhanced by the use of less traditional recruitment sources, such as community colleges, service organizations, and newsletters and networks of minority providers.

Along with professional qualifications and clinical skills, qualities that make a good HIV provider include cultural sensitivity, maturity, and the ability to focus on and work fully in the present. The desire to care, not cure, allows for long-term development and helps prevent burnout. Applicants who are motivated primarily by a sense of beneficence about working with the patient population are not helpful to women with HIV disease. The need is for staff who are willing to work alongside families in dealing with their disease, rather than staff who feel sorry for them.

Regularly scheduled full-staff meetings can assist in creating group coherence. In this forum, educational programs can be presented and the experiences of team members synthesized to create the best plans for challenging patient problems.

Staff training and staff support are important to the success of the multidisciplinary team. Staff members encounter the emotional difficulties associated with HIV illness as well as the effect of the deaths and hospitalizations of multiple family members. Mental health support for staff is very important and may include flexible hours, staff support groups, mental health days, retreats, and exercise or meditation groups. Attendance at education programs is a must for staff to appreciate the changing field of HIV care and to improve their skills by learning new techniques and information.

A means of preventing burnout is to allow staff members who have become successful and well skilled at their jobs to present talks to others about their work. This accomplishes several important tasks: The expertise of the staff is legitimized and shared with others, staff can feel that they are contributing to HIV education by sharing their experiences with professionals and community groups, and a human face is given to the health workers involved with HIV infection and often to people with HIV, as well.

## ❖ Summary

The social epidemiology of HIV disease in women and children requires that a wide variety of preventive, diagnostic, therapeutic, social, psychological, and ancillary services be readily available. The primary health care model, with emphasis on family-centered care, is ideal for providing services to this patient population, whether in dedicated HIV clinics or primary care clinics.

As outlined, these suggestions place the patient at the center of the model of care and necessitate many staff and financial resources for implementation. Although the ideal service program for women and children with HIV includes a wide range of services, depending on the number of patients in a community, a clinic may opt to pick and choose which services can be included on site and which require liaisons and referral.

## ❖ References

Carr, A. (1990). *Changes in the health care and social services needs of HIV+ women and children in metropolitan Chicago.* Chicago: Visiting Nurse Association of Chicago.

Engel, G. L. (1980). The clinical application of the biopsychosocial model. *American Journal of Psychiatry, 137*(5), 535–544.

Starfield, B. (1992). *Primary care: Concept, evaluation, and policy.* New York: Oxford University Press.

World Health Organization. (1978). *Primary health care.* Geneva: Author.

# ❖ Chapter 3

# Epidemiology and Natural History of HIV Infection in Women

SHELDON H. LANDESMAN

SUSAN HOLMAN

HIV disease first came to the world's attention in 1981 with reports of severe immunodeficiency and Kaposi's sarcoma in gay men living in New York and San Francisco (Centers for Disease Control [CDC], 1981). Ensuing reports documented the presence of this disease in injection drug users, (IDUs), infants born to women with risk factors, recipients of blood transfusion and anti-hemophiliac factor, and sexual partners of people with risk factors (CDC, 1982a, 1982b, 1983a, 1983b). By the middle of the decade, HIV had gained widespread acceptance as the infectious cause of this acquired immunodeficiency. Receptive sexual intercourse, most often among men, and exchange or transfer of infected blood products were established as principal modes of acquisition of the disease. Initially, the focus of the epidemic was on men: gay men, intravenous drug users (75% male), and hemophiliacs (100% male). Little attention was paid to women in general and heterosexual transmission in particular.

Additional studies also documented the presence of HIV disease in central Africa (Nkowane, 1991), the Caribbean, and other developing regions, albeit with a different pattern of transmission. In these less developed areas of the world, HIV was transmitted largely through heterosexual intercourse. Prostitution played a major role in the transmission, as did the cultural and sexual mores of local populations (Piot et al., 1987). Gay men and injection drug users were a small part of the problem in these developing regions, though transmission via blood transfusion was common until screening of blood became available after 1985.

When HIV transmission occurs principally among gay men and injection drug users, it is termed Pattern I. This type of transmission is seen largely in the industrialized countries of the West. Pattern II transmission, characterized by an equal* gender distribution and the predominance of heterosexual transmission, affects central African and Caribbean countries. More recently, a new pattern (Pattern III) has been described in Thailand, India, and the Middle East, where commercial sex workers and injection drug users are introducing and spreading the virus via heterosexual transmission. Although not as severely affected as Pattern II countries, these new areas are unfortunately moving toward widespread dissemination of HIV disease (Mann, Tarantola, & Netler, 1992).

This chapter focuses on the epidemiology and natural history of HIV disease in women living in the United States, a largely Pattern I country. Although gay men and injection drug users are still the groups most affected by HIV disease in this country, women have been increasingly affected over the last decade.

## ❖ Epidemiology of HIV in Women

Early in the epidemic in the United States, women were infected with HIV almost exclusively through injection drug use. Only a small percentage had contracted the disease via heterosexual transmission, and these were women who, by and large, were sexual partners of infected injection drug users.

During the last several years, increasing attention has been paid to the epidemiology of HIV acquisition among women. A useful, but admittedly incomplete, view of the prevalence of HIV disease in women is obtained from the population-based studies of newborns that began in 1986. These anonymous serological surveys of newborns, commonly done as part of a larger, standard newborn screening program (PKU, hyperthyroidism), allow for measurement of the prevalence of HIV in women who have delivered a live child by testing newborn blood for the presence of maternally transferred anti-HIV immunoglobulins.

Newborn screening for HIV is ongoing in nearly all of the 50 states and U.S. territories. Consistent with the data on HIV infection in general, HIV disease among childbearing women is concentrated in specific localities. The rates of HIV antibody positivity in newborns range from a low of 0.0/1,000 in New Hampshire to 5.8/1,000 in New York. Other localities reporting a high prevalence rate include the District of Columbia (5.5/1,000), Maryland (3.1/1,000), New Jersey (4.9/1,000), Florida (4.5/1,000), and Connecticut (3.0/1,000). Most other states have a rate of 1.0/1,000 or less (Gwinn et al., 1991).

The incidence of HIV infection in childbearing women is even more localized than suggested by the above data. For example, in New York State, the greatest density of disease is in New York City, where 12.5/1,000 newborns test HIV positive. Hospitals in central Brooklyn have a 2.5% rate of infection in newborns, whereas one hospital in central Harlem has a rate of 4% (Novick et al., 1989). In other states, the results are similar. For example, in Florida, Miami is the epicenter; in Connecticut, New Haven; and in New Jersey, Newark and Jersey City. All of these urban areas (inner cities) have high concentrations of poor women, many of whom live in close social and sexual contact with drug users.

Using data from 39 nationwide newborn serosurveys, the Centers for Disease Control (CDC) estimated that 6,079 HIV-infected women delivered live births in 1989 (Gwinn et al., 1991). Based on the estimated 4 million deliveries in that year, the national prevalence of HIV infection among childbearing women is calculated to be 1.5/1,000. These estimates represent the minimal prevalence of HIV infection in the female population. Only approximately 10% of the women of childbearing age deliver infants annually (H. Minkoff, personal communication, 1992), and some women with HIV become too ill to have children, choose not to have children, or terminate a pregnancy when they discover they are HIV infected. For further discussion of the transmission and epidemiology of HIV in children born to women with HIV infection, see chapter 6.

According to data from the newborn surveys, the prevalence of HIV disease in childbearing women has remained relatively stable over the last several years. However, this does not mean that new infections are not occurring. For the reasons noted above, a static prevalence in this circumstance masks new cases and may hide an increasing incidence in certain populations. If the total number of infected women is decreased by death, disease, or reproductive choice while the prevalence rate is unchanged, the pool must have been replenished by an equal number of new cases.

Sexually transmitted disease (STD) clinics across the country document a significant rate of HIV infection in women. In a survey of 80,000 blood specimens taken from 77 STD clinics, the median seroprevalence was 0.8%. However, 20% of these clinics reported a seropositivity rate greater than 5%. Again, the clinics with the highest incidence were located on the East Coast in inner-city areas (Chu, Berkelman, & Curran, 1992).

Other epidemiologic measures also provide a partial picture of the prevalence of HIV in women. The CDC AIDS surveillance data indicate a rising percentage of AIDS in women. In 1985, 6.6% of all AIDS cases involved women; in 1990, 11.5% of AIDS cases involved women. The actual number of women diagnosed with AIDS increased from 538 in 1985 to 4,890 in 1989 (Ellerbrock, Bush, Chamberland, & Oxtoby, 1991). However, as seen in the data from newborn surveys, AIDS surveillance data indicate a very focal and spotty disease pattern, with the preponderance of cases in New York (New York City), Florida (Miami), New Jersey (Jersey City, Newark) and Puerto Rico. Of all women with AIDS, 52% are black, 27% are white, and 20% are Hispanic; similar percentages are seen in the newborn surveys and pediatric AIDS cases. These percentages reflect the disproportionate impact of HIV disease on women and children of color. The majority of women diagnosed with AIDS are from 15 to 44 years of age, that is, in their childbearing years.

In summary, the prevalence of HIV infection in women is greatest on the East Coast of the United States and in Puerto Rico. It is highest among women of childbearing age and is most common among inner-city blacks and Hispanics.

## ❖ Modes of Transmission

### Intravenous Drug Use

Intravenous drug use and the sharing of needles has been the dominant mode of HIV acquisition for women, who acquire the virus when they share needles contaminated with the blood of infected drug users. Cumulative AIDS surveillance data through 1990 indicate that 51% of all female cases were associated with injection drug use. Another 21% were attributed to heterosexual contact with an infected drug user. Thus, fully 72% of all AIDS cases diagnosed in women were associated in some way with substance abuse (Ellerbrock et al., 1991).

Drug-injection behaviors are associated with HIV infection. Areas in which needle sharing is common among drug users are the same areas in which the acquisition of HIV from drug use is most common. Novick and colleagues reported in their study of newborn screening of HIV that the zip codes that had the highest prevalence of newborn HIV positivity were identical to the geographic areas where injection drug use was most common (Novick et al., 1989). In one San Francisco study, intravenous cocaine use significantly increased the risk of HIV acquisition, with 35% of daily cocaine users infected as compared to 8% of nonusers (Chaisson et al., 1989). HIV infection has also been associated with injecting in a "shooting gallery" where needles and "works" are commonly shared. A study of drug users in New York found that HIV infection was directly correlated with the number of injections per month, injecting in a shooting gallery, and sharing needles (DesJarlais et al., 1989).

### Heterosexual Transmission

Heterosexual transmission of HIV is increasing at a faster rate than other modes of transmission. In 1989, AIDS cases classified as "acquired through heterosexual activity" were one tenth of the number of cases acquired exclusively through homosexual activity. By 1994, the ratio of heterosexual to homosexual cases was projected to be closer to 5:1 (CDC, 1992c). Because AIDS cases represent transmission that occurred 5 to 10 years earlier, an ever-increasing incidence of AIDS attributed to heterosexual transmission can be expected well beyond 1994. Because heterosexual acquisition of HIV usually represents transmission from an infected man to a previously uninfected woman, the increase in heterosexual transmission will ultimately be reflected in an increase in AIDS among women.

The women at greatest risk for heterosexual acquisition of HIV are those who live in urban areas in which drug use is common and women are in close social and sexual contact with men who currently or once used injection drugs. As the epidemic continues, more women will be infected through sexual contact with injection drug users who were largely infected early in the epidemic. Through repeated sexual exposure, women, whether or not themselves drug users, would eventually become infected. Over time, the reservoir of HIV-infected sexually active drug-using men would create a secondary pool of women infected via heterosexual intercourse.

The risk of heterosexual transmission from an infected man to a woman through vaginal intercourse cannot be accurately estimated. Summary data for the United States suggest a greater efficiency of man-to-woman HIV transmission than woman-to-man transmission (Handsfield, 1988; Haverkos & Edelman, 1988). Other factors, such as STDs (ulcerative and nonulcerative), lack of circumcision, and disease severity, may enhance transmission of the virus (Handsfield, 1988).

The infection of women through heterosexual contact went largely unnoticed during the early years of the epidemic. This was not unexpected given the relatively low numbers of infected women early on, the inability to detect HIV infection during the first years of the epidemic, the long latency period between HIV infection and clinical disease, and the lack of recognition of heterosexual HIV transmission of the virus.

## Woman-to-Woman Transmission

Published data indicate that woman-to-woman transmission through oral-genital sex is rare compared to heterosexual transmission. HIV has been isolated from vaginal secretions as it has been from semen (Vogt et al., 1987). Although a few anecdotal cases of woman-to-woman HIV transmission have been reported (Marmor et al., 1986; Monzon & Capellan, 1987), epidemiologic studies have not shown conclusive evidence of HIV transmission among women who were exclusively lesbian. Petersen and colleagues assessed 144 HIV-infected female blood donors from a pool of 960,000 donors at 20 large U.S. blood centers. Among the 106 lesbian women who were interviewed, none had had sexual contact exclusively with women, but all had had sexual contact with bisexual or drug-using men. The authors concluded, "We identified no woman who was infected with HIV through sexual contact with another woman" (Petersen et al., 1992). Additionally, in a review of AIDS cases among women who reported sex only with women, 95% of the 79 women with AIDS also reported a history of injection drug use. The remaining 5% acquired infection through HIV contaminated blood products (Chu, Birchler, Fleming, & Berkelman, 1990).

Another study by the CDC suggested that a principle modality of HIV acquisition among lesbian/bisexual women is heterosexual sex with male injection drug users (McCombs, McCray, Wendell, Sweeney, & Onorato, 1992). In a study of 15,685 women seen at STD clinics and women's health centers, 470 bisexual women, of whom 13 had HIV infection, were identified. Eleven of the 13 reported sex with male injection drug users. The other two women had equal numbers of male and female partners. In the same study, 41 lesbian women were identified, of whom none were HIV positive.

## Cofactors for Transmission of HIV

A variety of biological and behavioral factors increase the risk of heterosexual acquisition of HIV.

### Biologic Cofactors

Several biologic cofactors increase the rate of heterosexual transmission of HIV. Partner studies in the United States demonstrate more efficient transmission from men to women than from women to men. Most discordant partner studies show a 20% to 30% rate of man-to-woman transmission, compared to an 8% to 15% rate of woman-to-man transmission (Peterman & Curran, 1986).

Most, but not all, studies have identified an increased risk of transmission during late-stage disease (Holmberg, Horsburgh, Ward, & Jaffe, 1989). The probable biologic reason for this finding is the increased viral load, and therefore increased infectivity, commonly seen in late-stage disease.

Studies primarily from sub-Saharan Africa suggest that STDs, particularly genital ulcer disease, increase the infectivity of an HIV-infected individual and the susceptibility of a seronegative individual. Studies by Greenblatt and colleagues (1988) and Laga, Nzila, and Manoka (1990) reported an increased risk of transmission in association with nonulcerative and ulcerative STDs, respectively.

### Behavioral Cofactors

Cocaine use is an important social accelerant of HIV transmission, increasing the risk of HIV acquisition in several ways. Women who use cocaine, especially poor women in urban environs, are more likely to live in drug subcultures and have as sexual partners men who are intravenous drug users. These women may trade sex for drugs and thus expose themselves to HIV through an increased number of sexual partners. Cocaine itself impairs judgment and may contribute to less-cautious behavior in relation to the number and type of partners, the use of condoms, or both (Fullilove, Fullilove, Bowser, & Gross, 1990; Minkoff et al., 1990; National Research Council, 1989; Wolfe, Vranizan & Gorter, in press).

Latex condoms, a proven method of decreasing the risk of HIV acquisition, are not commonly used in the heterosexual populations that are most at risk for HIV disease. In areas in which injection drug use is common, the probability of having unprotected sex with an infected individual is substantially increased. In a recent prospective study of HIV acquisition among 630 sexually active inner-city women in Brooklyn, only 20% ever used a condom, and 10% always used them (Landesman, personal communication, 1991). In a CDC study of condom use among partners of injection drug users, fewer than 10% always used condoms during insertive vaginal intercourse, and 27% sometimes used condoms. Given 10 years of HIV prevention and education, these findings are discouraging from the point of view of preventing HIV transmission in this very high-risk group of individuals.

Many complex and poorly understood factors contribute to the low rate of condom use. Women and men do not perceive themselves at risk and therefore do not see the need for condoms. Many couples feel that condoms are uncomfortable and interfere with the enjoyment and spontaneity of sex. For many men, a request from a partner to wear a condom implies distrust or even that the woman herself is infected. There is also a differential use of condoms, depending on the emotional attachment of the woman to her partner. Condom use is more common with "casual" as opposed to "steady" partners (CDC, 1992a).

Clearly, more study is needed of the individual and societal factors that will enhance condom use. When reliably and properly used, condoms are highly effective in preventing HIV transmission. In one study of discordant couples (one partner HIV positive, the other negative), none of the 123 seronegative partners who consistently used condoms seroconverted (CDC, 1993b). In comparison, there were 12 seroconversions in the 122 partners who never only occasionally used condoms.

## ❖ Natural History

Initial epidemiologic and natural history studies of HIV disease concentrated on cohorts of men with the disease. Specifically, long-term natural history studies of gay men and intravenous drug users, such as the Multicenter AIDS Cohort Study and the San Francisco Gay Men's Health Study, chronicled and described the clinical and immunologic natural history of HIV disease among men. Table 3–1 summarizes the results of these and other studies. Infection with HIV is often heralded with a viral, infectious mononucleosis-like syndrome that lasts 1 to 2 weeks. It is followed by a long asymptomatic or minimally symptomatic period that may last 10 years or longer. As the T cell count drops below $250/mm^3$, and eventually below $100/mm^3$, multiple opportunistic infections and, ultimately, death ensue.

Until recently, no comparable prospective longitudinal study of HIV disease in women had been performed. It is therefore unclear what role hormonal and other gender-related factors may play in the natural history of HIV in women. Although the National Institutes of Health and the CDC recently initiated longitudinal studies of several thousand women with HIV infection, their results will not be available for several years. In the interim, our knowledge of HIV disease in women will continue to be extrapolated from studies of men and derived from smaller cohorts of women followed for relatively short periods of time.

TABLE 3–1    Stages of HIV Disease

| Stage | Clinical Features | Typical Duration | CD4 Range |
|---|---|---|---|
| Acute retroviral syndrome | Brief mononucleosis-like illness | 1–2 weeks | 1,000–500 |
| Asymptomatic | No signs or symptoms except lymphadenopathy | 10+ years | 750–500 |
| Early symptomatic | Non life-threatening infections, chronic or intermittent symptoms | 0–5 years | 500–100 |
| Late symptomatic | Increasingly severe symptoms, life-threatening infections, cancers | 0–3 years | 200–50 |
| Advanced | Increased hazard of death, less transferable "opportunistic infections" | 1–2 years | 50–0 |

*Source:* Reprinted with permission from Volberding, P. (1992). Clinical spectrum of HIV disease. In V. T. DeVita, S. A. Hellman, and S. A. Rosenberg (Eds.), *AIDS: Etiology, diagnosis, treatment and prevention* (3rd ed.). Philadelphia: J. B. Lippincott, p. 126.

## Progression of HIV Disease

Early studies of survival after an AIDS diagnosis suggested that women, as compared to men, had more a rapid progression of their disease and a shortened survival time after diagnosis (Stoneburner, 1988). However, the shorter survival appears to be related to poor access to care and later presentation at clinical facilities with more advanced disease and a greater number of symptoms (Brettle & Leen, 1991).

Studies in Europe and in San Francisco indicate no difference in survival rates for men and women. Analysis of more than 4,000 patients in San Francisco indicates no difference in survival of women as compared to men (Creagh, Doi, Andrews, & Nusinoff-Lehrman, 1988). A smaller study in Amsterdam found no significant difference in the one-year survival between men and women (Bindels et al., 1991).

Numerous studies of gay men have documented a fairly predictable rate of CD4 decline per year of HIV infection (Friedland et al., 1991; McDonnell, Chmiel, Wu, & Phair, 1990; Moss et al., 1988). Few comparable studies have been done on women. Carpenter and associates (1991) reported a rate of CD4 decline of 50 cells per year in women, a rate similar to that of men.

The spectrum of opportunistic infections seen in women is generally quite similar to that of men. Carpenter and associates (1991) found a 34% incidence of candida esophagitis, 18% herpes simplex, and 20% pneumocystis carinii pneumonia (PCP) in a cohort of 200 women. This reported incidence of PCP is lower than that reported for AIDS cases in men (Fleming, Ciesielski, Byers, Castro, & Berkelman, 1993). However, Guinan and Hardy, in a study of AIDS cases among women in the United States from 1981 to 1986, found no significant difference in the incidence of PCP (1987). The incidence of Kaposi's sarcoma in women is negligible compared to that in gay men and is similar to the rate seen in male nongay injection drug users men (Haverkos, Drotmen, & Morgan, 1990).

## Gynecologic Manifestations of Disease

During the first years of the epidemic, little attention was paid to gynecologic manifestations of HIV disease. More recently, there has been significant interest in HIV-related vaginal candidiasis, pelvic inflammatory disease, and cervical neoplasia.

### Vaginal Candidiasis

Oral-esophageal candidiasis has been a hallmark of severe HIV-related immunodeficiency, usually occurring in patients with fewer than 200 CD4 cells. Severe disease, manifested by the presence of extensive plaquelike lesions over the entire oral-pharynx and esophagus, is seen in patients with end-stage disease and CD4 counts of 50 or less.

There were few descriptions of vaginal candidiasis in the early AIDS literature. Recent studies document a high prevalence of vaginal candidiasis in HIV-infected women. Imam and colleagues (1990) noted a 50% incidence of new onset or increased frequency of vaginal candidiasis in otherwise asymptomatic HIV-infected women. The increased frequency of vaginal candidiasis was considered to be at least four episodes per year. Many of the women also noted an increased duration and severity of disease. At the onset of vaginal candidiasis in these women, their CD4 counts averaged 506 (±150). Women with oral candidiasis had a much lower CD4 count (230 ±80). Rhoads, Wright, Redford, and Burk (1987) also described seven women with chronic vaginal candidiasis for longer than 1 year who all had severe immunodeficiency and oral thrush. Similarly, in a prospective study of HIV-infected women in Brooklyn, 25% of the women had vaginal candidiasis, and the rate of symptomatic vulvovaginitis increased with the severity of immune dysfunction (Sierra, personal communication, 1992).

### Pelvic Inflammatory Disease

Pelvic inflammatory disease (PID) is an acute infectious process of the female genital tract. When severe, it can extend upward beyond the uterus and cause extensive inflammation of the fallopian tubes and ovaries. It is caused by a variety of pathogens, including N. gonorrhea and C. trachomatis. Vaginal flora, part of the native ecology of the female genitourinary tract, play a role in disease pathogenesis but are not the primary inciting agents of the process.

Several studies from San Francisco (Safrin, Dattel, Haver, & Sweet, 1990) and New York (Hoegsberg et al., 1990; Sperling, Friedman, Joyner, Brodman, & Dottino, 1991) suggest a high prevalence of HIV infection in patients who concurrently are diagnosed with PID, with rates ranging from 6.7% to 16.7%. Because *N. gonorrhea, C. trachomatis,* and HIV are all sexually transmitted, it is not surprising to find a second STD when diagnosing the first one.

The study by Hoegsberg and colleagues (1990) also suggested that HIV-positive women with PID may have a more severe course than those who are HIV negative. These findings are supported by those of Irwin, Rice, and O'Sullivan (1993) who found women with HIV infection and PID to have more severe symptoms and greater likelihood of admission than women who had negative HIV serostatus; Kamenga and coworkers (1993) found that HIV-positive women with PID had higher clinical scores and more severe illness presentation. Encouragingly, in the two latter studies, standard antibiotic therapy was adequate as treatment for resolution of symptoms.

All data on PID must be interpreted with caution. Long-term, prospective longitudinal studies with good follow-up of patients have not been done, and the numbers in published works are small. Recruitment or follow-up bias may lead to overreading of the significance of the interactions between the two STDs. Ongoing, multicenter prospective studies will help define the clinical history of PID in women with HIV infection.

## Human Papilloma Virus and Cervical Neoplasia

There is considerable evidence that human papillomavirus (HPV) is epidemiologically linked to cervical carcinoma (Koutsky et al., 1992; Maggwa, Hunter, Mbugua, Tukei, & Mati, 1993). Recent studies strongly suggest that immunosuppressed HIV-infected women are at a greater than normal risk for acquisition, persistence, and progression of HPV-related cervical lesions (Feingold et al., 1990; Maggwa et al., 1993; Maiman, 1991; Mandelblatt, Fahs, Senie, & Peterson, 1992). Clear answers as to the exact nature of the interaction between HIV, HPV, and cervical disease are not available. New technologies, applied to different and relatively small populations over short time periods, have given rise to a plethora of data, much of it confusing or contradictory. What is known is as follows:

1. Compared to HIV-negative women, those with HIV disease have higher rates of cervical HPV infection (Feingold, 1990).
2. The more severe the HIV-induced immunosuppression, the greater the rate of HPV infection (Vermund et al., 1991).
3. Compared to seronegative women, those infected with HIV had higher rates of cervical cytological abnormalities (Finegold et al., 1990; Vermund et al., 1991).

4. The greater the degree of HIV-induced immunosuppression, the more severe the cytological lesions (Finegold et al., 1990; Schafer, Friedman, Mielke, Schwartlander, & Koch, 1991; Vermund et al., 1991).

5. On occasion, women with HIV disease can develop severe, aggressive disseminated cervical cancer (Maiman et al., 1993).

6. Although uncommon, aggressive metastatic cervical carcinoma does occur in young HIV-infected women (Maiman et al., 1990). These aggressive neoplasms are thought to be associated with HIV-related immunosuppression, which induces an accelerated progression from mild cervical dysplasia to widespread malignancy. The immunosuppression may also enhance the replication of the oncogenic HPV strains that are causally linked to cervical cancer.

7. Women with cervical cancer and HIV infection have a higher reccurrence rate than HIV-negative women with comparable stages of disease (Maiman et al., 1993).

In a widely quoted paper, Maiman and colleagues (1991) noted cervical intraepithelial neoplasia (CIN) in 13 of 32 HIV-infected patients, only three of whom had abnormal Pap smears. This paper stimulated much discussion concerning the sensitivity of Pap smears for detecting cervical cytologic abnormalities in HIV-infected women. Other groups report contrary results and believe that the Pap smear is an adequate screening tool and that colposcopy is indicated only for HIV-infected women with an abnormal Pap result (Adachi, Fleming, Burk, Ho, & Klein, 1993). This issue raises clinical questions for the care of women with HIV infection, including whether Pap smears can be relied on as adequate to screen for cervical cancer, whether colposcopy should be performed as part of routine care, and the appropriate frequency of use for these diagnostic tools. These questions can only be answered by future studies.

## ❖ Changes in CDC Definition of AIDS

In response to a changing understanding of HIV disease, in 1992 the CDC revised its classification of HIV disease and expanded the surveillance case definition for AIDS among adolescents and adults (CDC, 1992b). These changes can be summarized as follows:

1. In addition to retaining the previously listed 23 clinical conditions of the previous surveillance definition of AIDS (e.g., toxoplasmosis, cryptococcal meningitis, cryptosporidiosis, etc.), the expanded definition for AIDS includes all HIV-infected people with pulmonary tuberculosis, recurrent bacterial pneumonia, and invasive cervical cancer.

2. In the revised classification system of HIV infection, those with persistent, frequent, or poorly responsive candida vulvovaginitis, moderate or severe cervical dysplasia, and cervical carcinoma were listed

in clinical category B, symptomatic HIV-related conditions that are not part of the AIDS surveillance definition. The changes related to candida vulvovaginitis and cervical dysplasia/cervical carcinoma provide recognition that these gynecologic conditions are exacerbated by coexisting HIV infection.

The revision of the case definition has resulted in a 142% increase in reported AIDS cases in men between 1992 and 1993 and a 182% increase in women (Chu, Ward, & Fleming, 1993). This preliminary finding suggests that the expanded AIDS case definition is more sensitive to disease manifestations in women.

## ❖ Summary

From a global perspective, HIV is principally a heterosexually transmitted disease affecting men and women in equal numbers. In the United States, the dominance of HIV-infected men partially blinded us to that fact. The unfortunate emergence of women infected largely from sexual contact with male injection drug users in certain areas of the country has returned us to reality. Careful research about the epidemiology and natural history of HIV disease in women has now started in earnest. It is hoped that these studies, along with the research from Africa and elsewhere in the world, will yield information to help us slow the epidemic among women as well as men.

## ❖ References

Adachi, A., Fleming, I., Burk, R. D., Ho, G. F., & Klein, R. S. (1993). Women with human immunodeficiency virus infection and abnormal Papanicolaou smears: Prospective study of colposcopy and clinical outcome. *Obstetrics and Gynecology, 81*(3), 372–377.

Bindels, P. J., Poos, R. M. J., Jong, J. T., Mulder, J. W., Jager, M. H. C., & Coutinho, R. A. (1991). Trends in mortality among AIDS patients in Amsterdam 1982–1988. *AIDS, 5,* 853–858.

Brettle, R. P. & Leen, C. L. The natural history of HIV and AIDS in women. *AIDS, 5*(11), 1283–1292.

Carpenter, C., Mayer, K. H., Stein, M. D., Leibman, B. D., Fisher, A., & Fiore, T. C. (1991). Human immunodeficiency virus infection in North American women: Experience with 200 cases and a review of the literature. *Medicine, 70,* 307–324.

Centers for Disease Control. (1981). Pneumocystis pneumonia—Los Angeles. *Morbidity and Mortality Weekly Report, 30,* 250–252.

Centers for Disease Control. (1982a). Pneumocystis carinii pneumonia among persons with hemophilia A. *Morbidity and Mortality Weekly Report, 31,* 365–367.

Centers for Disease Control. (1982b). Unexplained immunodeficiency and opportunistic infections in infants—New York, New Jersey, California. *Morbidity and Mortality Weekly Report, 31,* 665–667.

Centers for Disease Control. (1983a). Acquired immunodeficiency syndrome among patients with hemophilia—United States. *Morbidity and Mortality Weekly Report, 32,* 613–615.

Centers for Disease Control. (1983b). Immunodeficiency among female sexual partners of males with acquired immunodeficiency syndrome—New York. *Morbidity and Mortality Weekly Report, 31,* 697–698.

Centers for Disease Control. (1991). Drug use and sexual behavior among sex partners of injecting drug users—United States (1988–1990). *Morbidity and Mortality Weekly Report, 40,* 855–859.

Centers for Disease Control and Prevention. (1992a). Condom use among male intravenous drug users in New York City, 1987–1990. *Morbidity and Mortality Weekly Report, 41,* 617–620.

Centers for Disease Control and Prevention. (1992b). HIV infection and expanded surveillance case definition for AIDS among adolescents and adults. *Morbidity and Mortality Weekly Report, 41,* 1–14.

Centers for Disease Control and Prevention. (1992c). Projections of the number of persons diagnosed with AIDS and the number of immunosuppressed HIV infected persons—United States, 1992. *Morbidity and Mortality Weekly Report, 41,* 1–23.

Centers for Disease Control and Prevention. (1993a). Acquired immunodeficiency syndrome—United States—1992. *Morbidity and Mortality Weekly Report, 42,* 547–557.

Centers for Disease Control and Prevention. (1993b). Barrier protection against HIV infection and other sexually transmitted diseases. *Morbidity and Mortality Weekly Report, 42,* 588–591.

Centers for Disease Control and Prevention. (1993c). HIV prevention through case management for HIV-infected persons—selected sites—United States 1989–1992. *Morbidity and Mortality Weekly Report, 42,* 448–556

Centers for Disease Control and Prevention. (1993d). Mortality attributable to HIV infection/AIDS among persons aged 25–44 years—United States 1990–1991. *Morbidity and Mortality Weekly Report, 42,* 481–486.

Chaisson, R. E., Bacchetti, P., Osmond, D., Brodie, B., Sande, M. A., & Moss, A. R. (1989). Cocaine use and HIV infection in intravenous drug users in San Francisco. *Journal of the American Medical Association, 261*(11), 1471–1472.

Chu, S., Berkelman, R. L., & Curran, J. W. (1992). Epidemiology of HIV in the United States. In V. T. DeVita, S. Hellman, & S. A. Rosenberg (Eds.), *AIDS: Etiology, diagnosis, treatment and prevention* (3rd ed., pp. 99–110). Philadelphia: J. B. Lippincott.

Chu, S. Y., Birchler, J. W., Fleming, P. L., & Berkelman, R. L. (1990). Epidemiology of reported cases of AIDS in lesbians—United States, 1980–1989. *American Journal of Public Health, 80*(11), 1380–1381.

Chu, S., Ward, J., & Fleming, P. (1993, October). Impact of the expanded AIDS surveillance definition on the ascertainment of HIV morbidity in women. American Public Health Association 121st Annual Meeting, San Francisco.

Creagh, K. T., Doi, P., Andrews, E., & Nusinoff-Lehrman, S. (1988). Survival experience among patients with AIDS receiving zidovudine: Follow-up of patients in a compassionate plea program. *Journal of the American Medical Association, 260*(20), 3009–3015.

DesJarlais, D. C., Friedman, S. R., Novick, D. M., Sotheran, J. L., Thomas, P., Yancovitz, S. R., Mildvan, D., Weber, J., Kreech, M. J., & Maslansky, R.

(1989). HIV-1 infection among intravenous drug users in Manhattan, New York City from 1977–1987. *Journal of the American Medical Association, 261*(7), 1008–1012.

Ellerbrock, T. V., Bush, T. J., Chamberland, M. E., & Oxtoby, M. J. (1991). Epidemiology of women with AIDS in the United States—1981–1990. *Journal of the American Medical Association, 265,* 2971–2975.

Feingold, A. R., Vermund, S. H., Burk, R. D., Kelley, K. F., Schrager, L. K., Schreiber, K., Munk, G., Friedland, G. H., & Klein, R. S., (1990). Cervical cytologic abnormalities and papillomavirus in women infected with human immunodeficiency virus. *Journal of Acquired Immune Deficiency Syndromes, 3*(9), 896–930.

Fleming, P. L., Ciesielski, C. A., Byers, R. H., Castro, K. G., & Berkelman, R. L. (1993). Gender differences in reported AIDS-indicative diseases. *Journal of Infectious Diseases, 168*(1), 61–67.

Friedland, G. H., Saltzman, B., Vileno, J., Freeman, K., Schrager, L. K., & Klein, R. (1991). Survival differences in patients with AIDS. *Journal of Acquired Immune Deficiency Syndromes, 4,* 144–153.

Fullilove, R. E., Fullilove, M. T., Bowser, B. P., & Gross, S. A. (1990). Risk of sexually transmitted disease among black adolescent crack users in Oakland and San Francisco, Calif. *Journal of the American Medical Association, 263*(6), 851–855.

Greenblatt, R. M., Lukehart, S. A., Plummer, F. A., Quinn, T. C., Critchlow, C. W., Ashley, R. L., D'Costa, L. J., Ndinya-Achola, J. O., Corey, L., & Ronald, A. R. (1988). Genital ulceration as a risk factor for Human Immunodeficiency Virus infection. *AIDS, 2*(1), 47–50.

Guinan, M. E., & Hardy, A. (1987). Epidemiology of AIDS in women in the United States. *Journal of the American Medical Association, 257,* 2039–2042.

Gwinn, M., Pappaiganou, M., George, J. R., Hannon, W. H., Wasser, S. C., Redus, M. A., Hoff, R., Grady, G. F., Willoughby, A., & Novello, A. C. (1991). Prevalence of HIV infection in childbearing women in the United States. *Journal of the American Medical Association, 265*(13), 1704–1708.

Handsfield, H. H. (1988). Heterosexual transmission of human immunodeficiency virus. *Journal of the American Medical Association, 260,* 1943–1944.

Haverkos, H. W., & Edelman, R. (1988). The epidemiology of acquired immunodeficiency among heterosexuals. *Journal of the American Medical Association, 260,* 1922–1929.

Haverkos, H. W., Brotman, D. P., & Morgan, W. (1990). Kaposi's sarcoma in patients with AIDS: Sex, transmission mode, and race. *Biomedicine & Pharmacotherapy, 44*(9), 461–466.

Hoegsberg, B., Abulafia, O., Sedlis, A., Feldman, J., DesJalais, D., Landesman, S. H., & Minkoff, H. (1990). Sexually transmitted diseases and human immunodeficiency virus infection among women with pelvic inflammatory disease. *American Journal of Obstetrics and Gynecology, 163,* 1135–1139.

Holmberg, S. D., Horsburgh, R., Ward, J. W., & Jaffe, H. W. (1989). Biological factors in the sexual transmission of HIV. *Journal of Infectious Disease, 160,* 116–125.

Iman, N., Carpenter, C. C., Mayer, K. H., Fisher, A., Stein, M., & Danforth, S. B. (1990). Hierarchical pattern of mucosal candida infections in HIV-seropositive women. *American Journal of Medicine, 90*(2), 142–146.

Irwin, K., Rice, R., & O'Sullivan, M. (1993, June). *The clinical presentation and course of pelvic inflammatory disease in HIV+ and HIV- women: Preliminary results of a multicenter study*. Paper presented at the Ninth International Conference on AIDS, Berlin. (Abstract No.WS-BO7-1)

Kamenga, M., Toure, C. K., N'gbichi, J. M., (1993, June). *Human immunodeficiency virus (HIV) infection in women with pelvic inflammatory disease in Abidjan, Côte d'Ivoire*. Paper presented at the Ninth International Conference on AIDS, Berlin. (Abstract No. WS-BO7-2)

Koutsky, L. A., Holmes, K. K., Critchlow, C. W., Stevens, C. E., Paavonem, J., Beckman, A. M., DeRouen, T. A., Galloway, D. A., Vernon, D., & Kiviat, N. B. (1992). A cohort study of the risk of cervical intraepithelial neoplasia grade 2 or 3 in relation to papillomavirus infection. *New England Journal of Medicine, 327*(18), 1272–1278.

Laga, M., Nzila, N., & Manoka, A. T. (1990, June). *Nonulcerative sexually transmitted diseases (STD) as risk factors for HIV infection*. Paper presented at the Sixth International Conference on AIDS, San Francisco, CA. (Abstract No. Th-C97)

Maggwa, B. N., Hunter, D. J., Mbugua, S., Tukei, P., & Mati, J. K. (1993). The relationship between HIV infection and cervical intraepithelial neoplasia among women attending two family planning clinics in Nairobi, Kenya. *AIDS, 7*, 733–738.

Maiman, M. (1991). Human immunodeficiency virus infection and cervical neoplasia. *Postgraduate Obstetrics/Gynecology, 11*, 1–5.

Maiman, M., Fruchter, R., Guy, L., Cuthill, S., Levine, P., & Serur, E. (1993). Human immunodeficiency virus infection and invasive cervical carcinoma. *Cancer, 71*(2), 402–406.

Maiman, M., Fruchter, R. G., Serur, E., Remy, J. C., Feuer, G., & Boyce, J. (1990). Human Immunodeficiency Virus infection and cervical neoplasia. *Gynecology Oncology, 38*(3), 377–382.

Maiman, M., Tarricone, N., Vieira, J., Suarez, J., Serur, E., & Boyce, J. (1991). Colposcopy evaluation of HIV-seropositive women. *American College Obstetrics/Gynecology, 78*(1), 84–88.

Mandelblatt, J. S., Fahs, M., Senie, R. T., & Peterson, H. B. (1992). Association between HIV infection and cervical neoplasia. Implications for clinical care of women at risk for both conditions. *AIDS, 6*, 173–178.

Mann, J. M., Tarantola, D. J. M., & Netler, T. W. (Eds.). (1992). *AIDS in the world*. Cambridge, MA: Harvard University Press.

Marmor, M., Weiss, L. R., Lyden, M., Weiss, S. H., Saxinger, C. W., Spira, T. J., & Feorino, P. M. (1986). Possible female-to-female transmission of human immunodeficiency virus. (letter) *Annals of Internal Medicine, 105*, 969.

McCombs, S. B., McCray, E., Wendell, P. A., Sweeney, P. A., & Onorato, I. M. (1992). Epidemiology of HIV-1 infection in bisexual women. *Journal of Acquired Immunodeficiency Syndromes, 5*(8), 850–852.

McDonnell, K. B., Chmiel, J. S., Wu, S., & Phair, J. P. (1990). Predicting progression to AIDS: Combined usefulness of $CD_4$ lymphocyte counts and p24 antigenemia. *American Journal of Medicine, 89*, 706–712.

Minkoff, H. L., McCalla, S., Delke, I., Stevens, R., Salwen, M., & Feldman, J. (1990). The relationship of cocaine use to syphilis and Human Immunodeficiency Virus infections among inner city parturient women. *American Journal of Obstetrics and Gynecology, 163*(2), 521–526.

Monzon, O. T., & Capellan, J. M. B. (1987). Female-to-female transmission of HIV [letter to the editor]. *Lancet, 2*, 40.

Moss, A. R., Bacchetti, P., Osmond, D., Krampf, W., Chaisson, R. E., Stites, D., Wilber, J., Allain, J. P., & Carlson, J. (1988). Seropositivity for HIV and the development of AIDS or AIDS-related condition: Three year follow-up of the San Francisco General Hospital cohort. *British Medical Journal, 296*, 45–50.

National Research Council. (1989). *AIDS: Sexual behavior and intravenous drug use.* Washington, DC: National Academy Press.

Nkowane, B. M. (1991). Prevalence and incidence of HIV infection in Africa: A review of data published in 1990. *AIDS, 5*(Suppl.), 57–74.

Novick, L. F., Berns, D., Stricof, R., Stevens, R., Pass, K., & Wethers, J. (1989). HIV seroprevalence in newborns in New York State. *Journal of the American Medical Association, 261*, 1704–1708.

Peterman, T. A., & Curran, J. W. (1986). Sexual transmission of human immuno-deficiency virus. *Journal of the American Medical Association, 256*, 2220–2226.

Petersen, L. R., Doll, L., White, C., Chu, S., & the HIV Blood Donor Study Group. (1992). No evidence for female to female transmission among 960,000 female blood donors. *Journal of Acquired Immune Deficiency Syndromes, 155*, 853–855.

Piot, P., Plummer, F. A., Reu, M. A., Ngugi, E. N., Rouzioux, C., Ndinya-Achola, J. O., Veracauteren, G., D'Costa, L. J., Laga, M., & Nsanze, H. (1987). Retrospective seroepidemiology of AIDS virus infection in Nairobi prostitutes. *Journal of Infectious Disease, 155*(6), 1108–1112.

Rhoads, J. L., Wright, D. C., Redfield, R. R., & Burke, D. S. (1987). Chronic vaginal candidiasis in women with human immunodeficiency virus infection. *Journal of the American Medical Association, 257*(22), 3105–3107.

Safrin, S., Dattel, B. J., Haver, L., & Sweet, R. L. (1990). Seroprevalence and epidemiologic correlates of human immunodeficiency virus infection in women with acute pelvic inflammatory disease. *Journal of Obstetrics and Gynecology, 75*, 666–670.

Schafer, A., Friedman, W., Mielke, M., Schwartlander, B., & Koch, M. A. (1991). The increased frequency of cervical dysplasia neoplasia in women infected with HIV is related to the degree of immunosuppression. *American Journal of Obstetrics and Gynecology, 164*, 593–599.

Sperling, R. S., Friedman, F., Jouner, M., Brodman, M., & Dottino, P. (1991). Seroprevalence of human immunodeficiency virus in women admitted to the hospital with pelvic inflammatory disease. *Journal of Reproductive Medicine, 36*(2), 122–124.

Stoneburner, R. L., DesJarlais, D. C., Benezra, D., Gorelkin, L., Sotheran, J. L., Firedman, S. R., Schultz, S., Marmor, M., Mildvan, D., & Maslansky, R. (1988). A larger spectrum of severe HIV-1 related disease in intravenous drug users in New York City. *Science, 242*(4880), 916–919.

Vermund, S. H., Keller, K. F., Klein, R. S., Feingold, A. R., Schreiber, K., Munk, G., & Burk, R. D. (1991). High risk of human papillomavirus infection and cervical squamous intraepithelial lesions among women with symptomatic human immunodeficiency virus infection. *American Journal of Obstetrics and Gynecology, 165*(2), 392–400.

Vogt, M. W., Witt, D. J., Craven, D. E., Byington, B. S., Crawford, D. F., Hutchinson, M. S., Schooley, R. T., & Hirsch, M. S. (1987). Isolation patterns of the human immunodeficiency virus from cervical secretions during the menstrual cycle of women at risk for the Acquired Immunodeficiency Syndrome. *Annals of Internal Medicine, 106*(3), 380–382.

Wolfe, H., Vranizan, K. M., & Gorter, R. G. (in press). Epidemiology of women with AIDS in the United States, 1981–1990. *Journal of the American Medical Association.*

## ❖ Chapter 4

# Care of Women
# with HIV Disease

CATHERINE LYONS
JACK A. DEHOVITZ

The medical care of women with HIV disease includes an intertwining of the management of HIV and non-HIV medical problems, health maintenance, and psychosocial needs. This chapter focuses on the specifics of comprehensive medical care as it is combined with the provision of other services.

Women with HIV infection seek care at a variety of sites. Specialty and general medical clinics provide HIV medical services but often are not equipped to provide basic gynecologic care. Family practice clinics can generally deliver general and HIV-related services to both women and children. Bringing a child to a medical visit may provide an entrée for the woman into the health care system. Family planning clinics are often the only place women (especially young women) interact with the health care community. Although it may be out of the scope of their practice to establish full HIV care, these clinics can usually implement HIV education, counseling, testing, and referral. Some methadone maintenance clinics in areas of high HIV prevalence and where adequate staff training exists have set up primary HIV care clinics (Genser & Schlenger, 1993). In these settings, the medical needs of patients can be efficiently met. Clinics that provide services to homeless people, often set up in shelters, have expanded their medical services to include HIV care.

In communities where gay men still make up a large percentage of those affected by HIV, a woman may be uncomfortable sitting in a waiting room full of men. When the number of patients makes it possible, a separate women's clinic, a dedicated session, or a special provider can ease the comfort level of patients, provide a context for addressing psychosocial needs, and encourage networking. In the same way that education, counseling, and testing programs are creative in reaching out to women who are at risk for HIV, care providers must work to comfortably integrate women into care systems and to assist the systems to meet fully the needs of women with HIV disease.

## ❖ Initial Evaluation

The initial evaluation of women with HIV infection includes a full medical and psychosocial assessment. For all women, but particularly those who have recently learned of their HIV infection, emotional and educational needs can be monumental. The provider should consider doing the initial evaluation over two or more visits and sharing with the patient decisions about what will be included or completed at each visit. In addition to completing as much as possible of the initial evaluation, the provider can assess what the patient feels are her most pressing needs and try to meet at least one item on her agenda.

### Chief Complaint

Assess the patient's reason for coming into treatment at this time: Was she referred, or did she self-refer? Are there pressing psychosocial problems? Is there an acute medical complaint? If yes, one goal of the visit will be to start to address the specified problem. If no acute complaint is offered, a directed interview regarding the signs and symptoms of HIV should be done as part of the review of symptoms. Assess the patient's awareness of her risk, her knowledge of HIV disease, and her ability to be proactive in her care, by determining when, where, and why HIV testing was done.

### Past Medical History

The medical history (Figures 4–1 and 4–2) should include information about both HIV- and non-HIV-related processes. Inquire about hospitalizations. Be specific about illnesses that the patient may not identify as HIV related, such as bacterial pneumonia or pelvic inflammatory disease. (PID). Specifically ask about a history of (1) tuberculosis (TB), exposure to TB, or a positive skin test for TB (if the patient reports a recent negative TB skin, inquire about the placement of an anergy panel to determine if the test was a true negative); (2) hepatitis, including type and dates; (3) herpes

---

- Hospitalizations
- Significant non-HIV medical problems
- Tuberculosis, exposure to TB, positive PPD
- Hepatitis: date and type
- Herpes zoster
- Herpes simplex: location(s)
- Syphilis, positive VDRL
- Other sexually transmitted diseases

---

FIGURE 4–1   Past medical history (non-OB-GYN).

- Menstrual history
    Age at menarche
    Cycle interval and length
    Intermenstrual bleeding
    Associated symptoms
    Last normal period and any changes from normal
- Pregnancies and outcome
- Diethylstilbestrol (DES) exposure
- Sexual history
- Contraceptive history and HIV prevention
- History of sexually transmitted diseases, pelvic inflammatory disease, and undiagnosed vaginal ulcers and discharge
- Vaginal candidiasis: number of episodes in the last 6 months and treatment
- History of abnormal Pap smears and treatment
- History of breast problems
- History of sexual assault and rape

FIGURE 4–2    OB-GYN history.

simplex, including location and frequency of outbreaks; (4) herpes zoster; (5) syphilis and its treatment; (6) allergies; and (7) immunizations for influenza, pneumococcus, hepatitis, and diphtheria/tetanus.

Areas specific to women should be explored in some detail. Obstetric, gynecologic, and sexual histories are important for HIV management and for psychosocial and educational interventions. Although the relationship between HIV and menses is unclear and numerous other problems may affect the menstrual cycle of women with HIV infection, such as drug use or chronic disease, a complete menstrual history should be collected. It should include age at menarche, cycle interval, length and amount of flow, intermenstrual bleeding, associated symptoms, last normal menses, and recent changes. The basic obstetrical history should include the number and dates of pregnancies, abortions (spontaneous and therapeutic), and births; the status of living children (alive and well? HIV infected? HIV tested?); and any prenatal, delivery, or postpartum problems. The gynecologic history should include any history of sexually transmitted diseases (gonorrhea, syphilis, chlamydia, warts, PID, and others), genital ulcers (diagnosed or self-reported), vaginal discharge, vaginal candidiasis (including the number of episodes in the past 6 months and their treatment). In addition, the date of the last Pap smear, the history of abnormal Pap smears, and the recommended or received treatments are essential to appropriately tailor gynecologic care to the woman with HIV infection. Other useful information includes the patient's current contraceptive method, her history of breast problems (such as masses or infections), and her history of sexual assault or rape.

## Medications

Question patients about all current medications, regularly or occasionally used, including prescription drugs, over-the-counter drugs, drugs received from friends, creams/lotions, and nontraditional treatments, such as herbs, vitamins, and homeopathic remedies. To ensure open communication, phrase questions and receive answers about all of these topics in a nonjudgmental manner.

## Family History

Obtaining a family history helps to determine familial medical problems and gives clues to social patterns like substance abuse. The presence or lack of family support and the extent of HIV as a family disease can also be determined.

## Social History

The goal of obtaining the patient's social history is to determine as thoroughly as possible what social service, educational, psychological, and financial needs a woman has. HIV is a complex medical process, yet ultimately the patient will pay little attention to her medical needs if her psychosocial needs are not concomitantly addressed. Consequently, the integration of psychosocial services with medical services is important both for the patient-provider rapport and to address some of the barriers to maintaining primary care.

Where does the woman live? How long has she been there, and with whom does she live? Are her children in her custody? Is anyone else in the household known to be HIV positive or at risk for HIV? Who in her life knows that she is HIV positive? Many women have withheld this information even from those closest to them. All of these questions will determine what supports she has and what demands are placed on her.

All women should be asked about past or present drug use, including alcohol. Specific questions should be asked about the use of injection drugs, and if the patient is currently using them, an assessment should be made about her knowledge and use of safer needle techniques. Determine any history of drug treatment. For those currently in recovery, it is helpful to identify what program or support she uses to maintain sobriety. If the patient is currently using drugs, ask her if she identifies this as a problem, and if so whether she is interested in any intervention. In most settings (primary care within drug-treatment programs is an exception), it is appropriate to clearly let the patient know that her medical care is not contingent on her remaining drug-free. Questions should be asked in a nonjudgmental way. Substance abusers may feel guilty or be secretive about their behaviors; open, honest communication on the part of the provider is a necessity.

A sexual history should gather information on the gender of partners and on past and present sexual practices. Never assume the sexual orientation of the patient, but ask specifically whether she has been sexually active with women, men, or both. This information is important in providing appropriate safer sex counseling. Determine whether the woman desires pregnancy, what safer-sex practices she uses, what contraception methods she employs (for women who are sexually active with men), and whether there are impediments to the use of contraceptives.

Other specific areas to inquire about include the patient's cultural background, employment history, current means of income, educational history, and travel history. Ask also about the last grade completed in school. If there is any question about the patient's literacy, ask her directly about her ability to read and write.

## Review of Symptoms

In the review of symptoms (Table 4–1), it is important to ask specific HIV-focused questions. These will enable you to consider specific diagnoses, and it will give some clue as to the level of immune suppression. Assess the woman's level of well-being, energy level, and fatigue, and if there has been a change from what she considers normal, determine over what period of time the change occurred. If fevers and night sweats are present, determine the time course and frequency of occurrence. Memory impairment and other mental status changes may be very troubling to patients. In some cases, patients may be unwilling to acknowledge or be unaware of such a problem. In this case, a friend or family member might be a better source for this information.

Multiple skin problems are common with HIV, and the presence and character of recent skin rashes, discolorations, or other changes should be explored. Visual changes should be described in detail and a diagnosis of cytomegalovirus (CMV) retinitis specifically ruled out in those with CD4 counts lower than 50. Ask about the presence of swollen glands and white patches in the mouth. Dysphagia, odynophagia, or both may suggest candida esophagitis or an ulcerative process in the esophagus.

The presence of cough and dyspnea must again be characterized in detail; an alert provider can diagnosis pneumocystis carinii pneumonia (PCP) in its early, indolent form when it presents with a dry cough and mild dyspnea on exertion before it progresses to severe respiratory symptoms. Questions regarding gastrointestinal problems include weight loss, appetite changes, nausea and vomiting, diarrhea, and abdominal pain. Specifically ask about the presence of vaginal discharge or vaginal lesions, which suggest an acute gynecologic problem that should be assessed thoroughly on the present visit. Pain, numbness, or burning in the hands or feet suggest a peripheral neuropathy.

TABLE 4–1   Symptoms and Possible Diagnoses

| Symptom | Possible Diagnosis |
| --- | --- |
| Fatigue, lack of energy | New opportunistic infection(OI)<br>Anemia |
| Fever, night sweats | Mycobacterium avium complex (MAC)<br>Tuberculosis (TB) |
| Headache | Central nervous system (CNS)<br>   toxoplasmosis or lymphoma<br>Cryptococcal meningitis<br>Aseptic meningitis<br>Progressive multifocal<br>   leukoencephalopathy (PML) |
| Memory loss,<br>cognitive deficits | AIDS dementia complex<br>PML<br>CNS toxoplasmosis |
| Light-headedness | Adrenal insufficiency |
| Visual changes | Cytomegalovirus (CMV) retinitis |
| Dysphagia, odynophagia | Esophageal candidiasis<br>Herpes simplex virus (HSV)  or<br>   cytomegalovirus (CMV) esophagitis |
| Enlarged, tender lymph nodes | Infection<br>Lymphoma |
| Cough, dyspnea | Pneumocystis carinii pneumonia (PCP)<br>Bacterial pneumonia<br>TB |
| Poor appetite | New OI<br>MAC<br>Wasting syndrome |
| Diarrhea | Parasitic infection<br>Bacterial infection<br>CMV gastritis/colitis<br>MAC |
| Vaginal discharge, pruritus | Vaginal candida |
| Vaginal/perianal/anal ulcer, pain | HSV |
| Dry, flaky skin | Seborrheic dermatitis |
| Rash | Folliculitis<br>Drug reaction |
| Pain, numbness, burning in<br>   hands, feet | Peripheral neuropathy |

## Physical Exam

A complete physical exam should be done for the specific problems that may be revealed and to determine a baseline for future comparison. As with the history, findings on the physical exam can give important clues as to the level of immune functioning. Vital signs are an important initial piece of every physical exam; the weight is of particular value for future comparisons and interventions should be taken for even small losses.

Evaluation of the oral cavity should be done, noting dentition and presence of gingivitis. White, cottage cheese-like plaques on any surface that are easily removable are most likely candida, as are erythematous plaques on the palate; confirmation can be done with a potassium hydroxide (KOH) prep. Nonremovable white plaques on the lateral aspects or ventral surface of the tongue are hairy leukoplakia. The diagnosis is generally made based on clinical appearance, but a biopsy can be done for confirmation.

Lymph node examination should include evaluation of all chains. Specific note should be made of the presence, size, tenderness, and mobility of nodes greater than 1 cm. This is especially important for future comparison.

A thorough evaluation of the skin must be done, and skin pathologies must be noted. Dry, flaking skin on the face is most likely seborrheic dermatitis, which is common, as are fungal infections and bacterial processes like folliculitis (Berger, 1992). All lesions should be biopsied; HIV-related infections, such as cryptococcus, can present systemically, and only a biopsy is definitive (DeVita, Hellman, & Rosenberg, 1992).

A fundoscopic exam should be done. The ability to find retinal lesions consistent with CMV retinitis permits treatment before the onset of visual symptoms; however, the ability of a generalist primary provider to diagnose such lesions, even with pupil dilatation, may be limited, and prompt referral to an ophthamologist should be made if any uncertainties exist.

A screening neurologic exam might include evaluation of gait, deep tendon reflexes, and brief mental status determination. A more detailed exam should be done if any complaints were elicited during the history.

Auscultation of the heart and lungs and palpation of the abdomen for masses or organomegaly should be a part of the comprehensive and follow-up examinations. Do not underestimate the therapeutic importance of the hands-on examination for the patient. Remember that women with HIV infection often feel stigmatized or contaminated, and a physical exam can work to counter these feelings.

Unless there is a specific complaint, consider allowing the woman to decide if the breast and pelvic exams should be performed at this or a subsequent visit. The pelvic should include inspection of the external genitalia for the presence of condylomata or other lesions; internal speculum exam, noting the condition of the vagina and cervix; bimanual exam of the uterus; and rectal exam. All specimens should be collected before the bimanual exam and the introduction of the lubricant, which can ruin Pap smears and cultures.

## Diagnostic Tests

Laboratory analyses serve several purposes: obtaining baseline clinical data, assessing immune status, and screening for past or present evidence of infectious processes. It is helpful to arrange for patients to have their phlebotomy prior to their initial visit so that this information will be available to provide appropriate education and prompt intervention when required.

Routine clinical laboratory data (Figure 4–3) for women with HIV infection include complete blood count with differential and platelets. Although anemia and leukopenia may indicate more advanced HIV disease, the presence of any anemia should be thoroughly worked up. A complete chemistry panel, including blood urea nitrogen (BUN), creatine, liver function tests, and electrolytes should be done to determine baseline values. Elevated liver function tests will be seen in someone with chronic hepatitis, abnormal renal function in someone with HIV nephropathy, and decreased albumin in malnutrition or wasting syndrome. An increased globulin count and a low cholesterol count may be nonspecific indicators of HIV disease progression.

Evaluation of immune status involves primarily T lymphocyte subsets. The lowering of both absolute number and percentage of CD4 cells is reflective of immune destruction. Normal CD4 counts range from 600 to 1,200, vary from laboratory to laboratory, and can vary significantly (in both HIV-infected and uninfected people) based on various factors, including the time of day and the presence of infection (Gorter, Vranizan, Osmond, & Moss, 1992). Although the percentage may be a more stable measure, clinical decisions are commonly based on absolute CD4. It is important to inform patients that many things may affect the result, which may fluctuate from one occasion to another, and that there may even be significant interlaboratory variability. The CD4/CD8 ratio is normally 2:1; it is inverted to 1:2 as disease progresses. Beta 2 microglobulin, p24 antigen, and serum neopterin are tests that give some nonspecific indication of disease progression. They are not universally available, and they are of questionable clinical value.

---

- Complete blood count with differential and platelets
- Erythrocyte sedimentation rate
- Chemistry panel
- T lymphocyte subsets
- Syphilis serology
- Hepatitis serology
- Toxoplasmosis titer
- Tuberculosis screen (PPD with controls)
- Pap smear (if not done in last 6 months)
- Gonorrhea culture
- Chlamydia culture

---

FIGURE 4–3   Diagnostic tests.

Laboratory tests that will provide information about other past or present problems include the following: syphilis serology (screening with a rapid plasma reagin [RPR] or venereal disease research laboratory [VDRL] test and confirmed by the fluorescent treponemal antibody-absorption [FTA] test), hepatitis-B antibody and antigen screen, toxoplasmosis titer, Pap smear (if not done in the last 6 months), gonorrhea culture, and chlamydia culture. Wet mounts and herpes virus culture should be done if clinically indicated.

A tuberculosis screening panel should be planted with five units of intradermal purified protein derivative (PPD) given intradermally (Mantoux test) in one forearm and one or two delayed-type hypersensitivity antigens, usually mumps, candida, or tetanus toxoid, given in the other forearm as a control. The panel should be read 48 to 72 hours after placement. There are three possible biological responses to the TB panel:

1. *Positive PPD, positive control antigen response.* A reaction of 5 mm or greater on the PPD arm and any response on the control arm is read as a positive test. This indicates a functioning cell-mediated immune response and exposure at some point in the past to the tuberculosis bacilli. An evaluation consisting of chest x-ray and three sputum cultures should be done on these patients to rule out active disease. In the absence of active disease, patients with HIV infection and a positive PPD should be prophylaxed for 1 year with isoniazid 300 mg daily, along with vitamin B6/pyridoxine 25 to 50 mg daily. Repeat PPD testing is not indicated.

2. *Negative PPD, positive control antigen response.* This finding indicates a functioning immune system and is a fairly reliable indication of no tuberculosis infection at this time. Tests on these patients should be repeated every 6 months.

3. *Negative PPD, negative control antigen response.* This response indicates anergy or lack of cell-mediated immunity. It is evidence that the body cannot respond to antigens to which it has been previously exposed. This response occurs at variable points in the progression of HIV infection but generally with CD4 of 500 or less. It is not a true indicator of a lack of tuberculosis exposure. Because of the high risk of active TB in patients with HIV infection (Selwyn et al., 1992), all patients who are anergic should have a chest x-ray to rule out active TB and have the PPD and control panel testing repeated every once.

## Identification of Problems

After obtaining all pertinent data, including history, physical exam, and diagnostic test results, make a list of identified problems. This list should include health care maintenance needs, staging of HIV disease, active infections, current medical processes, positive laboratory values, and significant social problems (e.g., substance abuse, homelessness).

The staging of HIV disease is generally done by the level of CD4 cells and related disease manifestations. Some clinics use categories such as mild, moderate, and severe HIV disease (corresponding to CD4 cells >500, 500–201, and <200, respectively), symptomatic and asymptomatic disease, or other agreed-on classification categories.

## ❖ HIV Disease Intervention

Drug treatment for HIV disease takes three forms: antiretroviral therapy, prophylaxis against opportunistic infections (OIs), and treatment of OIs. Although basic treatment protocols have been established, drug therapy is a rapidly changing field. Clinical practice often precedes the publication of data in peer-review journals and changes based on information exchanged at conferences, clinical anecdotes, and impressions of providers with large populations of HIV-positive patients. Medical information for primary care providers is available from the following sources, which have turnarounds more rapid than those of most peer-reviewed journals:

- ❖ *AIDS Clinical Care,* published by the Massachusetts Medical Society, 1440 Main St., Waltham, MA 02154 (1-800-843-6356)
- ❖ *Treatment Issues,* available from the Gay Men's Health Crisis, Department of Medical Information, 129 W. 20th St., New York, NY 10011 (212-807-6664)
- ❖ *AIDS Treatment News,* P.O. Box 411256, San Francisco, CA 94141 (415-255-0588)

### *Antiretroviral Therapy*

Antiretroviral drugs, such as zidovudine (ZDV, Retrovir), didanosine (ddi, Videx), and zalcitabine (ddc, HIVID), have helped people with HIV infection achieve improved morbidity and mortality rates. Such treatment is a rapidly changing field, and many questions abound. Although antiretroviral treatment has been recommended for all patients with CD4 cells of less than 500, a number of recent studies have questioned the role of therapy in patients with early disease (asymptomatic with CD4 > 200) (Aboulker & Swart, 1993; Cotton, 1993). The role of and timing for initiation of combination therapy (zidovudine plus didanosine or zalcitabine) is also under study.

There are several agreed-on principles that should be used in considering initiation of antiretroviral therapy in women with HIV infection:

1. The choice to accept or decline antiretroviral therapy ultimately rests with the patient.
2. The decision to treat should be based on at least two CD4 counts, taken on separate occasions, as these counts have great variability.
3. There are no studies that show positive effects of treatment in patients with CD4 counts greater than 500.

4. All patients with CD4 counts of less than 200 should be offered antiretroviral therapy.
5. Patients with CD4 counts between 200 and 500 should be informed of the uncertainties of therapy. Decisions about initiating or delaying this therapeutic intervention should be made with the patient's input and based on a combination of clinical indicators and laboratory values.
6. Zidovudine should be considered as first-line therapy in patients who have received no prior antiretroviral therapy.
7. Patients who are intolerant of zidovudine or who have disease progression despite zidovudine therapy should be offered the option of didanosine or zalcitabine, according to the most current treatment guidelines. The most recent guidelines from a 1993 National Institute of Allergy and Infectious Diseases State-of-the-Art Conference (Sande, Carpenter, Cobbs, Holmes, & Sanford, 1993) are summarized in Table 4–2.
8. Regular laboratory monitoring is indicated for patients maintained on antiretrovirals according to the specific drug therapies.

## Prophylaxis of Opportunistic Infections

Prophylaxis against Pneumocystis carinii pneumonia (PCP) has been one of the most successful interventions of HIV therapy and should be given to any patient with a CD4 count of less than 200 or a percentage of less than 20 (Centers for Disease Control [CDC], 1992) whether or not she has had PCP. There are currently three options available for PCP prophylaxis:

1. Trimethoprim-sulfamethoxazole (TMP-SMX), one double-strength tablet taken daily or three times a week, is the drug of choice for PCP prophylaxis. There is a high rate of allergy to TMP-SMX in people with HIV, and rash, fever, neutropenia, and elevated liver function tests (LFTs) are common. Desensitization to TMP-SMX has been done successfully for some patients (Torres, 1992). Patients on TMP-SMX should have regular laboratory monitoring of complete blood counts (CBC) and liver function tests (LFTs).
2. Dapsone 100 mg per day is an alternative. Patients should have documentation of a functional level of the enzyme G6PD before initiation of dapsone therapy; deficiency with concurrent drug administration can result in a hemolytic crisis.
3. Aerosolized pentamidine (AP) is also available for PCP prophylaxis. However, its cost, the evidence of more breakthrough episodes of PCP with AP than with TMP-SMX or dapsone (Safrin, 1992) (in part, a result of improper administration), the need for specialized administration facilities, the fear of tuberculosis spread during administration, and AP's lack of protection against extrapulmonary Pneumocystis

TABLE 4–2    Antiretroviral Therapy for HIV-Infected Adults: Recommendations from the 1993 NIAID State-of-the-Art Conference

| Clinical Status | CD4+ Range, Cell Count × 10⁹/L | Recommendation |
|---|---|---|
| *No Previous Antiretroviral Therapy* | | |
| Asymptomatic | >0.50 | No therapy |
| Asymptomatic | 0.20–0.50 | Zidovudine or no therapy |
| Symptomatic | 0.20–0.50 | Zidovudine |
| Asymptomatic | <0.20 | Zidovudine |
| Symptomatic | <0.20 | Zidovudine |
| *Previous Antiretroviral Therapy* | | |
| Stable | ≥0.30 | Continue zidovudine |
| Stable | <0.30 | Continue zidovudine or change to didanosine |
| Progressing | 0.05–0.50 | Change to didanosine or zalcitabine |
| Progressing | <0.05 | Change to didanosine or zalcitabine |
| *Intolerant to Zidovudine* | | |
| Stable or progressing | <0.50 | Change to didanosine or zalcitabine |

*Source:* Reprinted with permission from Sande, M. A., Carpenter, C. J., Cobbs, G., Holmes, K. K., & Sanford, J. P. (1993). Antiretroviral therapy for adult HIV-infected patients. *Journal of the American Medical Association, 270*(21), 2583–2589. Copyright © 1993, American Medical Association.

carinii infection make this only a third choice for prophylaxis. It should be considered only when there is documentation of a patient's inability to take oral regimens.

Prophylaxis against Mycobacterium avium complex (MAC), a major contributor to morbidity and mortality in late-stage HIV disease, is recommended for all patients with HIV infection and CD4 counts below 100 (CDC, 1993b). Rifabutin 300 mg daily is available, and clarithromycin 500 mg bid and clarithromycin in combination with rifabutin are under evaluation. In placing a patient on MAC prophylaxis, providers must carefully weigh the possible benefits (Nightingale et al., 1993) with the multiple problems of drug interactions, compliance difficulties with the addition of another medicine to an already complicated regimen, and the unknown risk of drug resistance.

There are currently no established recommendations for primary prophylaxis of other OIs. In clinical practice, some providers prophylax against systematic fungal infections with fluconazole 100 mg daily if the CD4 count is under 100. Clinical trials are currently under way to evaluate the benefit of and most appropriate regimen for primary prophylaxis for candidiasis, toxoplasmosis (for those with positive toxoplasma antibody tests), and CMV infections. A new drug used in the treatment of pneumocystis, atovaquone, also has activity against toxoplasmosis and is being studied for its protective effect against both; TMP-SMX is currently believed to provide some protection against toxoplasmosis, as well.

Tuberculosis has emerged as a significant threat to people with HIV and their contacts (Braun, Cote, & Rabkin, 1993; Small et al., 1993), and certain modifications in prophylaxis are suggested for this population. All patients with HIV infection and a positive TB skin test (PPD) (5 mm of induration) should take isoniazid (INH) 300 mg daily for 12 months (CDC, 1989). People who are anergic and have chest x-ray evidence of past TB infection should also receive a 12-month course of INH. Preventive therapy of one year of INH should be considered for patients with HIV infection with no evidence of TB infection who are from groups that have a TB prevalence of greater than 10% (CDC, 1991). These groups include injection drug users, prisoners, migrant farm workers, homeless people, and those born in countries with a high prevalence of TB.

To prevent relapse in patients with HIV disease, secondary prophylaxis against opportunistic infections like PCP, cryptococcoses, other fungal infections like histoplasmosis, and toxoplasmosis must be done (see Table 4–3). Recurrent herpes simplex virus outbreaks should be treated with acyclovir (Zovirax) 200-400 mg tid-qid, working with the patient to establish the most effective regimen for prophylaxis (Drew, Buhles, & Erlich, 1992). Oral candidiasis, which occurs frequently, can often be controlled with local antifungals like clotrimazole troches or nystatin oral solution, taken up to five times a day. If there is no response, ketoconazole 200 to 400 mg per day may be effective.

## Treatment of Opportunistic Infections

Women with HIV infection are at increased risk for a variety of bacterial, viral, fungal, and parasitic infections. The most common infections seen by primary care providers are those that might present in essentially asymptomatic patients. These include community-acquired pneumonia (which can easily spread to become disseminated disease), tuberculosis, oral and vaginal candidiasis, genital herpes simplex virus infection, pelvic inflammatory disease, sinus infections, shingles, folliculitis, and molluscum contagiosum. Drugs used to treat some of the most common OIs are presented in Table 4–4.

**TABLE 4–3**    Prophylaxis against Opportunistic Infections

| Opportunistic Infection | CD4 Count | Primary Prophylaxis | Secondary Prophylaxis/ Maintenance |
|---|---|---|---|
| Pneumocystis carinii | <200 | TMP-SMX DS qd or TMP-SMX DS 3x week or Dapsone 100 mg qd or Aerosolized Pentamidine 300 mg q month | Same |
| Mycobacterium avium complex | <100 | Rifabutin 300 mg qd or Investigational: Clarithromycin 500–1,000 mg bid or Rifabutin plus clarithromycin | Maintain treatment for life |
| Cytomegalovirus | <50–100 | Investigational: Oral gancyclovir High dose acyclovir (ACV) | Gancyclovir or foscarnet for life |
| Candida, frequent or chronic | Any | None | Fluconazole 100–200 mg 1–7 days week |
| Toxoplasmosis | <200 | TMP-SMX DS qd | Pyrimethamine 25–50 mg qd and folinic acid 10–20 mg qd plus Sulfadiazine 2 g qd or Clindamycin 300 mg q 6 hours |

*Source:* CDC, 1993b; Fineberg, 1993; Sande & Volberding, 1992; Volberding & Sande, 1992.

In addition to the opportunistic infections, nutritional deficiencies with wasting syndrome are frequently seen in the later stages of HIV disease. This condition can result from several factors, including dysphagia secondary to esophagitis, anorexia secondary to medications, diarrhea, and the increased metabolic rate that accompanies chronic infectious disease. Interventions include nutritional consultation, supplements, and, occasionally, appetite stimulants. Megastrol (Megace) has been used successfully in many patients to enhance their appetites.

**TABLE 4–4**   Treatment of Opportunistic Infections

| Opportunistic Infection | Treatment |
| --- | --- |
| Pneumocystis carinii pneumonia | TMP-SMX 15–20 mg/kg/day of TMP po or IV for 21 days in 3–4 divided doses<br>*or*<br>Dapsone 100 mg/day plus TMP 15–20 mg/kg/day po in 3–4 divided doses for 21 days<br>*or*<br>Clindamycin 300–900 mg/day po or IV in 4 divided doses plus primaquine 30 mg/day po for 21 days<br>*or*<br>Pentamadine 4 mg/kg/day IV for 21 days<br>*or*<br>Atovaquone |
| Candida esophagitis | Fluconazole 100–200 mg qd po for 5–10 days<br>*or*<br>Amphotericin 0.7 mg/kg/day IV |
| Toxoplasma encephalitis | Pyrimethamine 200 mg po loading dose, then 50–75 mg qd with folinic acid 10–50 mg qd plus sulfadiazine 4–6 g qd po for 6 weeks, followed by maintenance therapy<br>*or*<br>Pyrimethamine plus clindamycin 600 mg q 6 hours po or IV for 6 weeks, followed by maintenance therapy |
| Cryptococcal meningitis | Amphotericin 0.7 mg/kg/day IV until stable, followed by fluconazole 400 mg qd po for 8–10 weeks, followed by maintenance therapy<br>*or*<br>Fluconazole 400 mg qd po for 8–10 weeks, followed by maintenance therapy |
| Mycobacterium avium complex | Clarithromycin 500–1,000 mg po bid plus ethambutol 400 mg qd with or without one or more of the following: clofazamine 100 mg qd po, ciprofloxacin 750 mg qd po |
| Bacterial infection | Appropriate antibiotics |

*Source:* Sande & Volberding, 1992; Volberding & Sande, 1992.

## Clinical Trials

Clinical trials should be an integral part of the care offered to women with HIV disease. The advantages of participating in a clinical trial go beyond the bounds of contributing to science. Enrollment offers a woman access to the latest medical treatment and represents a proactive move on behalf of her own health. In broadening their network of providers, women find that research staff can offer important caring relationships. Even the act of refusing trial participation affords a woman the chance for self-efficacy. Primary care providers can call 1-800-TRIALS to obtain information about the where and how of clinical trial availability for women and children in their practice.

## Adjunctive, Nontraditional Therapy

Although little research has been done on the benefits of the numerous nontraditional therapies available to women with HIV disease, there is no uncertainty about the important psychological advantages that they impart. The use of acupuncture, Chinese herbs, massage, psychotherapy, and culture-specific modalities may provide significant support and stress reduction for women with HIV infection (see chapter 13). Primary care providers should be aware of the limitations of the biomedical model and should be open and supportive of a patient's move to take her care into her own hands. A nonjudgmental attitude allows traditional medical care to be provided along with other treatment modalities without forcing the patient to chose one or the other.

## ❖ Gynecologic Infections and Sexually Transmitted Diseases

Most gynecologic infections and sexually transmitted diseases can be treated identically for women with and without HIV; however, some adjustments must be made in particular situations.

## Vaginal Candidiasis

Vaginal candidiasis should initially be treated by intravaginal antifungal therapy for 3 to 7 days. Some women with HIV may find that the infection either recurs frequently or does not fully resolve; oral antifungal agents, such as ketoconazole or fluconazole are indicated in these situations (Minkoff & Dehovitz, 1991). Ketoconazole 200 to 400 mg qd may be used in the short term, but drug interactions are common. Fluconazole, though expensive, has fewer toxicities and drug interactions. Women with relatively high CD4 counts may have a problem with frequently recurring vaginal candidiasis, and secondary prophylaxis may need to take place early in the disease process with the use of systematic antifungals, such as imidazole 200 mg daily or fluconazole 100 mg one to three times a week, to prevent outbreaks.

## Herpes Simplex Virus

Manifestations of Herpes simplex virus infection can become more recurrent and persistent in women with HIV infection. Attacks are treated with acyclovir 200 mg, five times a day for 10 days. Women who experience recurrent infections can generally be maintained on doses of acyclovir 200 mg tid (Drew et al., 1992).

## Syphilis

The evaluation, treatment, and follow-up of syphilis must be adapted for those with HIV infection. HIV appears to alter the natural history of syphilis such that the disease pursues a more aggressive course in the patient with HIV infection. Therefore, a thorough neurological exam must be done on anyone with serological evidence of syphilis, and a lumbar puncture is indicated for patients with any abnormal findings, regardless of the stage of the syphilis. In addition, all patients with latent syphilis (early or late) should have a lumbar puncture. Penicillin regimens are recommended for treatment, and in the case of documented penicillin allergy, desensitization can be done (CDC, 1993a). Treatment for early syphilis (primary, secondary, and early latent) is benzathine penicillin G 2.4 million units IM in one dose. Treatment for late latent syphilis is benzathine penicillin G 2.4 million units IM given on 3 consecutive weeks (7.2 million units total). Neurosyphilis is treated with aqueous penicillin G 2.4 million units every 4 hours IV for 10 to 14 days. Serological follow-up should be done at 1, 2, 3, 6, 9, and 12 months. Nontreponemal antibody titers (RPRs) should decline fourfold in 3 months with primary and secondary syphilis and by 6 months with early latent syphilis. If titers fail to decrease, a lumbar puncture should be done, and the patient should be retreated. A fourfold increase in titers at any time is indication for a lumbar puncture and treatment with the neurosyphilis regimen. Sexual partners must be evaluated for syphilis and other STDs (CDC, 1993a).

## Pelvic Inflammatory Disease

Pelvic inflammatory disease (PID) in women with HIV infection may be clinically more severe and refractory to treatment and have an increased risk of complications than in noninfected women (Hoegsberg et al., 1990). A high index of suspicion about the diagnosis of PID is indicated in evaluating lower abdominal pain in a sexually active woman, especially one with HIV infection. The outpatient regimen is contained in Table 4–5. Some clinicians recommend hospitalizing all women with HIV infection who develop PID, although in reality, mild cases are treated on an outpatient basis if there is assurance of close follow-up. After initiation of treatment, women must be seen for evaluation within 72 hours. Sexual partners of women with PID should be evaluated for STDs (CDC, 1993a).

## Other Sexually Transmitted Diseases

Other STDs are treated according to current recommendations, which are contained in Table 4–5. All partners of women who have gonorrhea, chlamydia, or trichomoniasis should be evaluated and treated (CDC, 1993a).

## Treatment of Cervical Disease

The association between HIV disease and cervical neoplasia is probably the result of reactivation of previous acquired human papilloma virus infection (HPV). The odds of an HIV-infected woman having cervical neoplasia is 4.9 times that of an HIV-negative woman (Mandelblatt, Fahs, Garibaldi, Senie, & Peterson, 1992), and the association is stronger for women with more advanced immunosuppression (Vermund et al., 1991). Questions about the adequacy of Pap smear screening and the possible need for rou-

TABLE 4–5  Outpatient Management of Pelvic Inflammatory Disease and Other Sexually Transmitted Diseases

| Infection | Treatment |
| --- | --- |
| Pelvic inflammatory disease | Ofloxacin 400 mg bid plus clindamycin 450 mg qid or metronidazole 500 mg bid for 14 days *or* Cefoxitin 2 g IM plus probenecid 1 g po concurrently or ceftriaxone 250 mg IM *plus* Doxycycline 100 mg po bid for 14 days |
| Gonorrhea | Cefixime 400 mg po x 1 *or* Ofloxacin 400 mg po x 1 *or* Ciprofloxacin 500 mg po x 1 *plus* Doxycycline 100 mg po bid for 7 days |
| Chlamydia | Azithromycin 1 g po x 1 *or* Doxycycline 100 mg po bid for 7 days |
| Syphilis | |
| <1 year duration | Benzathine penicillin G 2.4 million units IM x 1 |
| >1 year duration | Benzathine penicillin G 2.4 million units IM weekly x 3 |
| Trichomoniasis | Metronidazole 2 g po x 1 |
| Bacterial vaginosis | Metronidazole 500 mg po bid for 7 days |

Source: CDC, 1993a.

tine colposcopic examination in this patient population (Maiman et al., 1990) are still under study. The CDC recommends a Pap smear yearly for all HIV-positive women after two normal Pap smears at 6-month intervals. If the Pap smear shows severe inflammation with reactive squamous cellular changes, another Pap smear should be done in 3 months (CDC, 1993a). Some clinicians feel that Pap smears should continue to be done at 6-month intervals, in particular for those women with low CD4 counts (less than 200) or a history of HPV or abnormal Pap smears. All abnormalities should be referred for colposcopic evaluation, biopsy, and treatment. Aggressive follow-up is indicated even after initial colposcopy and treatment, as recurrence rates are high. Patients may become discouraged about the lack of success of the often uncomfortable treatments, and the primary care provider has an important role in encouraging them to continue treatments and follow-up exams.

## ❖ Health Maintenance in HIV Disease

Health maintenance, both routine and HIV specific, is important in providing comprehensive care for people with HIV (Jewett & Hecht, 1993). In a woman who has no acute disease process, follow-up visits, scheduled every 1 to 6 months, are determined by stage of HIV disease and medication regimen.

Immunizations are important for women with HIV infection. Pneumococcal bacteremia and pneumonia are a major threat to women with HIV (Janoff, Breiman, Daley, & Hopewell, 1992), and a one-time dose of pneumococcal vaccine is recommended for all women with HIV infection. Influenza vaccine should be given yearly. Because some studies have shown that patients with a CD4 count of less than 200 may not mount an adequate immune response, some clinicians choose to prioritize immunizations to patients with CD4 counts greater than 200. Women without antibodies to hepatitis B should be evaluated for ongoing risk and the vaccine series offered. The standard adult recommendations are valid for tetanus and diphtheria booster immunizations every 10 years. Measles, mumps, and rubella (MMR) should be considered for women with asymptomatic HIV disease born between 1957 and 1968. Because of the potential risk in giving live vaccines to immunocompromised patients, the decision to give MMR is left to the discretion of the provider.

A Pap smear is recommended every 6 months for women with CD4 counts of less than 200 or with CD4 counts greater than 200 and with a history of an abnormal Pap smear. All other women can get Pap smears yearly after two normal Pap smears at 6-month intervals. Breast exam should be done yearly, and breast self-exam should be taught. Women over 50 should receive mammogram screening every 1 to 2 years, as recommended by the American Cancer Society.

As previously noted, the risk of tuberculosis to people with HIV and their contacts is enormous. Purified protein derivative testing or chest x-rays for patients who are anergic should be performed yearly and perhaps twice a year for patients at high risk.

## ❖ Counseling

Directed counseling and teaching about the health- (not illness-) related components of HIV disease are indicated for primary care providers. Food safety is important to prevent infections with gastrointestinal pathogens, which can be prolonged and severe. All meat, fish, poultry, and eggs should be thoroughly cooked. Milk products should be pasteurized, and raw milk should be avoided. Organic foods should be eaten only if they can be peeled or are cooked. Other areas of care include careful hand washing, thorough cleaning of food preparation surfaces, and avoidance of chipped dishes and cups.

Although there are no data regarding alcohol, cocaine, heroin, or other substance use and enhanced HIV progression, common sense and anecdotal clinical observation suggest that an overall life-style of substance abuse has an adverse effect on health. Counseling regarding drug use should focus on the importance of maintaining proper nutrition and compliance with medical treatment, not on the morality of the issue.

Contraceptive and pregnancy counseling should be addressed within the context of primary care. Pregnancy counseling should include a discussion of the risk to the woman, the risk of transmission to the baby, and an evaluation of economic and psychosocial support systems. Contraceptive counseling and safer sex counseling need to be discussed in tandem because contraceptives other than condoms do not afford adequate protection against STDs. Oral contraceptives are problematic for women on multiple medications because of potential drug interactions. Intrauterine devices (IUDs) are contraindicated in HIV-infected women because of the increased risk of PID and because the increased blood loss caused by IUDs during menses increases the risk of anemia. Safer sex counseling must be appropriate to the woman's situation; a woman who has sexual contact with other women must be counseled accordingly.

Collaboration on psychosocial issues between the primary provider and a social worker, substance abuse programs, community agencies, and other support programs is essential. Adequate time should be allowed at clinic visits to meet emotional needs, provide support, and educate.

## ❖ Summary

The care of women with HIV is a complex medical and psychosocial undertaking. The primary provider is frequently in the position of coordinating the various aspects of the care. Knowing the appropriate medical interventions is obviously essential, but unless the primary provider can address the patient's psychosocial needs, the patient may be unable to manage her medical care appropriately. The rapidly changing field of HIV requires frequent adaptations in medical management. The patient-provider relationship is crucial to ensuring that every HIV-infected woman will receive optimal education, support, and medical care.

## ❖ References

Aboulker, J. P., & Swart, A. M. (1993). Preliminary analysis of the Concorde trial. *Lancet, 341*(8849), 889–890.

Berger, T. (1992). Dermatologic care in the AIDS patient. In M. A. Sande & P. A. Volberding (Eds.), *The medical management of AIDS* (pp. 145-160). Philadelphia: W. B. Saunders.

Braun, M. M., Cote, T. R., & Rabkin, C. S. (1993). Trends in death with tuberculosis during the AIDS era. *Journal of the American Medical Association, 269*(22), 2865–2868.

Centers for Disease Control. (1989). Tuberculosis and human immunodeficiency virus infection: Recommendations of the Advisory Committee for the Elimination of Tuberculosis (ACET). *Morbidity and Mortality Weekly Report, 38*(14), 236–238, 243–250.

Centers for Disease Control. (1991). Purified protein derivative (PPD)-tuberculin anergy and HIV infection: Guidelines for anergy testing and management of anergic persons at risk of tuberculosis. *Morbidity and Mortality Weekly Report, 40*(RR-5), 27–33.

Centers for Disease Control and Prevention. (1992). Recommendations for prophylaxis against Pneumocystis carinii pneumonia for adults and adolescents infected with human immunodeficiency virus. *Morbidity and Mortality Weekly Report, 41*(RR-4), 1–11.

Centers for Disease Control and Prevention. (1993a). 1993 sexually transmitted disease treatment guidelines. *Morbidity and Mortality Weekly Report, 42*(RR-14), 1–102.

Centers for Disease Control and Prevention. (1993b). Recommendations on prophylaxis and therapy for disseminated Mycobacterium avium complex for adults and adolescents infected with Human Immunodeficiency Virus. *Morbidity and Mortality Weekly Report, 42*(RR-9), 17–20.

Cotton, D. (1993). Disappointing assessment of current antiretrovirals. *AIDS Clinical Care, 5*(7), 51–58.

DeVita, V. T., Hellman, S., & Rosenberg, S. A. (Eds.). (1992). *AIDS: Etiology, diagnosis, treatment, and prevention.* Philadelphia: J. B. Lippincott.

Drew, W. L., Buhles, W., & Erlich, K. S. (1992). Management of herpes virus infections. In M. A. Sande & P. A. Volberding (Eds.), *The medical management of AIDS* (pp. 359–382). Philadelphia: W. B. Saunders.

Genser, S. C., & Schlenger, W. (1993, June). *Linking drug abuse treatment and primary medical care to optimize service delivery for HIV risk intervention.* Paper presented at the Ninth International Conference on AIDS, Berlin.

Gorter, R. W., Vranizan, K. M., Osmond, D. H., & Moss, A. R. (1992). Differences in laboratory values in HIV infection by sex, race, and risk group. *AIDS, 6*(11), 1341–1347.

Hoegsberg, B., Abulafia, O., Sedlis, A., Feldman, J., DesJarlais, D., Landesman, S., & Minkoff, H. (1990). Sexually transmitted diseases and immunodeficiency virus infection among women with pelvic inflammatory disease. *American Journal of Obstetrics and Gynecology, 163*(4), 1135–1139.

Janoff, E. N., Breiman, R. F., Daley, C. L., & Hopewell, P. C. (1992). Pneumococcal disease during HIV infection: Epidemiologic, clinical, and immunologic perspectives. *Annals of Internal Medicine, 117*(4), 314–324.

Jewett, J. F., & Hecht, F. M. (1993). Preventive health care for adults with HIV infection. *Journal of the American Medical Association, 269*(9), 1144–1153.

Maiman, M., Tarricone, N., Vieira, J., Suarez, J., Serur, E., & Boyce, J. (1990). Colposcopic evaluation of human immunodeficiency virus–seropositive women. *Obstetrics and Gynecology, 78*(1), 84–88.

Mandelblatt, J. S., Fahs, M., Garibaldi, K., Senie, R. T., & Peterson, H. B. (1992). Association between HIV infection and cervical neoplasia: Implications for clinical care of women at risk for both conditions. *AIDS, 6*(2), 173–178.

Minkoff, H. L., & DeHovitz, J. A. (1991). Care of women infected with the human immunodeficiency virus. *Journal of the American Medical Association, 266*(16), 2253–2258.

Nightingale, S. D., Cameron, D. W., Gordin, F. M., Sullam, P. M., Cohn, D. L., & Chaisson, R. E. (1993). Two controlled trials of rifabutin prophylaxis against mycobacterium avium complex infection in AIDS. *New England Journal of Medicine, 329*(12), 828–833.

Safrin, S. (1992, December). *Pneumocystis carinii pneumonia.* Paper presented at the meeting on Clinical Care of the AIDS Patient, San Francisco.

Safrin, S., Rush, J. D., & Mills, J. (1990). Influenza in patients with human immunodeficiency virus infection. *Chest, 98*(1), 33–37.

Sande, M. A., Carpenter, C. J., Cobbs, G., Holmes, K. K., & Sanford, J. P. (1993). Antiretroviral therapy for adult HIV-infected patients. *Journal of the American Medical Association, 270*(21), 2583–2589.

Sande, M. A., & Volberding, P. A. (Eds.). (1992). *The medical management of AIDS.* Philadelphia: W. B. Saunders.

Selwyn, P. A., Sckell, B. M., Alcabes, P., Friedland, G. H., Klein, R. S., & Schoenbaum, E. E. (1992). High risk of active tuberculosis in HIV-infected drug users with cutaneous anergy. *Journal of the American Medical Association, 268*(4), 504–509.

Small, P. M., Shafer, R. W., Hopewell, P. C., Singh, S. P., Murphy, M. J., & Desmond, E. (1993). Exogenous reinfection with multiple drug-resistant mycobacterium tuberculosis in patients with advanced HIV infection. *New England Journal of Medicine, 328*(16), 1137–1144.

Torres, G. (1992). Desensitization to sulfa drugs. *Treatment Issues, 6*(10), 6–10.

Vermund, S. H., Kelley, K. F., Klein, R. S., Feingold, A. R., Schreiber, K., & Munk, G. (1991). High risk of human papilloma virus infection and cervical squamous intraepithelial lesions among women with symptomatic human immunodeficiency virus infection. *American Journal of Obstetrics and Gynecology, 165*(2), 392–400.

Volberding, P. A., & Sande, M. A. (1992, December). *Clinical care of the AIDS patient.* Conference Proceedings. San Francisco.

# ❖ Chapter 5

# Pregnancy and Reproductive Concerns of Women with HIV Infection

ANN KURTH

HOWARD L. MINKOFF

In what has become a tragic equality, HIV disease is increasingly a mainstream cause of morbidity and mortality in women of reproductive age. AIDS is now the sixth leading cause of death in the United States for women aged 25 to 44 (Centers for Disease Control and Prevention [CDC], 1993a). Inevitably, over the next 10 to 15 years, women's reproductive care providers can expect to see a continuum of HIV disease in their practices. The incidence of HIV among women in the United States has been rising steadily since the first cases were identified in the early 1980s, reaching nearly 14% of total cases in 1992 (CDC, 1992a, 1992b). Because a majority of women with HIV are in their childbearing years, reproductive care, contraceptive methods, and factors affecting the practice of safer sex must be addressed in the context of HIV infection. It is important for primary care providers to understand perinatal HIV transmission, the effects of HIV on pregnancy, and the effects of pregnancy on HIV. This chapter addresses these topics as well as issues of obstetric management.

## ❖ Disease Progression and Pregnancy

Whether pregnancy modifies the natural history of HIV disease is still an unresolved issue. To understand the effect of pregnancy on the course of HIV disease, it is essential for the clinician to understand both the normal immune response to foreign antigens and the effect of pregnancy on that response (Nanda & Minkoff, 1989). The T4 lymphocyte has many functions, including the initiation of both humoral and cell-mediated immune responses (Claman, 1987; Nosal, 1987). T4 lymphocytes are also called CD4 cells, based on their "cluster designations" or reaction with various monoclonal antibodies. HIV has a predilection for T4 (helper) cells and results in a reduction in the T4 population. In the presence of a normal T8 (suppressor) population, a reversal of the T4-to-T8 ratio occurs. With a decrease in the proliferation of T4 cells, impairment of lymphokine production occurs, and defective cytotoxic activity by natural killer cells is observed. Various B cell abnormalities have also been observed. These multiple defects in the immune response render the host susceptible to the array of opportunistic infections seen in patients with AIDS.

Pregnancy may also influence immune function. Many studies support the hypothesis that a pregnant woman is more susceptible to various viral, bacterial, and fungal infections and is more prone to serious morbidity and mortality than a nonpregnant woman (Bowen, Lane, & Fauci, 1985; Freeman & Barno, 1969). However, because pregnant women can mount a satisfactory response to intradermal skin antigens and can reject skin grafts, it is likely that only certain selective functions of cell-mediated immunity are depressed during pregnancy. Lymphocytes have received the most attention in the latter regard.

It is not entirely clear in what manner T lymphocyte function is compromised in pregnancy. Studies have shown decreases in T4 cells during pregnancy (particularly in the last trimester), altered T4-to-T8 ratios, and decreased B cells (Bailey, Herrod, Younger, & Shaver, 1985; Fiddes et al., 1986; Glassman, Bennet, Christopher, & Self, 1985; Sridama et al., 1982; Vanderberken et al., 1982) Thus, there would appear to be a consensus that a decrease in cell-mediated immunity does occur during pregnancy, probably mediated through an altered ratio of T4 helper cells to T8 suppressor cells. Other factors may contribute to the immunosuppression of pregnancy, including increased levels of total steroids and other pregnancy-specific plasma proteins and hormones like human chorionic gonadotropin (HCG), alphafeto protein, and pregnancy-associated alpha 2-glycoprotein.

As noted, the multiple defects in the immune response seen in AIDS patients renders them susceptible to a variety of opportunistic infections. Concern has been expressed that pregnancy-induced depression of cell-mediated immunity could enhance the relative immune incompetence of HIV-infected women. The initial reports of pregnant women with AIDS seemed to confirm this impression (Jensen et al., 1984; Minkoff, DeRegt, Landesman, & Schwarz, 1986; Minkoff, Nanda, Menez, & Fikrig, 1987; Wetli, Roldan, & Fujaco, 1983). These early studies of pregnant women with AIDS or AIDS-related complex (ARC) showed a greater than expected disease progression than seen in nonpregnant patients, suggesting that pregnancy was responsible for disease acceleration.

More recent controlled studies have been performed in which HIV-positive mothers have been prospectively followed. Overall, these studies have found that pregnancy has only a minor effect on the course of HIV disease (Berrebi et al., 1990; Bigger, Pahwa, Landesman, & Goedert, 1988; MacCallum et al., 1988; Schaefer, et. al, 1988).

In sum, a significant influence of pregnancy on the course of HIV disease has not yet been documented. The available evidence suggests that pregnancy exerts, at most, a minor influence on the progression of disease. More prospective, long-term studies are needed to confirm this supposition.

## ❖ Vertical HIV Transmission

### *Perinatal Transmission*

Perinatal transmission of HIV was initially reported in the early 1980s (CDC, 1982; Joncas, Delage, Chad, & Lapointe, 1983; Rubin et al., 1983; Thomas et al., 1984). Although perinatal HIV transmission is now an accepted route of transmission, the rate and determinants of that transmission remain uncertain. Reported transmission rates have shown wide geographic variation. The lowest published rates come from the European Collaborative Study, which reported that only 14% of children born to infected mothers were eventually found to be HIV infected (European Collaborative Study, 1992). In Africa, conversely, transmission rates of approximately 50% have been reported (Ryder et al., 1989). North American authors have generally reported intermediate rates (Boylan & Stein, 1991).

Some of the reported variation in transmission rates can be attributed to differences in study methodologies. An additional factor, however, may be differences in the individuals under study. Preliminary reports summarized in Table 5–1 suggest that biological factors may contribute to differing transmission rates. A number of studies have shown that lower T4 counts and evidence of viremia, which includes p24 antigenemia, have also been related to higher rates of transmission. Recent seroconversion, which is associated with viremia, has also been linked to high transmission rates, as has advanced clinical illness in the mother. The level and specificity of maternal antibodies (e.g., gp 120) may play a role in determining transmission (Broliden et al., 1989; Devash, Calvelli, Wood, Reagen, & Rubinstein, 1990; Goedert, Duliege, Amos, Felton, & Biggar, 1989; Rossi, Moschese, & Broliden, 1989).

The timing of perinatal transmission also remains unclear; studies suggest that it can occur both early and late in pregnancy. HIV has been detected as early as the 12th week of pregnancy by Courgnaud and colleagues (1989). Soeiro, Rashbaun, Ruben, and Lyman (1991) studied human abortus tissue and suggested that up to 30% of HIV transmissions may occur by the second trimester of pregnancy. However, the possibility of contamination from maternal sources is difficult to exclude definitively in any study of aborted fetal tissues.

The presence of p24 antigen in newborn serum or a positive HIV culture shortly after birth also suggests that the infant was infected during pregnancy (Borkowski et al., 1989; Courportin, Israel, & Dubeaux, 1988). Miles and coworkers (1993) found five of eight cord samples from neonates with proven HIV infection to be positive for immune-complex-dissociated p24 antigen. These findings and rapidly rising antigen titers in the neonatal period are compatible with perinatal transmission.

The inability to detect evidence of HIV infection before 4 months of age in 50% to 70% of exposed infants ultimately proved to be infected suggests

TABLE 5–1   Summary of Reported Factors Associated with Perinatal Transmission of HIV

| Study | Year | No. of Women | Factors Associated With Transmission |
|---|---|---|---|
| D'Arminio et al. | 1991 | 66 | Advanced disease:<br>10/10 with CDC Class IV<br>7/56 with Class II or III<br>Maternal p24 antigenemia |
| Hague et al. | 1991 | 58 | Women with AIDS during<br>  or shortly after pregnancy<br>Acute viremia from maternal<br>  seroconversion just prior to or during<br>  pregnancy or breast feeding |
| European Collaborative Study | 1992 | 701 | Maternal p24 antigenemia<br>CD4 count <700/mm$^3$ |
| Kreiss et al. | 1991 | 59 | High proviral load >10/100,000<br>  lymphocytes = 72% transmission<br>  vs. low proviral load <10/100,000<br>  lymphocytes = 27% transmission |
| Boue et al. | 1990 | 490 | High p24 level = 78% transmission<br>  vs. low p24 level = 26% transmission<br>CD4 <150/mm$^3$ = 66% transmission<br>  vs. CD4 >150/mm$^3$ = 26%<br>transmission |
| St. Louis et al. | 1991 | 324 | Low CD4 percentage levels |
| Burn et al. | 1991 | 74 | Prepregnancy CD4 <20% = 42%<br>  transmission<br>  vs. prepregnancy CD4 >20% = 18%<br>  transmission |
| Tibaldi et al. | 1991 | 25 | CD4 <400/mm$^3$ and/or p24<br>  antigenemia = 71% transmission<br>  vs. CD4 >400/mm$^3$ and/or p24<br>  antigenemia = 6% transmission |
| Lindgren et al. | 1991 | 44 | Longer duration of HIV infection,<br>  symptomatic HIV disease,<br>  and/or low CD4 counts |

that the timing of transmission may be perinatal in the majority of cases (Ehrnst et al., 1991). Also, Goedert, Duliege, Amos, Felton, and Biggar (1991) have shown that HIV infection was significantly more common in firstborn than in second-born twins, leaving open the possibility that exposure to infected vaginal secretions in the hours preceding birth predisposes the infant to infection. The European Collaborative Study (1992) also found that infants born by cesarean section had lower infection rates. The timing of pediatric seroconversion to positive IgA status is also compatible with the concept of perinatal viral transmission because most infants subsequently found to be infected do not demonstrate antibody to IgA until months after birth (Landesman et al., 1991; Quinn et al., 1991). Despite these findings, there are no empirical data to support a protective effect of cesarean section.

Other pregnancy outcomes do not appear to be affected by serostatus, at least among asymptomatic patients. Birth weight and gestational age did not differ between HIV-infected drug-using women and seronegative controls in reports from Britain (Johnstone, MacCullum, Brettle, Inglis, & Peutherer, 1988) nor between seropositive and seronegative women from the United States, whether they had used drugs or not (Minkoff, Henderson, & Mendez, 1990). Studies that included more symptomatic women, however, have reported higher prematurity rates and lower birth weights among seropositive women (Ryder et al., 1989).

## Breast-Feeding Transmission

HIV has been isolated in both the cellular and liquid portion of breast milk (Ellerbrock & Rogers, 1990), though there is theoretical evidence from small studies that human milk factor, maternal IgM and IgA antibodies, or both may inhibit HIV binding to CD4 receptors and protect against postnatal HIV transmission (Newberg, Viscidi, Ruff, & Yolken, 1992; Van de Perre et al., 1993). There have been documented cases of breast milk transmission, often following postpartum seroconversion in women who received HIV-infected blood transfusions (Lepage et al., 1987; Van de Perre et al., 1991). Evidence also suggests that HIV can be transmitted via breast feeding in those women who were already infected at the time of the pregnancy (Dunn, Newell, Ades, & Peckham, 1992; European Collaborative Study, 1992; Palasanthiran et al., 1993; Peckham, 1993). Estimates of the additional risk due to breast feeding when the mother is already positive during this period are around 15% (range = 7–22%). For those women who become seropositive following delivery, breast-feeding transmission is thought to be around 30% (range = 16–42%) (Peckham, 1993). To date, there has been no large, randomized trial looking at breast-feeding risk because of ethical considerations (Berer & Ray, 1993).

## ❖ Management of HIV and Pregnancy

The golden rule in the care of pregnant women is to provide all necessary treatments unless there is compelling evidence that treatment presents an unacceptable risk to the fetus. The mother should be counseled as to the risks and benefits of treatments and alternatives and included in decision making. The same principle applies to the care of women with HIV infection. Even when pregnant, women with HIV infection should receive pneumococcal vaccine, influenza vaccine, and hepatitis vaccine, if indicated. Testing should be performed to detect any sexually transmitted diseases, such as syphilis, gonorrhea, and chlamydia. Tuberculosis (TB) should be ruled out, and baseline toxoplasmosis titers should be obtained (CDC, 1991).

Tuberculosis screening (CDC, 1991) and prophylaxis against and aggressive management of active disease are of particular importance in the HIV-infected gravida. The increased vulnerability of HIV-infected people to rapid disease manifestation of primary or reactivated tuberculosis has been well documented (Barnes, Bloch, Davidson, & Snider, 1991). Although no cohort studies in women with HIV infection have shown a particularly increased risk for TB disease during pregnancy, given the strong association between HIV and TB, health care workers will need renewed expertise in managing tuberculosis in pregnancy (Feinberg & Soper, 1992). Certain TB drugs are contraindicated during pregnancy, and management using a multidrug regimen requires multidisciplinary consultation (Frieden & Fujiwara, 1992; Mays, 1993).

## Sexually Transmitted Diseases in the Antepartum Period

It is important to remember that many women continue to have sex during pregnancy and that screening for sexually transmitted diseases (STDs) and reinforcement of the need for safer sex practices should not be neglected during this period. Also, many women with HIV present for care only during pregnancy (Johnstone, 1993) or only discover their HIV status during pregnancy, and so an opportunity to address their gynecologic needs should not be lost. The disease course of several of the STDs, such as human papilloma virus (HPV), normally can be exacerbated by pregnancy. Condyloma acuminata, for example, can become hyperplastic under the hormonal influence of pregnancy, and persistent monilial vulvovaginitis is also more common during pregnancy (Burrow & Ferris, 1988). Gynecologic screening protocols are described in chapter 4 and are summarized in Figure 5–1. The use of podophyllin, autogenous vaccine, and topical interferon for treatment of HPV during pregnancy is contraindicated (Burrow & Ferris, 1988).

## Antepartum Management

During the antepartum period, clinicians must be wary of nonspecific symptoms that may, in other circumstances, be attributed to pregnancy. Fatigue and weight loss are common in early pregnancy but may be early manifestations of HIV disease. Upper respiratory tract symptoms (e.g., fever and tachypnea), in particular, warrant aggressive investigation. Patients should be encouraged to report all symptoms immediately. Nutritional counseling should be instituted if difficulty is encountered in maintaining appropriate weight gain. Although no cofactors have proved to affect adversely the rate of disease progression, it seems prudent to advise

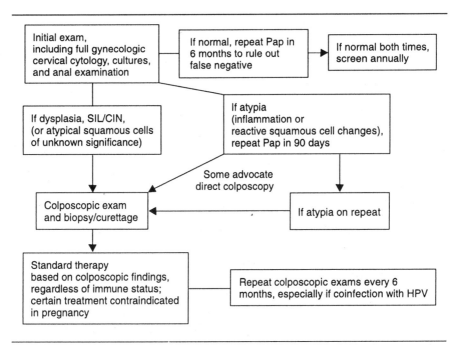

**FIGURE 5–1**  Gynecological screening in HIV.

*Source:* Allen & Marte, 1991; Ellerbrock, 1993; LaGuardia, 1993.

patients to avoid factors shown to alter T4-to-T8 ratios (sleep deprivation, stress) or to enhance viral replication in vitro (e.g., antigenic stimulus, infections). Alcohol and illicit drugs should be prohibited (Nanda & Minkoff, 1989).

The institution of many drug therapies used in the management of HIV infection is determined by an individual's T cell count. During pregnancy, T cell counts should be monitored regularly to evaluate the need for therapeutic agents (American College of Obstetricians and Gynecologists [ACOG], 1992; Biggar et al., 1989; Nanda & Minkoff, 1989). Although some component of the decline of T4 counts during pregnancy may be attributable to pregnancy itself (as opposed to viral effect), it should not be assumed that the prognostic significance of a low count is less reliable than in nonpregnant populations (Minkoff, Willoughby, et al., 1990).

Standard approaches to prophylaxis against pneumocystis carinii pneumonia should be maintained during pregnancy. Women whose CD4 counts drop below 200 mm³ should receive either pentamidine or trimethoprim-sulfamethoxazole (TMP-SMX) therapy. Although pentamidine has the advantage of less frequent side effects and extremely low blood levels, the aerosol form may not be readily available to all women, and its use can be associated with breakthrough infection. TMP-SMX is readily available and highly effective and may be continued to term. Although adverse maternal reactions are common (most often comprising a rash), neonatal consequences have not been serious, and kernicterus has not been reported in settings in which sulfa derivatives were discontinued during the neonatal period. The specific agent that is used is probably less important than the fact that some therapy is prescribed during gestation.

There is current disagreement about the benefits of initiating antiretroviral therapy for nonpregnant individuals with T4 cell counts between 200 and 500. There is, however, general agreement that antiretroviral therapy is beneficial for individuals with T4 cell counts of less than 200. Considerations about the use of antiretrovirals during pregnancy include the possible adverse fetal effects and the potential beneficial effects on vertical transmission as well as on the mother's health. Pharmacokinetic studies have shown that zidovudine (ZDV, ZDV) crosses the placenta and achieves relatively high concentrations in the fetus and placenta within several hours of maternal dosing (Little, Bawdon, Christmas, Sobhi, & Gilstrap, 1989). Although studies of teratogenicity in animals are on the whole reassuring, one study has caused concern. It was reported that among rats exposed to ZDV throughout their lives, approximately 10% of the females had nonmetastasizing vaginal tumors at the time of their deaths. However, several factors make the relevance of these findings to humans highly tenuous, including the fact that rats, unlike humans, excrete ZDV and its metabolites in their urine and that rats soil the vaginal vault with urine. It is doubtful, therefore, that in utero exposure to ZDV has the same potential for adverse sequelae as that seen in the rat model. The reported experience among humans exposed to ZDV during pregnancy, though small, has not been worrisome. Sperling and colleagues (1992) reported on 43 women who took varying doses of ZDV for varying periods of time during gestation. No teratogenic effects were noted. The most common adverse neonatal sequela was anemia, which often took place in a context in which that finding might have been anticipated in any event (e.g., prematurity). Given the small sample size and the short follow-up, however, the possibility of teratogenicity must still be entertained.

Conversely, because ZDV acts to prevent reverse transcription of ribonucleic acid (RNA), the possibility also exists that its use in pregnancy could lower the rate of perinatal viral transmission. This possibility is the basis for an ongoing placebo control trial, which is discussed in the section on the prevention of perinatal transmission.

## Intrapartum Management

The intrapartum management of the mother with HIV infection is not substantively altered by her serostatus, although to some extent the care of all mothers and neonates in the labor and delivery suite has been influenced by the HIV epidemic. The introduction of universal precautions into the labor and delivery area, for example, has changed some of the standards in that setting. Airway cleaning of the newborn is no longer performed with DeLee suction generated by a clinician. The mucus trap should be attached to wall suction with pressure less than 140 mm/Hg to prevent damage to the neonate's gut.

Fetal scalp electrodes and scalp clips may be potential vectors of viral transmission. This concern is based on the presence of the virus in the vaginal secretions with which the fetus has prolonged contact after the membranes have ruptured. Piercing the skin to obtain a scalp blood sample or placing an electrode into the skin could pose a theoretical risk of inoculating the fetus with virus. There are scant empirical data that address this concern. Some investigators have reported that infants who underwent the types of invasive procedures described were no more likely to become infected than infants who were not so exposed, but the sizes of those cohorts were too small to have the requisite statistical power to rule out the level of risk generally associated with needle-stick injuries. Thus, clinicians must continue to balance the theoretical risk of these procedures with the clinical benefit of their performance. Nevertheless, "routine" use should be avoided.

Current obstetric standards for choosing a route of delivery should not be modified on the basis of serostatus. Many HIV-infected children have been delivered by cesarean section. It should be noted, however, that few of the reports on infection and mode of delivery have commented on the status of membranes or the duration of labor, and none had a sufficient sample size to rule out the possibility of some ameliorating effect of operative delivery. Recent reports have suggested a trend toward some protective effect associated with operative delivery. Given the previously discussed effect of birth order on neonatal infection among twins and the presence of the virus in vaginal secretions, the possibility that cesarean section could be protective cannot be ruled out. Nor is it implausible that some form of vaginal antisepsis could also be beneficial (Peckham, 1993). Pending the documentation of benefit from these approaches, standard obstetric indications for cesarean section seem warranted.

## Substance Use

As discussed by Williams and O'Conner in chapter 14, many addicted women are motivated to seek medical and drug treatment during pregnancy. This is true even for women who continue to use cocaine or crack (Mitchell, Loftman, & Williams, 1992). In one study of 146 crack-addicted women in New York, the major motivation for women to seek drug treatment was concern for their children (cited by 70%), yet a majority of national experts on drug treatment surveyed in the same study cited lack of access (71%) and lack of child care (59%) as the two major barriers to treatment (Paone & Chavkin, 1991). Women who are actively using drugs may not go for prenatal care or may relapse into drug use on learning of their HIV-positive status (Faltz & Madover, 1988), particularly if this is discovered during pregnancy.

Substance use is a significant cause of morbidity and mortality for women in the United States, whether complicated by HIV infection or not. Though women are historically underrepresented in research, service, and literature on substance use, 20% of the estimated 500,000 heroin users in the United States were women (1988 estimate), and an additional 1 million women were thought to be intermittent users (Wells & Jackson, 1992). Many crack users are female and may have additional health risks from multiple sexual partners due to the exchange of sex for drugs.

Many studies have focused on female injection drug users in relation to vertical HIV transmission. Some of the original studies looking at the impact of maternal HIV status on obstetric and perinatal outcome failed to control for confounding factors like maternal substance use. Selwyn, Schoenbaum, and colleagues (1989) compared the pregnancies of HIV seropositive and seronegative injection drug users and found no differences between the groups in terms of frequency of spontaneous or elective abortion, ectopic pregnancy, preterm delivery, stillbirth, or low birth weight. Seropositive women were more likely to be hospitalized for bacterial pneumonia and had an increased tendency for breech presentation; otherwise, there were no differences between the groups in the occurrence of prenatal, intrapartum, or neonatal complications. A recent analysis of the Women and Infants Transmission Study (WITS) of 162 HIV-positive mother-infant pairs found that women tended to underreport their drug use. When only these self-reported data were used, there was a spurious association between HIV infection status and birth weight. Multivariate regression analysis adding urine toxicology test data showed that cocaine use—not HIV status—accounted for the differences seen (Rodriguez et al., 1993). Studies like these point out the need to separate the significant impact of drug use on perinatal outcomes.

Guidelines for managing addiction during pregnancy have been published elsewhere (Ronkin, FitzSimmons, Wapner, & Finnegan, 1988) and should be followed, regardless of whether the pregnancy is complicated by HIV. The ideal intrapartum pain management for the addicted parturient is regional anesthesia, which is not contraindicated by HIV seropositivity (Mitchell et al., 1992).

## ❖ Postpartum Management

### Maternal and Infant Care

In the postpartum period, the clinician's responsibilities include the continuation of universal precautions, which should be extended to the neonate, a proscription of breast feeding (in developed countries), and appropriate referral of mother and child to physicians with expertise in the management of HIV disease. As soon as the child is born, universal precautions should be exercised by pediatric care providers. Gloves should be worn until all secretions have been removed from the skin. Secretions should be washed off the baby immediately following delivery and before administration of any skin-breaking procedure, such as vitamin K shots or heel sticks. Care should be taken to maintain the baby's thermoregulation.

Infection control policies in the form of universal precautions should be explained to every woman prior to delivery so that she will not be unduly concerned about interactions with her baby or with her care providers. The HIV-positive woman needs to know to alert staff for cleanup following blood spills and to properly dispose of soiled peripads. As with any patient, staff members should use barrier protection, such as latex gloves, when conducting perineal care or when otherwise in contact with visibly bloody fluids. There is no reason to isolate an HIV-positive woman after delivery unless she has active pulmonary tuberculosis.

All efforts should be made to enhance bonding between the mother and child. This may be more problematic in the face of previous or current substance use. Infants addicted in utero may be difficult to soothe, straining the mother's attempts to develop effective parenting skills; concern about transmission of cocaine or other lipid-soluble substances via breast milk likewise may be an issue. At Harlem Hospital, New York City, women perceived to be at potential risk for HIV infection due to substance use but who do not wish to know their HIV status are encouraged not to breast feed as a preventive measure (Mitchell, Brown, Loftman, & Williams, 1990). Methadone use is not a contraindication to breast feeding (Mitchell et al., 1992).

Women should be reassured that it is all right for them, family members, and friends to cuddle, kiss, and play with the infant; simple instructions regarding universal precautions in the home should be given prior to discharge (Kurth, 1993). All other referrals for postpartum, contraceptive, and HIV care should be made as needed, including concrete assistance with housing, child care, and transportation if these will be impediments to obtaining ongoing care for the woman or for her child. Instructions on safer sex and condom use should be stressed because women are at risk during this time for postpartum endometritis (Hatcher et al., 1992).

## Recommendations Regarding Breast Feeding

Breast feeding—a cornerstone of maternal-infant bonding and a contributor to infant health—is a topic that has been fraught with concern in the context of HIV positivity. In the United States, where safe, affordable alternatives to breast feeding are presumed to exist, it has been recommended that women with HIV infection be encouraged not to breast-feed (CDC, 1985).

Because the risks of not breast feeding in areas without safe alternatives include infant morbidity and mortality due to malnutrition and diarrheal diseases (Heymann, 1990), which may affect millions of children in the developing world as well as in poor areas of so-called developed countries, a blanket recommendation for all women regarding breast feeding in the presence of HIV is not possible. In 1992, the World Health Organization (WHO) issued a recommendation that HIV-positive women should (a) breast-feed in those areas where infectious diseases and malnutrition are a high cause of infant morbidity and mortality; (b) use a safe feeding alternative where these are not main causes and where infant mortality is low; (c) seek advice from health care professionals about how to safely feed their infants in those settings where safe alternatives exist; and (d) not be subjected to commercial pressures regarding infant formula choice or sales (WHO/UNICEF, 1992).

## ❖ Contraception Considerations

### Contraceptive and Safer Sex Options

Discussions with patients about safer sex must be realistic in terms of the context of their lives. To date, many of the safer sex messages have placed the burden of risk reduction on women. This approach has persisted despite the fact that women often do not hold the balance of power or have the ability to negotiate terms of sexual conduct in their relationships. Ironically, many women are at risk from their primary relationship. In many cultures, male infidelity is expected, whereas the same behavior in women faces condemnation, including in some cases economic consequences and physical threat. (This does not mean that no women have sex outside their primary relationships. It does mean, however, that they face greater biological and social risks in doing so.) In parts of Africa and Latin America, for example, large proportions of HIV-positive women had only one lifetime sexual partner. This has led some to state that the simple fact of being married can be a risk factor for women (PANOS, 1993).

The initiation and maintenance of safer sex practices for women with HIV infection must be reinforced. Women with HIV need to be counseled about the risks of reinfection with different viral strains as well as the need to avoid other STDs that can seriously complicate their health or stimulate HIV replication. These health risks include pelvic inflammatory disease (PID), cervical intraepithelial neoplasia (CIN), herpes simplex infection, and neurosyphilis, all of which can be difficult to treat and control in women already immunocompromised by HIV (Shannon & Hutchison, 1993). Older, postmenopausal women with HIV infection may face an increased risk of STDs because their vaginal mucosa is atrophic and may facilitate organism entry (Elias & Heise, 1993).

Changing sexual behaviors can be difficult, especially in long-term relationships in which, over time, a "consolidation of the silent norm" regarding sexual patterns has occurred (Mhloyi, 1993). Many women—with or without HIV—are financially dependent on their male partners and may fear repercussions in changing to barrier protection and safer sex practices.

For these reasons, some workers have called for the promotion of exist-ing, and the development of new, female-controlled methods (Rosenberg & Gollub, 1992; Stein, 1990). Examples of existing methods that do not depend on male involvement include spermicides, cervical caps, diaphragms, and sponges; the latter two have shown some effectiveness when used alone against bacterial STDs like cervical gonorrhea and chlamydial infections (Louv, Harland, Alexander, Stagno, & Cheeks, 1988; Rosenberg, Davidson, Chen, Judson, & Douglas, 1992). However, others have cautioned that "cur-rent data remain inconclusive regarding the absolute level of protection against HIV infection that these methods can provide, as well as their relative level of protection (as compared to that of the condom) against other sexually transmitted diseases" (Cates, Stewart, & Trussell, 1992). Nonethe-less, these authors came to the same conclusion reached by others about the use of female-controlled methods in a hierarchy of risk reduction options: Where condom use is not possible as the first line of defense, female meth-ods can be used as fallback protection (Stein, 1992).

Another potential impediment to safer sex is that when practiced effec-tively, no conception will occur (PANOS, 1993). For HIV-positive women or couples who want a child, this creates an unresolvable tension, which may lead to denial and unsafe behavior. Researchers are beginning to investigate new antimicrobials that will have virucidal but not spermicidal properties (Elias & Heise, 1993). The use by HIV-positive women of current methods for the prevention of conception and STD transmission are reviewed in Table 5–2 and discussed below.

## Barrier Methods

### Condoms

The use of barriers during sex is critical for prevention of STD transmission. It is important to point out that HIV can be transmitted through cervical cells, through breaks in vaginal epithelium, and through intact vaginal mucosa (Elias & Heise, 1993). Available methods for the prevention of both conception and STD transmission must be evaluated against this understanding of HIV transmission risk.

The latex male condom remains the best studied and most effective method of STD protection. Natural-membrane condoms are contraindicated because their pore size allows passage of the virus. The CDC now recom-mends the use of latex condoms with or without spermicide because "no studies have shown that nonoxynol-9 used with a condom increases the protection provided by condom use alone against HIV infection" (CDC, 1993b, p. 590). The first female condom for sale in the United States (Real-ity©), a polyurethane pouch, was finally approved by the Food and Drug Administration in December 1992. Despite the possibility that this method, as with other female-controlled methods, might be seen as a technological fix that allows men to take less responsibility for sexual behavior, its avail-

TABLE 5–2  Pregnancy Prevention and Safer Sex for People with HIV

| | Failure rates[a] | Side Effects | Indications |
|---|---|---|---|
| *Barrier Methods* | | | |
| Female condom[b] | 5–26% | Latex allergy (rare) | Use with non-oxynol-9 for STD and improved pregnancy protection |
| Male condom[b] | 2–12% | Irritation (wash powder off or use latex condom) | Female condom and dams cover perineum in oral sex |
| Dental dams | STD protection unknown | | |
| Cervical barrier methods: | | | |
| Diaphragm | 6–18% | ↑ risk urinary tract infection, toxic shock syndrome, microabraisions | Use with latex condom and/or spermicide for improved STD and pregnancy protection |
| Cervical cap | 6–18% | ↑ risk micro-abrasions, possible abnormal Pap smear | |
| Contraceptive sponge | 6–18% nulliparous 9–28% multiparous | ↑ risk micro-abrasions, candida, possible TSS | Limit long-term use; use with condom and/or spermicide |
| *Antimicrobials* | | | |
| Spermicides with nonoxynol-9 | 3–21% / in vitro and circumstantial evidence against STDs | Allergy; high-dose use can cause mucosal irritation, microabrasions | Use for STD protection, ideally with barrier method |
| Spermicides with octoxynol | Only other U.S.-approved spermicide; in vitro data only | Less documentation of anti-STD effectiveness | Use nonoxynol-9 unless allergies exist |
| *Hormonal Methods* | | | |
| Combination pills | 0.1–3% | Ectopy with ↑ risk STD, possible ↑ risk CIN | Condom and spermicide essential for anti-STD |
| Progestin-only: | | | |
| Pills | 0.5–3% | ↑ intermenstrual bleeding | Monitor OC use in HIV+ women closely |
| Implants (Norplant) | 0.03–0.4% | ↑ intermenstrual bleeding for first few months | Use condom/spermicide; monitor |
| Injectables (DMPA, NET) | 0.3–0.4% | Menstrual irregularities, including amenorrhea, weight gain | Use condom/spermicide; monitor |

TABLE 5–2    (Continued)

|  | Failure rates[a] | Side Effects | Indications |
|---|---|---|---|
| *Postcoital* | | | |
| Therapeutic abortion | 0.1–0.3% completeness | Safer than pregnancy; trauma, infection, bleeding | Should be available in timely manner choice |
| Combination pills | 0.16–1.6% | Usual OC risks | Within 72 hours of intercourse |
| RU-486 | 15% within 3 weeks | None serious seen so far | Unknown in HIV+; not yet available in United States |
| *Other* | | | |
| Abstinence | 0% unless involuntary/rape | None | Options for sexual expression other than intercourse |
| Coitus interruptus | 4–18% | Risk of pregnancy and STDs | Use condom/ spermicide |
| Fertility-aware- ness methods | 1–20% | Risk of pregnancy and STDs | Use condom/ spermicide |
| Intrauterine device (IUD) | 2–3% | ↑ risk PID, inter- menstrual bleeding | Contraindicated |
| Voluntary sterilization, male/female | 0.1–0.15%/ 0.2–0.4% | No STD protection | Use condom/ spermicide |

[a]Percentage of women experiencing accidental pregnancy in first year of use. Range = lowest typically expected to be seen.

[b]Rates without concurrent spermicide use.

*Source:* Elias & Heise, 1993; Hatcher et al., 1992; Shannon & Hutchinson, 1993.

ability to U.S. women represents a victory (Gollub & Stein, 1993). No clinical (i.e., in vivo) studies have been completed to define protection against HIV or other STD infection; however, a 6-month trial showed contraceptive failure rates that are comparable to other methods (CDC, 1993b).

HIV transmission has been linked in several case reports to receptive oral sex with men (fellatio) and, in one case, with women (cunnilingus) (Williams, 1993). HIV transmission is likely to be at least in part dose-response related. Due to the higher number of lymphocytes in semen, higher amounts of HIV are found in semen than in cervico-vaginal fluids (Laga, 1993). In a risk reduction hierarchy, then, HIV-positive and at-risk patients should be informed of the clear risk from unprotected anal or vaginal sex and of the possible risks from unprotected oral sex. Dental dams (latex squares available from dental supply houses), an unlubricated latex condom cut in half, or even household plastic wrap can be placed over the perineum during cunnilingus, and an unlubricated latex condom can be used for fellatio.

## Female Barrier Methods

Other barrier methods, such as the diaphragm, the cervical cap, and the contraceptive sponge, provide protection of the upper reproductive tract by covering the cervix. The cervix is an important site of entry (or reentry) of HIV and is the preferred site for gonorrhea, chlamydia, trichomonas, herpes simplex virus (HSV), and HPV. However, STD transmission through vaginal mucosa is still possible. It is not clear whether these methods are protective against HIV infection or reinfection, and it is advised that women use latex condoms and spermicide for additional protection. The use of the cervical cap was associated in one study with an increased incidence of abnormal Pap smears, though this finding was not replicated by others (Hatcher et al., 1992; Shannon & Hutchison, 1993). The diaphragm does protect against cervical neoplasia, an advantage of particular benefit to HIV-positive women. The risks of diaphragm and contraceptive sponge use include a low but increased incidence of toxic shock syndrome (TSS) (Hatcher et al., 1992). These disadvantages must be weighed when being considered for use in women with HIV infection.

## Spermicides/Microbicides

The two spermicides licensed for use in the United States are nonoxynol-9 and octoxynol. Both are surfactant agents that have demonstrated in vitro effectiveness against a number of STD-causing organisms, including HIV (Elias & Heise, 1993). Use of nonoxynol-9 in high doses has been reported to cause genital ulceration and microabrasions, with risk of HIV seroconversion (Kreiss, Datta, & Willerford, 1991). More recent studies using lower, "typical-use" doses of spermicide in non-sex-worker populations have shown that the mucosal irritation effect may be dose-dependent and that nonoxynol-9 use can provide HIV protection (Elias & Heise, 1993).

## Hormonal Methods

The interaction between exogenous hormone use—oral contraceptives (OCs), implants, and injectables—and HIV disease has not been well defined, and further study is needed (Celum, 1993). However, to date no association has been found between OC use in women with HIV infection and increased risk of disease progression (Minkoff & DeHovitz, 1991).

The use of progestin-only injectables (such as Depo-Provera©/DMPA or NET) and implants (such as Norplant©) in combination with latex condoms may be a beneficial regimen for women with HIV infection. The potential advantages of Norplant include a low, constant dose of hormone (no surge, as with OC cycles or injection) and highly effective pregnancy prevention. Although menstrual changes following Norplant insertion can include prolonged bleeding in the first few months and an increase in the number of bleeding/spotting days, overall blood loss is stable, and hemoglobin levels in long-term users show an increase or no average change over time (Hatcher et al., 1992). Anemia can occasionally result from the use of injectables like DMPA and should be monitored for when this method is used by women with HIV infection.

## Other Methods

Complete abstinence is 100% effective against STDs but is not achievable or desirable for many women. Coitus interruptus does not provide protection against STDs or pregnancy, and again the use of barrier protection for the health of the woman who is HIV positive and her partner should be stressed. Fertility-awareness methods ("natural family planning" using calendar, ovulation, symptothermal, or postovulation methods) will not protect against STDs.

Several concerns pertain to the use of intrauterine devices (Progestasert®, Copper T 380A) in HIV-positive women. These include the risk of PID, which is greatest at the time of insertion, and the fact that the increased bleeding associated with IUDs may make HIV transmission to a partner more likely (Hatcher et al., 1992). For these reasons, placement of new IUDs is contraindicated in women with HIV infection. However, clinicians can individually evaluate whether to remove an IUD in a woman with a regular partner who has had no problems with her previously placed IUD.

## ❖ Pregnancy Decisions

### Reproductive Decision Making

Numerous studies have found that HIV-positive women make reproductive decisions that are very similar to those of HIV-negative women; these are summarized in Table 5–3. These studies have identified multiple factors as influencing the pregnancy decisions of women with HIV infection. Among these factors involved in pregnancy-continuation decisions are strong ethical feelings against abortion, the desire to leave a legacy or to have a child, an unwillingness to reveal HIV status to the partner, denial of infection, a chance to "start anew," good maternal health, the perception of risk, the influence of the partner and family, barriers to abortion service, and the inability to follow through on an abortion. The factors involved in pregnancy-termination decisions include the perception of risk, the influence of the partner and family, the fear of accelerating HIV disease or of infecting the infant, long-term care or child-care concerns, and poor maternal health.

Very little research has been conducted on male reproductive decision making despite the fact that many similar variables may be at play. In one German study of HIV-discordant couples (seropositive males), for example, the study authors explored the motivations of both partners, finding that the wish that "a part of myself should live on" was more apparent in men than in women (Sonnenberg-Schwan, Jaeger, Reuter, & Hammel, 1993).

TABLE 5–3   Summary of Reported Reproductive Decision Making in Women with HIV Infection

| Study | Date | No. of Women | Findings |
|---|---|---|---|
| Sunderland et al. | 1992 | 98 HIV+, 108 HIV– | Index pregnancy terminated by 19% of HIV+, 3% of HIV– women (p ≤ 0.05); subsequent pregnancies terminated by 23% of HIV+ and 19% of HIV– |
| Selwyn, Carter, et al. | 1989 | 28 HIV+, 36 HIV– | The two groups had similiar termination rates |
| Jason & Evatt | 1990 | 280 pregnancies in 2,276 hemophiliac couples | Fertility rate comparable to U.S. population |
|  |  | 24 pregnancies in 20 HIV+ partners of HIV+ men | 9 planned pregnancies, 15 unplanned pregnancies |
| Johnstone et al. | 1990 | 69 HIV+, 94 HIV– injection drug users | 45% HIV+ and 35% HIV– terminated pregnancies; no statistically significant difference |

The nondirective genetic counseling model has been cited as a useful approach in helping women with HIV infection work though their reproductive decisions (Kass, 1992; Sunderland, 1990). Unlike many inheritable diseases, however, the diagnosis of HIV holds profound and certain maternal implications as well as potential fetal ones (Marte & Anastos, 1990). For many women, adaptation to their own HIV diagnosis involves a grief process, one that may become subsumed by childbearing (Hutchison & Kurth, 1991). A recent study of 50 mothers with HIV infection in New Haven, Connecticut, found that most women experienced great isolation in their lives; for many, their children were the single greatest source of both social support and of psychological stress (Williams & Andrews, 1993).

The desire to bear children and to parent cuts across divides of socioeconomic and health status. HIV-positive women, like their HIV-negative counterparts, make their decisions based on a number of factors, both internal and external, cognitive and affective, HIV related and non-HIV related. For these reasons, the genetic counseling model may be helpful but not sufficient, and health provider attention must also focus on the psychological and medical needs of the woman herself. Reproductive decision counseling should have several goals: (1) to provide accurate information (acknowledging that much is still unknown about HIV and pregnancy); (2) to explore options through discussion of the woman's own values and goals (internal and external factors); (3) to become attuned to the woman's stage of adaptation to her HIV diagnosis, addressing both cognitive and affective factors (Hutchison & Kurth, 1991); and (4) to support the woman in her decision (Holman et al., 1989; Sunderland, 1990). Counseling must take into account the social and behavioral context in which such decisions take place (Selwyn, Carter, et al., 1989), while avoiding assumptions about what any given woman may decide. It is also important for counselors to be aware of their own feelings about substance use, HIV, pregnancy, and abortion (Williams, 1990).

## Other Reproductive Options

### Therapeutic Abortion

Women with HIV have been subject to both pressure to have abortions and restrictions in obtaining them. A phone survey of abortion providers in New York City, conducted at three different times between 1988 and 1992, found that, in the first two surveys, 42% and 31% of the providers refused services but that this discrimination was significantly reduced (4%) after the Commission on Human Rights issued letters and subpoenas (de Jung, Holman, Carrino, Caplan-Cotenoff, & de Leon, 1993). Abortion complications, though rare, increase with gestational age (Hatcher et al., 1992); women with HIV infection need timely access to abortion services.

### Voluntary Sterilization

Surgical sterilization (tubal ligation in women, vasectomy in men) is the most commonly used method of contraception (Hatcher et al., 1992). One study comparing 83 HIV-positive and 213 HIV-negative women's postpartum contraceptive choices found that seropositive women were significantly more likely to elect to have tubal ligation (Lindsay, Grant, Peterson, Nelson, & Klein, 1993). Although voluntary surgical contraception is efficacious in pregnancy prevention, women with HIV infection must be counseled to use barrier methods to minimize HIV/STD transmission risk.

### Artificial Insemination

Artificial, or assisted, insemination may be sought by couples who are infertile, HIV-discordant, or same-sex as well as by single women who wish to become mothers. Each case must be discussed individually, addressing not only the biological risks involved, but also the psychosocial issues.

HIV is found as both an extracellular (in seminal fluid) and an intracellular (within the white cells) component of ejaculate (WHO, 1992). There is some evidence that the virus may attach to the sperm itself (Scofield, 1992), though other studies have failed to document this (Elias & Heise, 1993). HIV transmission has occurred following artificial insemination with cryopreserved and fresh semen from HIV-positive donors (Ellerbrock & Rogers, 1990). Transmission has occurred in cases in which an effort was made to separate motile sperm from other cells and seminal plasma via centrifuging and washing (CDC, 1990). All donor semen should be screened according to established recommendations (CDC, 1988).

Some couples may desire parenting so strongly that they will have unprotected intercourse in order to conceive. Studies of HIV-discordant couples have shown that the wish for a child is a commonly cited reason for abandoning condom-protected intercourse even though the use of a condom has been strongly urged (Sonnenberg-Schwan et al., 1993). Fertility awareness—that is, knowledge of when the woman is ovulating—may be important to minimize exposure for those couples who choose to have unprotected sex. Where this is the case, these couples should be advised on how to minimize the risk involved, having unprotected sex only on the day of ovulation (natural family planning). Referrals can also be made to adoption agencies. Some researchers are continuing to study semen-processing techniques in an attempt to reduce the risk of artificial insemination when the donor is known to be HIV-positive (Semprini et al., 1992; Sonnenberg-Schwan et al., 1993).

## ❖ Therapeutic Regimens for Women with HIV

Despite dramatic improvements in the therapies available for the care of HIV-infected children, the prognosis for pediatric AIDS remains grim. Research interest therefore continues to focus on mechanisms to prevent the vertical transmission of HIV from the infected mother. Many of the theoretical underpinnings of a well-designed assault on perinatal transmission still need to be fully developed, however. The rates, timing, and determinants of transmission must all be known to optimize the design of intervention studies.

Even in the absence of definitive answers to the questions raised above, drug trials are already under way that are designed to measure the efficacy of several interventions, and other trials are under active development. The AIDS Clinical Trials Group study 076, a trial comparing placebo to zidovudine given in pregnancy, intrapartum, and the early neonatal period, had a goal of enrolling approximately 700 women to assess the effect of ZDV on perinatal transmission. An interim alalysis of data from this trial showed a significant reduction in mother-to-child transmission in the group treated with ZDV. These results are discussed in chapters 6 and 9.

Another agent that should be entering large-scale trials in the near future will be HIV immunoglobulin (HIVIG). HIVIG, an immunoglobulin obtained from HIV-infected, asymptomatic volunteers, has no p24 antigen and has high titers of antibody against p24 and other portions of the viral envelope. Studies of nonpregnant individuals have documented some beneficial effects on the rates of decline of CD4 cell counts with the administration of HIVIG. The perinatal trials of HIVIG will enroll women who are already taking ZDV for maternal indications, and they will be randomized to receive either HIVIG and ZDV or intravenous immunoglobulin (IVIG) and ZDV. One concern about the use of HIVIG is a "rebound" phenomenon that has been seen in the CD4 cell counts of nonpregnant women after their course of therapy has been completed.

Soluble CD4 is a molecule similar to the receptor found on the surface of CD4 cells to which HIV binds. This molecule has been engineered to bind to IgG to prolong its half-life and to facilitate transport across the placenta. In theory, it would act as a "false receptor" for HIV so that the virus will not be free to bind to fetal cells. However, Phase I trials (safety and pharmacokinetics) of soluble CD4 have not been encouraging, failing to demonstrate substantial levels of agent in fetal circulation over time. At the moment, no further perinatal studies are planned.

Other areas of investigation into potential "intervention" strategies are ongoing. These include vaccines and monoclonal antibodies. It is hoped that these modalities will result in fetal protection by utilizing either passive or active immunity against key components of the virus. It is unclear at the moment which, if any, specific portion of the virus must be blocked to prevent fetal infection.

Efforts to minimize transmission rates are one necessary branch of therapeutic research. The other important consideration is the use of effective treatment regimens for HIV disease manifestations in women. Wofsy and coworkers (1992) have pointed out that of 26 therapies commonly used to treat OIs or HIV, none has been demonstrated to pose no fetal risk in controlled trials in pregnant women. Nevertheless, the fetal risk of untreated disease in the mother remains serious and in most cases will outweigh the theoretical risk of pharmaceutical treatment (Mitchell et al., 1990).

## ❖ Summary

Nearly half of all new HIV infections in the world are estimated to occur among women (Merson, 1993), most of whom are of reproductive age. In the coming years, health care workers must be prepared to assess risk, provide HIV counseling and testing, and manage and support HIV-infected women (and their partners) in their need for reproductive services. Advances in diagnostics and preventive treatment may lead to increasing benefit for women with HIV infection and their children. Nonetheless, reproductive decisions regarding such benefits and risks are necessarily those of the woman with HIV infection, with the informed support of her health care provider.

## ❖ References

Allen, M., & Marte, C. (1991). Primary care of women infected with the human immunodeficiency virus. *Obstetrics and Gyneology Clinics of North America, 17*(3): 557–559.

American College of Obstetricians & Gynecologists (ACOG). (1992). Human immunodeficiency virus infection. *Technical Bulletin (Revised), 162,* 1–11.

Bailey, K., Herrod, H. G., Younger, R., & Shaver, D. (1985). Functional aspects of T-lymphocytes subsets in pregnancy. *Obstetrics and Gynecology, 66*(2), 211–215.

Barnes, P., Bloch, A., Davidson, P., & Snider, D. (1991). Tuberculosis in patients with human immunodeficiency virus infection. *New England Journal of Medicine, 324*(23), 1644–1650.

Berer, M., & Ray, S. (1993). *Women and HIV/AIDS: An international sourcebook.* London: Pandora.

Berrebi, A., Kobuch, W. E., Puel, J., Tricoire, J., Herne, P., Grandjean, H., & Pontonnier, G. (1990). Influence of pregnancy on human immunodeficiency virus disease. *European Journal of Obstetrics and Gynecology, 37*(3), 211–217.

Biggar, R. J., Pahwa, S., Minkoff, H., Mendes, H., Willoughby, A., Landesman, S., & Goedart, J. J. (1989). Immunosuppression in pregnant women infected with human immunodeficiency virus. *American Journal of Obstetrics and Gynecology, 161*(5), 1239–1244.

Bigger, R. J., Pahwa, S., Landesman, S., & Goedert, J. J. (1988, June). *Helper and suppressor lymphocyte changes in HIV-infected mothers and their infants.* Paper presented at the Fourth International Conference on AIDS, Stockholm.

Borkowski, W., Krazinski, K., & Paul, D. (1989). Human immunodeficiency virus type 1 antigenemia in children. *Journal of Pediatrics, 114,* 940–945.

Boue, F., Pons, J. C., & Keros, L. (1990, June). *Risks for HIV-1 perinatal transmission vary with the mother's stage of HIV infection.* Paper presented at the Sixth International Conference on AIDS, San Francisco.

Bowen, D. L. Lane, H. C., & Fauci, A. S. (1985). Immunopathogenesis of the acquired immunodeficiency syndrome. *Annals of Internal Medicine, 103,* 704–709.

Boylan, L., & Stein, Z. A. (1991). The epidemiology of HIV infection in children and their mothers—vertical transmission. *Epidemiologic Reviews, 13,* 143–177.

Broliden, P. A., Moschese, V., Junggren, K., Rosen, J., Fundaro, C., Plebani, A., Jondal, M., Rossi, M., & Wahren, B. (1989). Diagnostic implications of specific immunoglobulin G patterns of children born to HIV infected women. *AIDS, 3*(9), 577–582.

Burn, D., Muenz, L., & Walsh, J. (1991, October). *Correlation of perinatal transmission of HIV-1 with mother's lowest prepartum CD4 level.* Paper presented at the 31st Interscience Conference on Antimicrobial Therapy and Chemotherapy (ICACC). Chicago.

Burrow, G. N., & Ferris, T. F. (1988). *Medical complications during pregnancy.* Philadelphia: W. B. Saunders.

Cates, W., Stewart, F., & Trussell, J. (1992). The quest for women's prophylactic methods—Hopes vs. science [Commentary]. *American Journal of Public Health, 82,* 1479–1481.

Celum, C. (1993). Women and HIV: Epidemiology and clinical features. *STD Bulletin, 12*(1), 3–11.

Centers for Disease Control. (1982). Unexplained immune deficiency and opportunistic infection in infants, New York, New Jersey and California. *Morbidity and Mortality Weekly Report, 31,* 665.

Centers for Disease Control. (1985). Recommendations for assisting in the prevention of perinatal transmission of human T-lymphotrophic virus type III/lymphadenopathy-associated virus and acquired immunodeficiency syndrome. *Morbidity and Mortality Weekly Report, 34,* 721–726, 731–732.

Centers for Disease Control. (1988). Semen banking, organ and tissue transplantation, and HIV antibody testing. *Morbidity and Mortality Weekly Report, 37,* 57–58, 63.

Centers for Disease Control. (1990). HIV-1 infection and artificial insemination with processed semen. *Morbidity and Mortality Weekly Report, 39*(15), 249–255.

Centers for Disease Control. (1991). Purified protein derivative (PPD)-tuberculin anergy and HIV infection: Guidelines for anergy testing and management of anergic persons at risk of tuberculosis. *Morbidity and Mortality Weekly Report, 40*(RR-5), 27–33.

Centers for Disease Control and Prevention. (1992a). Acquired immunodeficiency syndrome—1991. *Morbidity and Mortality Weekly Report, 41,* 463–468.

Centers for Disease Control and Prevention. (1992b). Monthly Surveillance Reports: December.

Centers for Disease Control and Prevention. (1993a). *Facts about women and HIV/AIDS.* Atlanta: Author.

Centers for Disease Control and Prevention. (1993b). Update: Barrier protection against HIV infection and other sexually transmitted diseases. *Morbidity and Mortality Weekly Report, 42,* 589–597.

Claman, H. N. (1987). The biology of the immune response. *Journal of the American Medical Association, 258*(20), 2834–2840.

Courgnaud, V., Laure, F., & Barin, F. (1989, June). *In utero HIV-1 transmission identified through PCR.* Paper presented at the Fifth International Conference on AIDS, Montreal.

Courpotin, C., Israel, G., & Dubeaux, D. (1988). Predictive value of HIV replication in cell culture in babies born to seropositive mothers. *Lancet, 2,* 1074–1075.

D'Arminio, M. A., Ravizza, M., & Muggiasca, M. L. (1991, June). *HIV-infected pregnant women: Possible predictors of vertical transmission.* Paper presented at the Seventh International Conference on AIDS, Florence.

de Jung, T., Holman, S., Carrino, A. F., Caplan-Cotenoff, S., & de Leon, D. (1993, June). *HIV-related discrimination in abortion clinics, New York City, USA: 1988–1992.* Abstract presented at the Ninth International Conference on AIDS, Berlin.

Devash, Y., Calvelli, T., Wood, D. G., Reagen, K. J., & Rubinstein, A. (1990). Vertical transmission of HIV is correlated with absence of high affinity/avidity maternal antibodies to the gp120 principal neutralizing domain. *Proceedings of the National Academy of Science USA, 87*(9), 345–349.

Dunn, D. T., Newell, M. L., Ades, A. E., & Peckham, C. (1992). Risk of human immunodeficiency virus type 1 transmission through breastfeeding. *Lancet, 339,* 585–588.

Ehrnst, A., Lindgren, S., Dictor, M., Johansson, B., Sonnerborg, A., Czajkowski, J., Sundin, G., & Bohlin, A. B. (1991). HIV in pregnant women and their offspring: Evidence for late transmission. *Lancet 338*, 203–207.

Elias, C. J., & Heise, L. (1993). *The development of microbicides: A new method of HIV prevention for women.* (Working Paper No. 6). New York: The Population Council.

Ellerbrock, T. (1993, June). Preliminary announcement of expected CDC guidelines, made at the Ninth International Conference on AIDS, Berlin.

Ellerbrock, T. V., & Rogers, M. (1990). Epidemiology of human immunodeficiency virus infection in women in the United States. *Obstetrical and Gynecology Clinics of North America, 17*(3), 523–544.

European Collaborative Study. (1992). Risk factors for mother to child transmission of HIV-1. *Lancet, 339*, 1007–1012.

Faden, R., Geller, G., & Powers, M. (Eds.). (1992). *AIDS, women and the next generation.* New York: Oxford University Press.

Faltz, B. G., & Madover, S. (1988). Treatment of substance abuse in patients with HIV infection. In L. Siegal (Ed.) *AIDS and substance abuse.* New York: Haworth Press.

Feinberg, B. B., & Soper, D. E. (1992). Miliary tuberculosis: Unusual cause of abdominal pain in pregnancy. *Southern Medical Journal, 85*(2), 184–186.

Fiddes, T. M., O'Reilly D. B., Cetrulo, C. L., Miller, W., Rudders, R., Osband, M., & Rocklin, R. E. (1986). Phenotypic and functional evaluation of suppressor cells in normal pregnancy and in chronic aborters. *Cellular Immunology, 97*(2), 407–418.

Freeman, D. W., & Barno, A. (1969). Deaths from influenza epidemic associated with pregnancy. *American Journal of Obstetrics and Gynecology, 78*, 1172.

Frieden, T., & Fujiwara, P. (1992). Tuberculosis treatment. New York City Department of Health *City Health Information, 11*(3), 1–3.

Glassman, A. B., Bennet, C. E., Christopher, J. B., & Self, S. (1985). Immunity during pregnancy: Lymphocyte subpopulation and mitogen responsiveness. *Annals of Clinical Laboratory Science, 15*(5), 357–362.

Goedert, J., Mendez, H., Drummond, J. E., Robert-Guroff, M., Minkoff, H. L., (1989). Maternal infant transmission of HIV type 1: Association with prematurity or low anti-gp120. *Lancet, II*, 1351–1353.

Goedert, J. J., Duliege, A. M., Amos, C. I., Felton, S., & Biggar, R. J. (1991). High risk of HIV-1 infection for first born twins. *Lancet, 338*, 1471–1475.

Gollub, E., & Stein, Z. (1993). The new female condom—Item 1 on a women's AIDS prevention agenda [Commentary]. *American Journal of Public Health, 83*, 498–500.

Hague, R. A., Mok, J. Y. Q., & MacCallum, L. (1991, June). *Do maternal factors influence the risk of HIV?* Paper presented at the Seventh International Conference on AIDS, Florence.

Hatcher, R., Stewart, F., Trussell, J., Kowal, D., Guest, F., Stewart, G., & Cates, W. (1992). *Contraceptive technology 1990–1992* (15th rev. ed.). New York: Irvington.

Heymann, D. (1990, November–December). Mother to child. *World Health*, 13–14.

Holman, S., Berthaud, M., Sunderland, A., Moroso, G., Cancellieri, F., Mendez, H., Beller, E., & Marcel, A. (1989). Women infected with human immunodeficiency virus: Counseling and testing during pregnancy. *Seminars in Perinatology, 13*(1), 7–15.

Hutchison, M., & Kurth, A. (1991, February). "I need to know that I have a choice": A study of women, HIV, and reproductive decision-making. *AIDS Patient Care, 17–25.*

Jensen, L. P., O'Sullivan, M. J., Gomez-del-Rio, M., Setzer, E. S., & Gaskin, C. (1984). Acquired immune deficiency syndrome in pregnancy. *American Journal of Obstetrics and Gynecology, 148*(8), 1145–1146.

Johnstone, F. D. (1993). Pregnancy outcome and pregnancy management in HIV-infected women. In M. A. Johnson & F. D. Johnstone (Eds.), *HIV infection in women* (pp. 187–198). London: Churchill Livingstone.

Johnstone, F. D., Brettle, R., MacCallum, L., Mok, J., Peutherer, J. & Burns, S. (1990). Women's knowledge of their HIV antibody state; Its effect on their decision whether to continue the pregnancy. *British Medical Journal, 300*, 23–24.

Johnstone, F. D., MacCullum, L., Brettle, R., Inglis, J. M., & Peutherer, J. F. (1988). Does infection with HIV affect the outcome of pregnancy? *British Medical Journal, 296*, 467–471.

Joncas, J. H., Delage, G., Chad, Z., & Lapointe, N. (1983). Acquired or congenital immune deficiency syndrome in infants born to Haitian mothers. *New England Journal of Medicine, 308*, 842–846.

Kass, N. (1992). Reproductive decision making in the context of HIV: The case for nondirective counseling. In R. Faden, G. Geller, & M. Powers (Eds.), *AIDS, women and the next generation.* New York: Oxford University Press.

Kreiss, J., Datta, P., & Willerford, D. (1991, June). *Vertical transmission of HIV in Nairobi: Correlation with maternal viral burden.* Paper presented at the Seventh International Conference on AIDS, Florence.

Kurth, A. (1993). Reproductive issues, pregnancy and childbearing in HIV-positive women. In F. Cohen & J. Durham (Eds.), *Women, children and AIDS.* New York: Springer.

Laga, M. (1993, June). *STD control for HIV prevention.* Speech presented at the Ninth International Conference for AIDS, Berlin.

LaGuardia, K. (1993). Other sexually transmitted disease: Cervical intraepithelial neoplasia. In M. A. Johnson & F. D. Johnstone (Eds.), *HIV infection in women* (pp. 247–262). London: Churchill Livingstone.

Landesman, S., Weiblem, B., Mendez, H., Willoughby, A., Goeddert, J. J., Ruben, A., Minkoff, H., Moroso, G., & Hoff, R. (1991). Clinical utility of HIV-lgA assay in the early diagnosis of perinatal HIV infection. *Journal of the American Medical Association, 266*, 3443–3446.

Lepage, P., van de Perre, P., Carael, M., Nsengumuremyi, F., Nkurunziza, J., Butzler, J., & Sprecher, S. (1987). Postnatal transmission of HIV from mother to child. *Lancet, 2*(8550), 400.

Lindgren, S., Anzen, B., Bohlin, A., & Lidman, K. (1991). HIV and childbearing: Clinical outcome and aspects of mother-to-infant transmission. *AIDS, 5*, 1111–1116.

Lindsay, L., Grant, J., Peterson, H., Nelson, P., & Klein, L. (1993, June). *A comparison of the contraceptive choices of HIV seropositive and seronegative parturients.* Abstract presented at the Ninth International Conference on AIDS, Berlin.

84     PREGNANCY AND REPRODUCTIVE CONCERNS WITH HIV

Little, B. B., Bawdon, R. E., Christmas, J. T., Sobhi, S., & Gilstrap, L. C.(1989). Pharmacokinetics of azidothymidine during late pregnancy in Long-Evans rats. *American Journal of Obstetrics and Gynecology, 161*, 732–734.

Louv, W. C., Harland, A., Alexander, W. J., Stagno, S., & Cheeks, J. (1988). A clinical trial of nonoxynol-9 for preventing gonococcal and chlamydial infections. *Journal of Infectious Diseases, 158*, 518–523.

MacCallum, L. R., France, A. J., & Jones, M. E. (1988, June). *The effects of pregnancy on the progression of HIV disease.* Paper presented at the Fourth International Conference on AIDS, Stockholm.

Marte, C., & Anastos, K. (1990, Spring). Women—The missing persons in the AIDS epidemic. *Health/PAC Bulletin,* 11–18.

Mays, M. (1993). Tuberculosis: A comprehensive review for the certified nurse-midwife. *Journal of Nurse-Midwifery, 38*(3), 132–139.

Merson, M. (1993, June). The HIV pandemic—Global spread and response. Plenary speech presented at the Ninth International Conference on AIDS, Berlin.

Mhloyi, M. (1993, June). Improving HIV prevention and care for women. Plenary speech presented at the Ninth International Conference on AIDS, Berlin.

Miles, S. A., Baldin, E., Magpantay, L., Wei, L., Leiblein, A., Hofheinz, D., Toedter, G., Stiehm, E. R., & Bryson, Y. (1993). Rapid serologic testing with immune-complex-dissociated HIV p24 antigen for early detection of HIV infection in neonates. *New England Journal of Medicine, 328*, 297–302.

Minkoff, H. L., & DeHovitz, J. A. (1991). Care of women infected with the human immunodeficiency virus. *Journal of the American Medical Association, 266*, 2253–2258.

Minkoff, H. L., DeRegt, R. H., Landesman, S., & Schwarz, R. (1986). Pneumocystis carinii pneumonia associated with acquired immunodeficiency syndrome in pregnancy: A report of three maternal deaths. *Obstetrics and Gynecology, 67*(2), 284–287.

Minkoff, H. L., Henderson, C., Mendez, H., Gail, M. H., Holman, S., Willoughby, A., Goedett, J. J., Rubinstein, A., Stratton, P., & Walsh, J. H. (1990). Pregnancy outcomes among women infected with HIV and matched controls. *American Journal of Obstetrics and Gynecology, 163*, 1598–1603.

Minkoff, H., Nanda, D., Menez, R., & Fikrig, S. (1987). Pregnancies resulting in infants with acquired immunodeficiency syndrome or AIDS related complex. *Obstetrics and Gynecology, 69*, 285–289.

Minkoff, H. L., Willoughby, A., & Mendez, H. (1990). Serious infections among women with advanced HIV infection. *American Journal of Obstetrics and Gynecology, 162*, 30-34.

Mitchell, J., Brown, G., Loftman, P., & Williams, S. (1990). HIV infection in pregnancy: Detection, counseling, and care. *Pediatric AIDS and HIV Infection: Fetus to Adolescent, 1*(5), 78–82.

Mitchell, J., Loftman, P., & Williams, S. (1992). HIV infection, chemical dependency, and pregnancy. *The AIDS Reader, 2*(2), 62–67.

Nanda, D., & Minkoff, H. L. (1989). Effect of HIV infection on immune status and transmission in pregnancy. *Clinical Obstetrics and Gynecology, 32*(3) 456–466.

Newberg, D. S., Viscidi, R. P., Ruff, A., & Yolken, R. H. (1992). A human milk factor inhibits binding of human immunodeficiency virus to the CD4 receptor. *Pediatric Research, 31*(1), 22–28.

Nossal, G. J. (1987). The basic components of the immune system. *New England Journal of Medicine, 316*(21), 1320-1325.

Palasanthiran, P., Ziegler, J. B., Stewart, G. J., Stuckey, M., Armstrong, J. A., Cooper, D. A., Penny, R., & Gold, J. (1993). Breast feeding during primary HIV infection and the risk of transmission from mother to infant. *Journal of Infectious Diseases, 167*(2), 441–444.

PANOS. (1993). *AIDS: The second decade* (PANOS Briefing No. 1). London: PANOS Institute.

Paone, D., & Chavkin, W. (1991, June). *Decreasing HIV disease among women drug-users.* Paper presented at the Seventh International Conference on AIDS, Florence.

Peckham, C. (1993, June). Mother-to-child transmission of HIV: Risk factors and timing. Plenary presentation at the Ninth International Conference on AIDS, Berlin.

Quinn, T. C., Kline, R. L., Halsey, N., Hutton, N., Ruff, A., Butz, A., Boulos, R., & Modlin, J. F. (1991). Early diagnosis of perinatal HIV infection by detection of viral specific IgA antibodies. *Journal of the American Medical Association, 266*(24), 3439–3442.

Rodriguez, E. M., Rich, K., Mofenson, L., Mendez, H., Diaz, C., Fox, H., Green, K., & Brambilla, D. (1993, June). *Maternal cocaine use predicts adverse neonatal outcome more strongly than does infant HIV infection: The Women and Infants Transmission Study (WITS).* Abstract presented at the Ninth International Conference on AIDS, Berlin.

Ronkin, S., FitzSimmons, J., Wapner, R., & Finnegan, L. (1988, March). Protecting mother and fetus from narcotic abuse. *Contemporary OB/GYN,* 178–187.

Rosenberg, M., Davidson, A., Chen, J. H., Judson, F., & Douglas, J. (1992). Barrier contraceptives and sexually transmitted diseases in women: A comparison of female-dependent methods and condoms. *American Journal of Public Health, 82,* 669–674.

Rosenberg, M., & Gollub, E. (1992). Methods women can use that may prevent sexually transmitted disease, including HIV [Commentary]. *American Journal of Public Health, 82,* 1473–1478.

Rossi, P., Moschese, V., & Broliden, P. A. (1989). Presence of maternal antibodies to human immunodeficiency virus 1 envelope glycoprotein gp120 epitopes correlates with the noninfective status of children born to seropositive mothers. *Proceedings of the National Academy of Science USA, 86,* 8055–8058.

Rubinstein, A., Sicklick, M., Gupta, A., Yang-Bernstein, L., Klein, N., Rubin, E., Spigland, I., Fruchter, L., Litman, N., Lee, H., & Hollander, M. (1983). Acquired immunodeficiency with reversed T4/T8 ratios in infants born to promiscuous and drug-addicted mothers. *Journal of the American Medical Association, 249*(17), 2350–2356.

Ryder, R. W., Nsa, W., Hassig, S. E., Behets, F., Rayfield, M., Ekungola, B., Mulenda, U., Francis, H., Mwandagalirwa, K. (1989). Perinatal transmission of the human immunodeficiency virus type 1 to infants of seropositive women in Zaire. *New England Journal of Medicine, 320*(25), 1637–1642.

Schaefer, A., Grósch-Woerner, I., Friedman, W., Kunzer, R., Mielke, M., & Jimenez, E. (1988, June). *The effect of pregnancy on the natural course of HIV disease*. Paper presented at the Fourth International Conference on AIDS, Stockholm.

Scofield, F. (1992). Sperm as vectors and cofactors for HIV-1 transmission. *Journal of NIH Research, 4*, 105–111.

Selwyn, P. A., Carter, R. J., Schoenbaum, E. E., Robertson, V. J., Klein, R. S., & Rogers, M. F. (1989). Knowledge of HIV antibody status and decisions to continue or terminate pregnancy among intravenous drug users. *Journal of the American Medical Association, 261*, 3567–3571.

Selwyn, P. A., Schoenbaum, E. E., Davenny, K., Robertson, V. J., Feingold, A. R., Shulman, J. F., Mayers, M. M., Klein, R. S., Friedland, G. H., & Rogers, M. (1989). Prospective study of human immunodeficiency virus infection and pregnancy outcomes in intravenous drug users. *Journal of the American Medical Association, 261*(9), 1289–1294.

Semprini, A. E., Levi-Setti, P., Bozzo, M., Ravizza, M., Taglioretti, A., & Sulpizio, P. (1992). Insemination of HIV-negative women with processed semen of HIV-positive partners. *Lancet, 340*(11), 1317–1319.

Shannon, M., & Hutchison, M. (1993). Reproductive health and counseling [Table 4.1]. In A. Kurth (Ed.), *Until the cure: Caring for women with HIV* (pp. 49–51). New Haven: Yale University Press.

Soeiro, R., Rashbaun, W. F., Ruben, A., & Lyman, W. D. (1991, June). *The incidence of human fetal HIV-1 infection as determined by the presence of HIV-1 DNA in abortus tissues*. Paper presented at the Seventh International Conference on AIDS, Florence.

Sonnenberg-Schwan, U., Jaeger, H., Reuter, U., & Hammel, G. (1993, June). *HIV-discordant couples: Artificial insemination with processed sperm—psychological and psychosocial implications*. Abstract presented at the Ninth International Conference on AIDS, Berlin.

Sperling, R. S., Stratton, P., and the OB/GYN Working Group of the AIDS Clinical Trials Group of the National Institutes of Health. (1992). Treatment options for HIV virus infected pregnant women. *Obstetrics and Gynecology, 79*, 443–447.

Sridama, V., Pacini, F., Yang, S. L., Moawad, A., Reilly, M., & DeGroot, L. J. (1982). Decreased level of helper T cells: A possible cause of immunodeficiency in pregnancy. *New England Journal of Medicine, 307*(6), 352–356.

Stein, Z. (1990). HIV prevention: The need for methods women can use. *American Journal of Public Health, 80*, 460–462.

Stein, Z. (1992). The double bind in science policy and the protection of women from HIV infection [Editorial]. *American Journal of Public Health, 82*, 1471–1472.

St. Louis, M. E., Kabagabo, U., & Brown, C. (1991, June). *Maternal factors associated with perinatal HIV transmission*. Paper presented at the Seventh International Conference on AIDS, Florence.

Sunderland, A., Minkoff, H. L., Handte, J., Moroso, G., & Landesman, S. (1992). The impact of influence of human immunodeficiency virus serostatus on reproductive decisions of women. *Obstetrics and Gynecology, 7*(6), 1027–1031.

Sunderland, A. (1990). Influence of human immunodeficiency virus infection on reproductive decisions. *Obstetrics and Gynecology Clinics of North America, 17*(3), 585–594.

Thomas, P. A., Jaffe, H. W., Spira, T. J., Reiss, R., Guerrero, I. C., Auerbach, D. (1984). Unexplained immune deficiency in children: A surveillance report. *Journal of the American Medical Association, 252*(5), 639–644.

Tibaldi, C., Palomba, E., & Ziarati, N. (1991, June). *Maternal factors influencing vertical HIV transmission.* Paper presented at the Seventh International Conference on AIDS, Florence.

Van de Perre, P., Simonon, A., Deo-Gratius, H., Dabis, F., Msellati, P., Mukamabano, B., Butera, J.-B., Van Goethem, C., Karita, E., & Lepage, P. (1993). Infective and anti-infective properties of breastmilk from HIV-1-infected women. *Lancet, 341,* 914–918.

Van de Perre, P., Simonon, A., Msellati, P., Hiltmana, D. G., Vaira, D., Bazubagira, A., VanGoethem, C., Stevens, A. M., Karita, E., & Sondag-Thull, D. (1991). Postnatal transmission of immunodeficiency virus type 1 from mother to infant: A prospective cohort study in Kigali, Rwanda. *New England Journal of Medicine, 325,* 593–598.

Vanderberken, Y., Vheghe, M. P., & Velespesse, G. (1982). *Clinical Experimental Immunology, 48,* 1118.

Wells, D., & Jackson, J. (1992). HIV and chemically dependent women: Recommendations for appropriate health care and drug treatment services. *International Journal of the Addictions, 27*(5), 571–585.

Wetli, C. V., Roldan, E. O., & Fujaco, R. M. (1983). Listeriosis as a cause of maternal death: An obstetric complication of acquired immune deficiency syndrome. *American Journal of Obstetrics and Gynecology, 147*(1), 7–9.

WHO/UNICEF Consultation on HIV Transmission and Breastfeeding. (1992, May). Consensus statement and press release. Geneva: Author.

Williams, A. (1990). Reproductive concerns of women at risk for HIV infection. *Journal of Nurse-Midwifery, 35*(5), 292–298.

Williams, A., & Andrews, S. (1993, June). *Mother-child relationship in the HIV-positive family.* Paper presented at the Ninth International Conference on AIDS, Berlin.

Williams, S. (1993, June). HIV transmission and oral sex linked. *Positively Aware,* 4.

Wofsy, C. B., Padian, N. S., Greenblatt, R., Coleman, R., & Korvick, J. (1992). Management of HIV disease in women. In P. Volberding & M. A. Jacobson (Eds.), *AIDS clinical review 1992.* New York: Marcel Dekker.

# ❖ Chapter 6

# Epidemiology and Natural History of HIV Infection in Children

ROBERT J. SIMONDS
MARGARET J. OXTOBY

The incidence of new AIDS cases is now increasing more rapidly among women and perinatally infected children than among any other exposure category in the United States. Several unique features of HIV infection in children are of both scientific and public health importance. First, most HIV-infected children have been infected by mother-to-child transmission, a transmission mode unique to children. Second, in children, HIV infects a naive, developing immune system and a growing body, resulting in somewhat different disease manifestations than are seen in adults. Finally, diagnosing HIV infection in young infants born to HIV-infected mothers can be difficult and often requires close monitoring during early infancy. In this chapter, we review important epidemiologic and clinical features of HIV infection in children, emphasizing those aspects unique to children.

## ❖ HIV Transmission to Children

Before 1985, many children were infected with HIV through receipt of blood and blood products; however, the introduction of heat treatment and monoclonal purification has eliminated transmission through clotting factor transfusion, and the screening of blood donors for HIV risk factors and antibody has greatly reduced the risk of transmission by blood and blood product transfusion. Consequently, mother-to-child transmission currently accounts for nearly all HIV transmission to children.

Of the 4,249 AIDS cases in children less than 13 years old reported through 1992, mother-to-child transmission accounted for 86%. Among the cases reported in 1992 alone, this proportion increased to 90%. Two percent of the cases reported in 1992 are attributed to the receipt of transfusion of blood or blood products and 3% to receipt of clotting factor from infected donors, representing children that were infected in 1985 or earlier. The remaining cases are either still under investigation or have inadequate information available to determine the mode of transmission (Table 6–1).

TABLE 6–1    AIDS Cases in Children[a]

| | 1992 | | 1981–1992 | |
|---|---|---|---|---|
| | No. | (%) | No. | (%) |
| *Exposure Category* | | | | |
| Mother-to-child | 697 | (90) | 3,665 | (86) |
| Exposure category of mother: | | | | |
| Injection drug use | 246 | | 1,698 | |
| Heterosexual contact | 240 | | 1,345 | |
| Other/undetermined | 211 | | 622 | |
| Treatment for hemophilia | 21 | (3) | 188 | (4) |
| Receipt of transfusion | 19 | (2) | 306 | (7) |
| Other/undetermined | 34 | (4) | 90 | (2) |
| *Age at AIDS Diagnosis* | | | | |
| <12 months | 311 | (40) | 1,711 | (40) |
| 12–23 months | 126 | (16) | 819 | (19) |
| 2–5 years | 207 | (27) | 1,099 | (26) |
| 6–12 years | 125 | (16) | 615 | (14) |
| *Race/Ethnicity* | | | | |
| Black | 468 | (61) | 2,311 | (54) |
| Hispanic | 166 | (22) | 1,027 | (24) |
| White | 128 | (17) | 871 | (20) |
| Other/unknown | 9 | (1) | 40 | (1) |
| *State of Residence* | | | | |
| New York | 199 | (26) | 1,153 | (27) |
| Florida | 119 | (15) | 631 | (15) |
| California | 59 | (8) | 316 | (7) |
| New Jersey | 47 | (6) | 403 | (9) |
| Puerto Rico | 27 | (4) | 214 | (5) |
| Texas | 27 | (4) | 183 | (4) |
| Other | 293 | (38) | 1,349 | (32) |
| Total | 771 | (100) | 4,249 | (100) |

[a]Cases reported in 1992 and reported cumulatively, 1981–1992, United States.

Transmission to children by other routes has been reported only rarely. These include several cases attributed to sexual abuse (Gutman et al., 1991), receipt of medical injections with unsterilized needles and other injection equipment (Hersh et al., 1991; Koenig, Gautier, & Levy, 1986) and from transplanted organs before antibody screening of donors became available in 1985 (Malekzadeh et al., 1987).

Except for the relatively large proportion of cases among male adolescents (ages 13–19 years) attributed to the treatment of hemophilia, behaviors leading to HIV transmission among adolescents with AIDS resemble those of adults. Among the 671 adolescent males with AIDS reported through 1992, infection was attributed to the receipt of clotting factor treatment for hemophilia in 41% of the cases, male-to-male sex in 34%, injection drug use in 7%, male-to-male sex and injection drug use in 6%, receipt of blood transfusion in 4%, and heterosexual contact in 3%. Among the 275 adolescent females with AIDS, transmission was attributed to heterosexual contact in 48% of the cases, injection drug use in 26%, receipt of transfusion in 11%, and receipt of clotting factor in 1%. In 5% of adolescent males and 14% of adolescent females, the transmission risk is undetermined or under investigation.

HIV transmission has not been reported in schools, day-care centers, or other child-care settings outside of the home. Transmission between sibling children has been suggested in only three cases; in two of these cases, needles were used for injections or infusion in the home (Centers for Disease Control and Prevention [CDC], 1992a; Koenig et al., 1986). In a third case, transmission was attributed to biting (Wahn et al., 1986), but this brief report did not address all other possible transmission modes. The risk of transmission in the home setting is extremely low. No transmission was found in 17 studies that monitored more than 1,100 household contacts of people with HIV infection for more than 1,700 person-years of contact (Simonds & Chanock, in press).

## ❖ Mother-to-Child Transmission of HIV

Mother-to-child HIV transmission, also termed vertical or perinatal transmission, includes transmission to a fetus during pregnancy, to a newborn during labor and delivery, or to an infant during breast feeding. Although mother-to-child transmission is the predominant mode of HIV transmission to children, many of the factors that facilitate transmission and affect the timing of transmission remain poorly understood.

The rates of mother-to-child transmission observed in a variety of prospective studies have ranged from 14% to 50%. Most studies in developed countries have reported rates between 15% and 30%. Higher rates have been reported in studies of African children (Report of a Consensus Workshop, 1992). These studies have identified several factors related to an increased likelihood of transmission. One is the stage of infection in the mother, as measured by clinical symptoms, the quantity of virus in her blood, and the numbers of circulating CD4+ and CD8+ lymphocytes. A higher likelihood of transmission has been suggested during very early and late stages of infection, both times when the amount of HIV in the blood may be high (Report of a Consensus Workshop, 1992). Secondly, the presence of chorio-amnionitis, which may disrupt the placental barrier, has been shown to increase the likelihood of transmission (Ryder et al., 1989; St. Louis et al., 1993).

Other factors that may affect mother-to-child transmission include the aggressiveness of the viral strain and the presence of antibodies in the mother to select portions of the HIV envelope, especially to those of the specific HIV strains that have infected the mother (Bryson et al., 1993; Parekh et al., 1991). Moreover, one study showed no higher rate of infection in subsequent children born to an infected mother if the first child was infected than if the first child was uninfected (Perinatal AIDS Collaborative Transmission Studies Group, 1992), suggesting that factors related to a particular pregnancy or delivery are important and may change from one pregnancy to the next.

Mother-to-child transmission of HIV can occur either during pregnancy through transplacental transmission, during labor and delivery though exposure to blood or vaginal secretions, or after delivery through breast feeding. Although there is evidence to support each of these routes, the relative contribution of each to mother-to-child transmission is unknown.

Transmission early in pregnancy has been documented by the detection of HIV in first- and second-trimester fetuses (Sprecher, Soumenkoff, Puissant, & Deguelde, 1986). Moreover, nearly half of all infected newborns test positive by HIV culture or polymerase chain reaction (PCR) soon after birth (Burgard et al., 1992), suggesting that infection occurred before labor and delivery in these children.

However, more than half of infected children do not demonstrate virologic or immunologic evidence of infection until after the first few days of life; thus, a substantial proportion of infected children may be infected close to or at the time of labor and delivery. One study reported a higher transmission rate to firstborn twins, especially those born vaginally, than to second-born twins (Goedert, Duliege, Amos, Felton, & Biggar, 1991), suggesting that factors related to labor and delivery play a role in transmission. A recent meta-analysis demonstrating that HIV transmission is somewhat less likely in children born by cesarean section supports the possibility that some events surrounding labor and delivery may be important for HIV transmission, although these events have yet to be delineated (Villari, Spino, Chalmers, Lau, & Sacks, 1993).

In early 1994, an interim analysis of data from the Pediatric AIDS Clinical Trials Group protocol 076 demonstrated the efficacy of zidovudine in reducing mother-to-child HIV transmission when administered to HIV-infected pregnant women who had CD4+ cell counts >200/µl (Centers for Disease Control and Prevention, 1994). Zidovudine given to the mother during pregnancy and at delivery, and to the newborn reduced the rate of HIV transmission from 26% to 8%. Based on these findings, the U. S. Public Health Service has recommended that all health-care workers providing care to women of childbearing age be informed of the results of this study, that HIV-infected pregnant women be informed of the potential benefits but unknown long-term risks of such preventive therapy with zidovudine, and that the decision to use zidovudine to reduce the risk of mother-to-child transmission be made in consultation with health-care providers.

HIV has been isolated from breast milk, and HIV transmission through breast feeding has been demonstrated (Thiry et al., 1985; Van de Perre et al., 1991). The additional risk of HIV transmission through breast feeding has been estimated at 14% (Dunn, Newell, Ades, & Peckham, 1992). For this reason, breast feeding is not recommended for HIV-infected women in the United States. However, breast feeding is considered the best option for infant feeding in areas where clean water to mix formula is not available and infant mortality due to infections and malnutrition is high (HIV transmission and breastfeeding, 1992).

## ❖ Scope of the Epidemic

Since the first reports of children with AIDS in 1982, nationwide AIDS surveillance has provided the most consistent picture of trends in the number of children with AIDS in the United States: their age, race, and geographic distribution and the means by which they became infected. Throughout the 1980s, the number of AIDS cases diagnosed in children increased steadily (Figure 6–1). In the past few years, however, the rate of increase of new AIDS cases has slowed somewhat. Because increasing numbers of children are born to infected women each year, this flattening of the epidemic curve is most likely due either to therapy prolonging the period between infection and the development of AIDS or to increased delays in reporting AIDS cases after diagnosis. Estimates indicate that approximately 7,500 children will have been diagnosed with AIDS attributed to mother-to-child transmission by the end of 1994 (CDC, 1992c).

The largest numbers of AIDS cases in children occur among those in the first two years of life, those who are black or Hispanic, and those living in high-incidence states (Table 6–1). Because most HIV-infected children acquired their infection from their mother, their race and geographic distribution reflect those of HIV-infected childbearing women.

Understanding how the mothers of children with perinatally acquired AIDS became infected provides insight into the risk factors that are determining the epidemic among children. Slightly more than one third of children with perinatally acquired AIDS reported in 1992 had mothers who were injection drug users. This proportion has declined over the past several years. In most of the remaining cases, the mothers were thought to have acquired their infections heterosexually (Table 6–1).

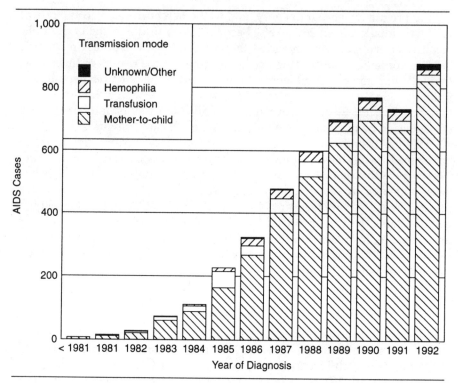

FIGURE 6–1   Number of AIDS cases diagnosed, 1981–1992.

*Source:* Centers for Disease Control and Prevention, Atlanta, GA 1993.

One of the best ways to monitor the incidence of new infections in children is to monitor births to women with HIV infection. Since 1988, the Centers for Disease Control (CDC) has coordinated a series of state-based, blinded serologic surveys on newborns using dried blood specimens left over from metabolic screening tests. Estimates based on data collected from this national serosurvey of childbearing women indicate that 0.17% of women who delivered in the United States in 1991 were HIV infected (Gwinn et al., 1991). The HIV seroprevalence among childbearing women varies greatly by state (Figure 6–2) and has increased slightly during the period of the survey (1988–1991), most notably in southern states (Gwinn, Wasser, Fleming, Karon, & Petersen, 1993). Higher seroprevalence rates have been reported in local serosurveys, even in rural areas of the South (Ellerbrock et al., 1992). Based on the serosurvey of childbearing women, it is estimated that approximately 7,000 children are born to HIV-infected women annually; because the mother-to-child transmission rate is estimated to be 20% to 30%, this number translates into approximately 1,500 to 2,000 HIV-infected children born each year.

HIV infection has had a major impact on mortality among children, especially in certain subpopulations. As of December 1992, 71% of the 1,854

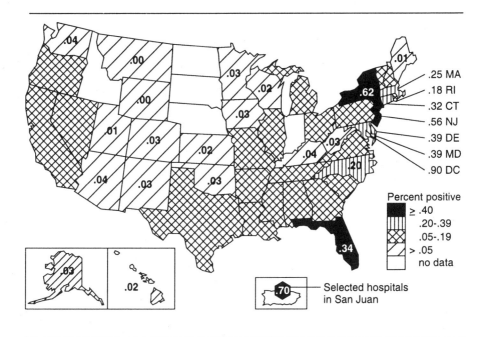

.25 MA
.18 RI
.32 CT
.56 NJ
.39 DE
.39 MD
.90 DC

Percent positive
≥ .40
.20-.39
.05-.19
> .05
no data

Selected hospitals
in San Juan

FIGURE 6–2   HIV servoprevalence among childbearing women.

*Source:* Centers for Disease Control and Prevention, Atlanta, GA 1993.

children diagnosed with AIDS before 1989 and 40% of the 2,395 children diagnosed since 1989 were reported to have died. Because these figures include only those deaths reported to the CDC, they probably underestimate the total deaths. By 1990, HIV/AIDS was the seventh leading cause of death among 1- to 4-year-old children in the United States. In New York and New Jersey, HIV/AIDS was surpassed only by unintentional injuries as the leading cause of death among black children in this age group (Chu, Buehler, Oxtoby, & Kilbourne, 1991).

In addition to precipitating the HIV epidemic in children through mother-to-child transmission, the HIV epidemic in adults has affected children in other ways. Largely as a result of parental HIV infection and parental drug use, many children born to HIV-infected mothers do not live with their biological parents. Among the 1,700 children in the CDC Pediatric Spectrum of Disease Project, 55% were living with a biological parent, 28% with foster parents, 10% with other relatives, 3% with adoptive parents, and 4% with other caregivers (Caldwell et al., 1992). Approximately 20,000 U.S. children have been orphaned as a result of their mothers having died from HIV infection, and this number is expected to reach 80,000 by the end of the decade (Caldwell, Fleming, & Oxtoby, 1992; Michaels & Levine, 1992). Additionally, children living in households with HIV-infected people may also be at higher risk for tuberculosis.

## ❖ Clinical Manifestations

Infants born to HIV-infected mothers present special diagnostic challenges. Because maternally derived anti-HIV IgG may persist in both infected and uninfected children for up to 15 months, measuring anti-HIV IgG, the most common test for HIV infection in adults, is not useful for diagnosis of infection in young infants. Recently, several other approaches to early HIV infection diagnosis in infants have been successful, including detecting HIV deoxyribonucleic acid (DNA) by polymerase chain reaction (PCR); measuring HIV p24 antigen, especially after disrupting antigen-antibody complexes; and measuring IgA antibodies to HIV, which are not passed from mother to infant. These tests can be used to diagnose HIV infection in many children by 6 months of age.

Most children with perinatally acquired HIV infection are asymptomatic at birth, but most will become symptomatic by 3 years of age. The most common initial symptoms of HIV infection in children are nonspecific, such as generalized lymphadenopathy, hepatosplenomegaly, failure to thrive, skin disease, or persistent thrush. Additionally, immunologic abnormalities are common. During the early stages of infection, hypergammaglobuline-mia is common, followed by a progressive decline in the number and percentage of CD4+ lymphocytes. Because CD4+ lymphocytes naturally decline during the first few years of life in uninfected children (Denny et al., 1992), interpreting CD4+ lymphocyte decline in children with HIV infection can be problematic. Moreover, the CD4+ lymphocyte counts that determine risk for opportunistic infections like pneumocystis carinii pneumonia (PCP) may be higher for HIV-infected infants than for adults.

Two distinct populations of children, those with rapid progression of illness (3-year survival of 48%) and those with slow progression of illness (3-year survival of 97%), have been described (Blanche et al., 1990). Most children remain asymptomatic or have only mild symptoms during early childhood. Many have survived much longer without severe symptoms; more than 50 perinatally infected children have been reported who did not develop AIDS until age 10 years or older. However, other children may develop severe opportunistic infection, such as PCP or cytomegalovirus infection, in the first year of life. The use of zidovudine has been shown to delay the progression of HIV-related symptoms in some children, though its effect on overall survival is less clear.

In children, as in adults, PCP is the most common of the serious HIV-related conditions that define AIDS, having occurred in 37% of children with AIDS. Among children, most cases of PCP occur between 3 and 6 months of age; the estimated risk of PCP in the first year of life for children with perinatally acquired HIV infection is 7% to 20% (Simonds, Oxtoby, Caldwell, Gwinn, & Rogers, 1993). Thus, it is extremely important to identify children at risk for perinatally acquired HIV infection as early as possible so that their need for PCP prophylaxis can be evaluated (CDC, 1991).

Although the AIDS case definition for adolescents and adults was modified in 1993 (CDC, 1992b), the definition for children has remained unchanged since 1987 (CDC, 1987b). Two conditions that are part of the AIDS definition for children, but not for adults, are also common in children: (1) lymphoid interstitial pneumonitis, a chronic lung condition marked by an interstitial lymphocyte infiltration and diagnosed in 20% of children with AIDS reported in 1992; and (2) recurrent serious bacterial infections, such as meningitis or septicemia, reported in 13% of cases.

Additionally, the manifestations of HIV encephalopathy and HIV wasting syndrome may be different in children than in adults. In children, encephalopathy may begin with the loss of developmental milestones before the onset of a variety of static or progressive neurological abnormalities (Diamond & Cohen, 1992), most prominently, impaired brain growth and motor dysfunction. Wasting syndrome may begin as a failure to thrive before actual weight loss occurs. Cancers occur much less frequently in HIV-infected children than in adults. Table 6–2 lists the 10 most common AIDS-defining conditions in children who were reported with AIDS in 1992.

To assist in standardizing the assessment of disease progression, the CDC is developing a new classification of HIV infection in children. This proposed new system uses two manifestations of HIV-related disease: the presence of clinical symptoms and immune dysfunction, as measured by age-stratified CD4+ lymphocyte counts and percentages. This system uses four clinical categories, ranging from no symptoms to severe manifestations of HIV infection, and three immune function categories to classify HIV

TABLE 6–2  Ten Common AIDS-Defining Conditions in Children (under 13) Reported with AIDS in the United States in 1992 (N = 771)

| AIDS-Defining Condition | Number | Percentage[a] |
| --- | --- | --- |
| Pneumocystis carinii pneumonia | 239 | 31 |
| Lymphoid interstitial pneumonitis | 158 | 20 |
| HIV wasting syndrome | 120 | 16 |
| HIV encephalopathy | 115 | 15 |
| Recurrent serious bacterial infections | 100 | 13 |
| Candida esophagitis | 82 | 11 |
| Cytomegalovirus disease | 57 | 7 |
| Mycobacterium avium infection | 35 | 5 |
| Herpes simplex disease | 30 | 4 |
| Pulmonary candidiasis | 27 | 4 |

[a]Children may have more than one condition reported.

infection in children. When completed, the new system should be simpler than the previous one (CDC, 1987a) and should allow HIV infection in children to be classified more specifically based on the severity of the illness.

## ❖ Summary

Several of the epidemiologic and clinical features of HIV infection in children have important consequences for the development of strategies to prevent or treat HIV infection and its manifestations. For instance, understanding how HIV is transmitted to children allows rational development of strategies to interrupt transmission. Observing that HIV infection progresses rapidly in many children highlights the need for early identification of HIV infection in children and their mothers so that interventions can be offered when most effective. Finally, determining the prevalence of HIV infection among childbearing women helps target screening programs to identify infected children as well as programs designed to help prevent HIV infection among women at highest risk.

## ❖ References

Blanche, S., Tardieu, M., Duliege, A. M., Rouzioux, C., Le Dist, F., Fukunaga, K., Caniglia, M., Jacomet, C., Messiah, A., & Griscelli, C. (1990). Longitudinal study of 94 symptomatic infants with perinatally acquired human immunodeficiency virus infection. *American Journal of Diseases of Children, 144,* 1210–1215.

Bryson, Y. J., Lehman, D., Garratty, E., Dickover, R., Plaeger-Marshall, S., & O'Rourke, S. (1993, April). *The role of maternal autologous neutralizing antibody in prevention of maternal fetal HIV-1 transmission.* Paper presented at the Keystone Symposium on HIV Pathogenesis in Infants and Children, Albuquerque. (Abstract No. QZ 005)

Burgard, M., Mayaux, M. J., Blanche, S., Ferroni, A., Guihard-Moscato, M. L., Allemon, M. C., Ciraru-Vigneron, N., Firtion, G., Floch, C., Guillot, F., Lachassine, E., Vial, M., Griscelli, C., Rouzioux, C., & the HIV Infection in Newborns French Collaborative Study Group. (1992). The use of viral culture and p24 antigen testing to diagnose human immunodeficiency virus infection in neonates. *New England Journal of Medicine, 327,* 1192–1197.

Caldwell, M. B., Fleming, P. L., and Oxtoby, M. J. (1992). Estimated number of AIDS orphans in the United States [Letter to the Editor]. *Pediatrics, 90,* 482.

Caldwell, M. B., Mascola, L., Smith, W., Thomas, P., Hsu, H. W., Maldonado, Y., Parrott, R., Byers, R., Oxtoby, M., & the Pediatric Spectrum of Disease Clinical Consortium. (1992). Biologic, foster, and adoptive parents: Care givers of children exposed perinatally to human immunodeficiency virus in the United States. *Pediatrics, 90,* 603–607.

Centers for Disease Control. (1987a). Classification system for human immunodeficiency virus (HIV) infection in children under 13 years of age. *Morbidity and Mortality Weekly Report, 36,* 225–236.

Centers for Disease Control. (1987b). Revision of the CDC surveillance case definition for acquired immunodeficiency syndrome. *Morbidity and Mortality Weekly Report, 36*(Suppl. 1S), 1S–13S.

Centers for Disease Control. (1991). Guidelines for prophylaxis against pneumocystis carinii pneumonia for children infected with human immunodeficiency virus. *Morbidity and Mortality Weekly Report, 40*(RR-2), 1–13.

Centers for Disease Control and Prevention. (1992a). HIV infection in two brothers receiving intravenous therapy for hemophilia. *Morbidity and Mortality Weekly Report, 41*, 228–231.

Centers for Disease Control and Prevention. (1992b). 1993 revised classification system for HIV infection and expanded surveillance case definition for AIDS among adolescents and adults. *Morbidity and Mortality Weekly Report, 41*(RR-17).

Centers for Disease Control and Prevention. (1992c). Projections of the number of persons diagnosed with AIDS and the number of immunosuppressed HIV-infected persons—United States, 1992–1994. *Morbidity and Mortality Weekly Report, 41*(RR-18), 1–29.

Centers for Disease Control and Prevention. (1994). Zidovudine for the prevention of HIV transmission for mother to infant. *Morbidity and Mortality Weekly Report, 43*, 285–287.

Chu, S. Y., Buehler, J. W., Oxtoby, M. J., & Kilbourne, B. W. (1991). Impact of the human immunodeficiency virus epidemic on mortality in children, United States. *Pediatrics, 87*, 806–810.

Denny, T., Yogev, R., Gelman, R., Skuza, C., Oleske, J., Chadwick, E., Cheng, S. C., and Connor, E. (1992). Lymphocyte subsets in healthy children during the first 5 years of life. *Journal of the American Medical Association, 267*, 1484–1488.

Diamond, G. W., & Cohen, H. J. (1992). Developmental disabilities in children with HIV infection. In A. C. Crocker, H. J. Cohen, & T. A. Kastner (Eds.), *HIV infection and developmental disabilities: A Resource for Service Providers* (pp. 33–42). Baltimore: H. Brookes.

Dunn, D. T., Newell, M. L., Ades, A. E., & Peckham, C. S. (1992). Risk of human immunodeficiency virus type 1 transmission through breastfeeding. *Lancet, 340*, 585–588.

Ellerbrock, T. V., Lieb, S., Harrington, P., Bush, T. J., Schoenfisch, S. A., Oxtoby, M. J., Howell, J. T., Rogers, M. F., & Witte, J. J. (1992). Heterosexually transmitted human immunodeficiency virus infection among pregnant women in a rural Florida community. *New England Journal of Medicine, 327*, 1704–1709.

Goedert, J. J., Duliege, A. M., Amos, C. I., Felton, S., & Biggar, R. J. (1991). International Registry of HIV-Exposed Twins: High risk of HIV-1 infection for first born twins. *Lancet, 338*, 1471–1475.

Gutman, L. T., St. Claire, K. K., Weedy, C., Herman-Giddens, M. E., Lane, B. A., Neimeyer, J. G., & McKinney, R. E. (1991). Human immunodeficiency virus transmission by child sexual abuse. *American Journal of Diseases of Children, 145*, 137–141.

Gwinn, M., Pappaioanou, M., George, J. R., Hannon, W. H., Wasser, S. C., Redus, M. A., Hoff, R., Grady, G. F., Willoughby, A., Novello, A. C., Peterson, L. R., Dondero, T. J., & Curran, J. W. (1991). Prevalence of HIV infection in childbearing women in the United States. *Journal of the American Medical Association, 265*, 1704–1708.

Gwinn, M., Wasser, S., Fleming, P., Karon, J., & Petersen, L. (1993, June). *Increasing prevalence of HIV infection among childbearing women, United States, 1989–1991* Paper presented at the Ninth International Conference on AIDS, Berlin. (Abstract No. PO-C16-2990)

Hersh, B. S., Popovici, F., Apetrei, R. C., Zolotusc, L., Beldescu, N., Calumfirescu, A., Jezek, Z., Oxtoby, M. J., Gromyko, A., & Heymann, D. L. (1991). Acquired immunodeficiency syndrome in Romania. *Lancet, 338,* 645–649.

HIV transmission and breastfeeding. (1992). *Bulletin of the World Health Organization, 70,* 667–669.

Koenig, R. E., Gautier, T., & Levy, J. A. (1986). Unusual intrafamilial transmission of human immunodeficiency virus [Letter to the Editor]. *Lancet, 2,* 627.

Malekzadeh, M. H., Church, J. A., Siegel, S. E., Mitchell, W. G., Opas, L., & Lieberman, E. (1987). Human immunodeficiency virus–associated Kaposi's sarcoma in a pediatric renal transplant recipient. *Nephron, 42,* 62–65.

Michaels, D., & Levine, C. (1992). Estimates of the number of motherless youth orphaned by AIDS in the United States. *Journal of the American Medical Association, 268,* 3456–3461.

Parekh, B. S., Shaffer, N., Pau, C. P., Abrams, E., Thomas, P., Pollack, H., Bamji, M., Kaul, A., Schochetman, G., Rogers, M., George, J. R., & the NYC Perinatal HIV Transmission Collaborative Study. (1991). Lack of correlation between maternal antibodies to V3 loop peptides of gp 120 and perinatal HIV-1 transmission. *AIDS, 5,* 1179–1184.

Perinatal AIDS Collaborative Transmission Studies Group. (1992, July). *Lack of increased risk of HIV perinatal transmission to subsequent siblings born to an HIV-infected mother.* Paper presented at the Eighth International Conference on AIDS, Amsterdam. (Abstract No. WeC 1057)

Report of a Consensus Workshop, Siena, Italy, January 17–18, 1992. (1992). Factors involved in mother-to-child transmission of HIV. *Journal of the Acquired Immune Deficiency Syndrome, 5,* 1019–1029.

Ryder, R. W., Nsa, W., Hassig, S., Behets, F., Rayfield, M., Ekungola, B., Nelson, A., Mulenda, U., Francis, H., Mwandagalirwa, K., Davachi, F., Rogers, M., Nzilambi, N., Greenberg, A., Mann, J., Quinn, T., Piot, P., & Curran, J. (1989). Perinatal transmission of human immunodeficiency virus type 1 to infants of seropositive women in Zaire. *New England Journal of Medicine, 320,* 1637–1642.

Simonds, R. J., & Chanock, S. (in press). Medical issues related to caring for HIV-infected children in and out of the home. *Pediatric Infectious Disease Journal.*

Simonds, R. J., Oxtoby, M. J., Caldwell, M. B., Gwinn, M. L., & Rogers, M. F. (1993). Pneumocystis carinii pneumonia among US children with perinatally acquired HIV infection. *Journal of the American Medical Association, 270,* 470–473.

Sprecher, S., Soumenkoff, G., Puissant, F., & Deguelde, M. (1986). Vertical transmission of HIV in 15-week fetus [Letter to the Editor]. *Lancet, 2,* 288–289.

St. Louis, M. E., Kamenga, M., Brown, C., Nelson, A. M., Manzila, T., Batter, V., Behets, F., Kabagabo, U., Ryder, R. W., Oxtoby, M., Quinn, T. C., & Heyward, W. L. (1993). Risk for perinatal HIV-1 transmission according to

Thiry, L., Sprecher-Goldberger, S., Jonckheer, T., Levy, J., Van de Perre, P., Henrivaux, P., Cogniaux-Leclerc, J., & Clumeck, N. (1985). Isolation of AIDS virus from cell-free breast milk of three healthy virus carriers. *Lancet, 2,* 891–892.

Van de Perre, P., Simonon, A., Msellati, P., Hitimana, D. G., Vaira, D., Bazubagira, A., Van Goethem, C., Stevens, A. M., Karita, E., Sondag-Thull, D., Dabis, F., & Lepage, P. (1991). Postnatal transmission of human immunodeficiency virus type 1 from mother to infant: A prospective cohort study in Kigali, Rwanda. *New England Journal of Medicine, 325,* 593–598.

Villari, P., Spino, C., Chalmers, T. C., Lau, J., & Sacks, H. S. (1993). Cesarean section to reduce perinatal transmission of human immunodeficiency virus. *Online Journal of Current Clinical Trials, 2,* Doc. 74.

Wahn, V., Kramer, H. H., Voit, T., Bruster, H. T., Scrampical, B., & Scheid, A. (1986). Horizontal transmission of HIV infection between two siblings [Letter to the Editor]. *Lancet, 1,* 694.

# ❖ Chapter 7

# Care of Children with HIV Infection

Mary Jo O'Hara

HIV infection in children is a serious, life-threatening illness that challenges the health care and related professions more and more each day. As a disease with more questions than answers about diagnosis, treatment, and disease progression, research and clinical interventions change on a daily basis. It requires a proactive response from primary care practitioners as more childbearing women become HIV infected and more children are thus exposed to this complex disease. The role of the primary care provider begins with early identification of children at risk for HIV and continues with their early prophylaxis and treatment. It must include consultation and collaboration with multiple health and social service providers, and it necessarily includes advocacy for children and families affected by this devastating disease.

This chapter discusses a proactive approach to evaluating and managing children at risk for HIV disease. Such an approach will provide timely and effective prophylaxis against opportunistic infections, promote early diagnosis and early treatment of infections, and, it is hoped, improve prognosis and life expectancy for the child living with HIV infection. In addition, this chapter reviews the impact of HIV disease on the normal growth and development of children and explores social concerns, such as school attendance and enhancing care for infected families.

## ❖ The HIV-Indeterminate Infant

The diagnosis of HIV infection in children under the age of 18 months is complicated by the passive transfer of maternal antibody. Virtually all infants born to women with HIV infection are themselves HIV seropositive. Previously, in the absence of an AIDS-defining condition, one had to wait until an infant reached 15 to 18 months of age before infection status could be determined. With the loss of maternal antibody, the exposed but not infected infant becomes a seroreverter; that is, he or she will lose maternal antibody by 15 to18 months of age. As shown in Figure 7–1, approximately 70% to 85% of children are not infected with HIV and will serorevert (test negative to an HIV ELISA and Western Blot) before 2 years of age.

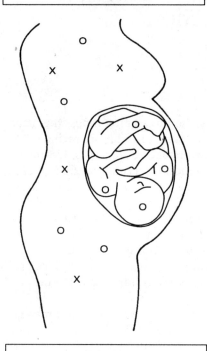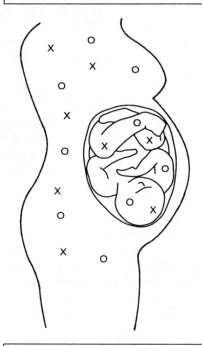

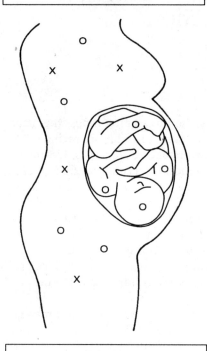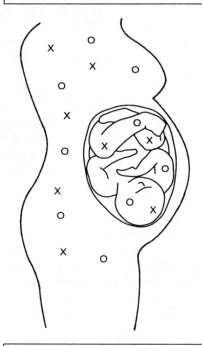

Mother 1:

HIV infection (XXX)
HIV antibody (OOO)

Mother 2:

HIV infection (XXX)
HIV antibody (OOO)

Baby 1:

• Has positive ELISA and Western Blot
• Has received HIV antibody only

• Does not have HIV infection

• Will serorevert before 2 years old

~ 70–85%

Baby 2:

• Has positive ELISA and Western Blot
• Has received HIV antibody and virus

• Does have HIV infection

• Is infected and will develop symptoms of illness over time

~ 15–30%

*Note:* Some percentage of HIV transmission occurs at the time of delivery.

FIGURE 7–1   Perinatal exposure to HIV and possible outcomes.

The remaining 15 to 30% of infants are HIV infected and will remain seropositive. Because perinatally acquired HIV infection is a relatively more rapidly progressive disease when compared to transfusion-acquired or adult disease, many infants develop symptoms before a definitive diagnosis of HIV can be made based on antibody status. Of those children with perinatally acquired infection, approximately 30% develop clinical symptoms within the first year of life, and their prognosis is poor (Delfraisy, Blanche, Rouzloux, & Mayaux, 1992). Recent advances in specific virological tests to detect HIV directly now permit diagnosis of infected infants as early as the first few days of life. These assays include HIV culture, HIV polymerase chain reactions (PCR), and immune complex dissociated (ICD) p24 antigen (Borkowsky et al., 1992; Burgard et al., 1992; Miles et al., 1993). HIV culture and PCR can identify up to 50% of infected infants in the first week of life and more than 95% of infected infants by 3 to 6 months of age. Although these tests have great specificity, their sensitivity varies by age (Consensus Workshop, 1992). Because of this variable sensitivity, negative test results, especially in young infants, must be interpreted cautiously. Young infants with negative culture or PCR test results may actually be HIV infected and therefore continue to require close monitoring, preferably in conjunction with a pediatric infectious disease specialist. ICD p24 antigen detection is currently emerging as a simple and promising technology for use in this age group (Miles et al., 1993). The important benefit of these testing advances has been the ability to confirm the diagnosis earlier and to intervene with specific antiretroviral and prophylactic therapies before symptoms appear, while providing families with appropriate supportive services (Figure 7–2).

The diagnosis of HIV infection may also be confirmed in infants and young children by the presence of nonspecific markers of immune dysfunction combined with specific clinical symptoms of HIV (Centers for Disease Control [CDC], 1987). Unfortunately, this requires that children have significant disease progression, and opportunities for early treatment and interventions may be lost ( Figure 7–3).

Passively acquired maternal antibody dissipates by 15 to 18 months of age. Older children can be diagnosed using standard tests for serum antibodies (HIV ELISA and Western Blot). These tests are highly sensitive and specific. In extremely rare instances, perinatally infected children have had such severe immune compromise that they never produce antibodies to HIV. However, these children are seriously ill, and the diagnosis can be made on clinical symptomatology alone.

Whenever a child is being evaluated for exposure to HIV infection, it is the responsibility of the practitioner to ensure that voluntary, informed consent has been obtained. Pretest and posttest counseling is never really complete with any family. Ongoing assessment of the family's interpretation of test results is necessary to clarify misinformation related to the possibility of children "outgrowing" the virus or being "carriers" of the virus but not infected. When the clinician has definitively diagnosed the infection, especially if the child is under 2 years old, the family needs to hear

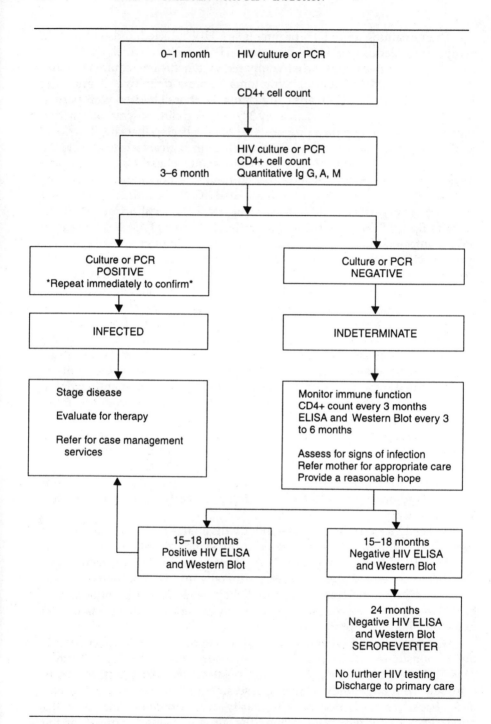

FIGURE 7-2  Laboratory schema for early diagnosis: HIV-exposed infants under 15 months.

**Diagnosis of HIV Infection in Children Younger Than 15 Months**

1. Virus in blood or tissue
2. HIV+ antibody *and* evidence of immune deficiency (cellular *and* humoral) *and* one or more class P-2 symptoms
3. Symptoms meeting CDC case definition for AIDS

**Diagnosis of HIV Infection in Children Older Than 15 Months**

1. Virus in blood or tissue
2. Persistent HIV antibody
3. Symptoms meeting CDC case definition for AIDS

FIGURE 7–3    Diagnosis of HIV infection in children.

that the child has HIV infection, that it will not go away, and that although there is no cure, there is hope and treatment. The connection between HIV infection and AIDS must be absolutely clear. Requesting that the family restate what they have heard is a helpful mechanism for determining any misinformation. Denial is a common response to shock and grief, and the clinician may need to repeat the facts more than once while continuing to provide hope for the family.

Regardless of the ultimate outcome, all HIV-exposed children and their families should receive anticipatory guidance, developmental assessments, health counseling, safety education, preventive-care services, and encouragement to lead as normal a life as possible. A shared approach between primary care providers and HIV subspecialists is ideal because primary care providers will know the child, the family, and the community and be able to individualize and implement any treatment plan but may not have access to all of the nuances of care and the specialty laboratory testing necessary for ongoing evaluation of the HIV-exposed infant.

## Identify and Test Family Members

Many children who have been HIV infected since birth live in families where there is no suspicion of HIV infection. The child may present with a variety of symptoms; the practitioner must be alert to the possibility of HIV as an etiology and must approach the family with these concerns.

The reluctance of parents to consider or to follow through on a practitioner's suggestion for HIV antibody testing for the child as well as for other family members is not an uncommon response. To health care providers, any delay or "unwillingness" to be tested may seem negligent or foolish. However, it may be overwhelming for a parent or caregiver to consider that both they and their baby may be HIV infected.

Families can be assisted by having a familiar provider available at the counseling and test-result visits. A realistic follow-up plan with a gradual implementation of the many other steps necessitated by a child's positive

HIV antibody test can provide a family with a concrete sense of not being abandoned.

On notification of a child's HIV seropositivity, many women will sacrifice their own care but be extremely attentive to the needs of the child. They may feel guilty or undeserving of care, and the pediatric provider may need to give reassurance and permission for them to care for themselves. The baby's father may or may not be infected, and women often need support to consider partner notification. Brothers and sisters of the HIV-exposed child present an additional challenge. It can be devastating for a parent or caregiver to consider that the other children may also have HIV infection, and efforts to have the children tested may be resisted.

A nonjudgmental approach, assessing the family's strengths and needs, may help clarify the best way for families to deal with each step of this process. In addition, it is essential that the care provider examine his or her own feelings about HIV infection, childbearing, and contact notification and be clear about the impact those beliefs may have on interactions with families.

## ❖ The HIV-Infected Child

### Signs and Symptoms of HIV Infection

The clinical spectrum of HIV disease is as varied as the children infected with it. The initial perception of HIV as an acute, rapidly fatal disease has changed to that of a chronic, multiorgan system disease, treatable though not curable, with prolonged periods of relative wellness.

Early in the epidemic, the Centers for Disease Control (CDC) issued a classification schema that was used to describe HIV infection along a continuum of increasing severity of symptoms. The classification P-0, or indeterminate, is used to describe infants born to women with HIV or whose HIV status is being evaluated. Class P-1, or asymptomatic infection, includes HIV-infected children with normal or abnormal immune function but minimal clinical symptomatology. Class P-2, or symptomatic infection, is then further subdivided into six subclasses, A to F, according to clinical findings. These subclasses include nonspecific findings (such as generalized lymphadenopathy, organomegaly, diarrhea, etc.), progressive neurological disease, lymphocytic interstitial pneumonitis, opportunistic infections, cancers, and other symptoms possibly related to HIV infection. Class P-2 includes those criteria that the CDC classifies as meeting the case definitions for AIDS (CDC, 1987). However, this disease classification system does not necessarily correlate with either prognosis or degree of illness. As described in the previous chapter, the CDC is presently considering revisions of this schema to more adequately identify and stage the course of HIV infection.

Since the beginning of the epidemic, clinicians have attempted to correlate different presentations of disease symptomatology with prognosis and survival. From the work of Scott and colleagues (1989) and Blanche and colleagues (1990), two distinct patterns of disease presentation have been observed. Approximately one third of children may exhibit rapid deterioration in neurological status, failure to thrive, and severe immune compromise, with a life expectancy of less than 4 years. The remaining children may be asymptomatic for long periods of time, perhaps not even needing HIV-related care until symptoms develop at 8 or 9 years of age. This latter cohort of children experiences the same childhood illnesses, has the same trips to the emergency room for broken bones and stitches, and is in the same public and private school systems as their uninfected peers.

With the notable exception of lymphocytic interstitial pneumonitis (LIP), the earlier in life that children develop AIDS-defining symptoms, the less hopeful the prognosis. Because many women with HIV infection may not consider themselves to be at risk for HIV infection, the primary care practitioner must be alert for the HIV-infected child born to a woman unaware of her HIV status.

The primary care provider must be alert to symptoms of HIV as well as any symptoms of opportunistic infections. Findings such as oral thrush, failure to thrive, fever, diarrhea, dermatitis, and generalized lymphadenopathy are not diagnostic but serve to increase the practitioner's suspicion of HIV infection. Recurrent bacterial infections, either resistant to usual therapies or presenting with abnormal symptoms, may further increase suspicion of HIV infection (Table 7–1).

TABLE 7–1   Indicators of Pediatric HIV Infection

| Medical History | Physical Examination | Laboratory Results |
| --- | --- | --- |
| Recurrent fever | Failure to maintain percentiles or to gain weight | Anemia |
| Serious bacterial infections | Failure to grow in length or head circumference | Thrombocytopenia |
| Recurrent otitis media | Loss of developmental milestones | Leukopenia |
| Recurrent sinusitis | | Liver function elevations |
| Recurrent or chronic oral thrush | Diaper dermatitis or condyloma | Hypergamma-globulinemia |
| Recurrent or chronic diarrhea | Candida or seborrhea | P24 antigen |
| Failure to thrive | Otitis media, rhinitis, parotitis | Reactive HIV culture |
| Poor feeding | Generalized lymphadenopathy (>0.5 cm), cervical, axillary, or inguinal | Reactive HIV polymerase chain reaction |
| Developmental delay | Hepatomegaly | Low CD4 count for age |
| | Splenomegaly | |
| | Clubbing | |

*Source:* Reprinted with permission from Boland, M., & Conviser, R. (in press). Nursing care of the child. In J. H. Flaskerud & P. J. Ungvarski (Eds.), HIV/AIDS: A guide to nursing care (3rd ed.). Philadelphia: W.B. Saunders.

## Pneumocystis Carinii Pneumonia

The most common serious opportunistic infection in HIV-infected children is Pneumocystis carinii pneumonia (PCP), which occurs in nearly 31% of pediatric AIDS cases reported to the CDC (CDC, 1992). PCP can occur at any time during the course of illness but is seen most frequently in infants between the ages of 3 and 6 months. Often, it is the presenting clinical manifestation of HIV infection. A recent review of documented cases of PCP determined that approximately 61% of these infants had not been evaluated for HIV infection (Simonds, Oxtoby, Caldwell, Gwinn, & Rogus, 1993). This alarming statistic emphasizes the need for voluntary HIV testing with informed consent as a standard of prenatal care so that a pregnant woman and her baby can receive optimal care.

Unlike adults with HIV infection, PCP in children is a primary infection, not a reactivation of disease. Despite the availability of effective treatment, PCP is associated with high morbidity and mortality. The median life expectancy for children who survive an episode of PCP is approximately 1 to 4 months (CDC, 1991).

However, PCP is preventable. Effective prophylaxis against PCP is available and recommended for HIV-infected infants and children, based on age-related CD4+ lymphocyte counts and percentages. Figure 7–4 shows the guidelines for the initiation of prophylaxis established by the CDC (CDC, 1991). A CD4+ cell count should be obtained at 1 month of age for all children born to women with HIV infection, followed by repeat counts every 3 to 4 months until the age of 2 years old. Due to the potentially life-threatening nature of PCP, any time a child's CD4+ count falls below the age-adjusted threshold, PCP prophylaxis should be initiated, including infants whose HIV status has not been determined. Children definitively diagnosed with HIV should continue to have CD4+ cell counts evaluated every 3 to 6 months. In addition, any child who develops PCP and recovers should receive PCP prophylaxis regardless of age or CD4+ cell count.

The specific PCP prophylaxis recommendations for children older than 1 month of age are as follows:

1. Trimethoprim/sulfamethoxazole (TMP-SMX; Bactrim, Septra) 75 mg/$kg^2$, bid, three times a week is the first choice. The side effects include anemia, neutropenia, and rash. Because antiretroviral agents and TMP-SMX can cause bone marrow suppression, a baseline and monthly complete blood count (CBC), with differential and platelet count, should be obtained.

2. Dapsone 1 mg/kg per day to a maximum dose of 100 mg is the second choice. The side effects include dermatitis and (rarely) methemoglobinemia. Assure that $G_6PD$ level is within normal limits before starting treatment.

3. Intravenous pentamidine 4 mg/kg every month is the third choice for children hypersensitive to or intolerant of other medications. The side effects include hypotension (rate-related) and hypoglycemia.

A CD4+ count and CD4+ % should be obtained for each child. Use test results and child's age as criteria for starting PCP prophylaxis.

| Age | CD4+ >20%, or unknown, with CD4+ count (cells per mm³) of: | | | | | | | | CD4+ <20% with any CD4+ count |
|---|---|---|---|---|---|---|---|---|---|
| | 200 | 300 | 500 | 600 | 750 | 1,000 | 1,500 | 2,000 | |
| 1–11 months | Start PCP prophylaxis | | | | | | | A    B | Start PCP prophylaxis |
| 12–23 months | Start PCP prophylaxis | | | | | A | B | | |
| 24 months 2–5 years | Start PCP prophylaxis | | | A | | B | C | | |
| ≥ 6 years | Start PCP prophy-laxis | A | B | | | C | | | |

A = No prophylaxis recommended at this time; recheck CD4+ count in 1 month.
B = No prophylaxis recommended at this time; recheck CD4+ count at least every 3 to 4 months.
C = No prophylaxis recommended at this time; recheck CD4+ count at least every 6 months.

*Note:* Any child who has had an episode of PCP should be started on PCP prophylaxis regardless of age or CD4+ count.

*Recommended regimen for PCP prophylaxis:*

Trimethoprim/sulfamethoxazole (TMP-SMX) 150 mg TMP/M²/day with 750 mg SMX/M²/day given orally in divided doses twice a day, three times a week, on consecutive days (e.g., Monday, Tuesday, Wednesday). When starting TMP-SMX prophylaxis

- Obtain baseline CBC, differential count, platelet count
- Monitor CBC, differential count, platelet count monthly
- Monitor CD4+ count at least every three months

FIGURE 7–4  Recommendations for Pneumocystis cainii pneumonia (PCP) prophylaxis.

Note that aerosolized pentamidine is not recommended for children under 5 years old, and data related to efficacy of intravenous or aerosolized pentamidine are lacking. PCP prophylaxis can be discontinued if the child is subsequently found not to be HIV infected or if CD4 cell counts rise to levels above the threshold on two subsequent evaluations at least 1 month apart, unless the child is receiving antiretroviral medications or other agents that may increase the CD4+ cell count (CDC, 1991).

## Immunizations

A modified immunization schedule is recommended for the HIV-exposed and HIV-infected infant, which includes substitution of enhanced potency inactivated polio vaccine (IPV) for trivalent oral vaccine (OPV). This recommendation is based on the rationale that live virus may be shed in secretions by the infant after vaccination and may pose a threat to immunocompromised household members as well as presenting a theoretical risk to the child (American Academy of Pediatrics, 1991).

Measles, mumps, and rubella (MMR) vaccine is also indicated. In epidemic areas, MMR may be given at 6 or 12 months to HIV-exposed as well as HIV-infected infants and should be repeated at 15 months of age. Over time, children with HIV infection may lose vaccine-associated antibodies. Pre- and post-MMR titers are useful in determining the child's ability to make functional antibody and should be monitored every 6 to 12 months for the lifetime of the child. Those children who receive MMR and do not maintain protective antibody titers (evaluated by measles titers 6 to 8 weeks after immunization) should receive a second booster vaccination. If antibody titers remain negative after a second boost, the child may be considered a candidate to receive intravenous immunoglobulin (Working Group on Retroviral Therapy, 1993).

Death from measles in HIV-infected children has been documented (Palumbo, Hoyt, Demasio, Oleske, & Connor, 1992), and prevention requires vigilance in monitoring the child's changing immune function. The practitioner needs to convey to the family that what may appear to be a harmless childhood illness can in fact become a dangerous disease for an HIV-infected child. The measles-exposed child with HIV infection whose immune status is unknown should receive passive immunization with intramuscular human immunoglobulin at a dose of 0.25 ml/kg (maximum dose of 15 ml) within 72 hours of exposure.

Children with HIV infection who have been exposed to varicella (chicken pox) should receive varicella zoster immune globulin (VZIG) as soon after exposure as possible, but no longer than 96 hours after exposure. Passive protection against varicella is not guaranteed to prevent infection, and the practitioner should be aware that the incubation period for children who have received VZIG may be prolonged. Varicella infection in the immunocompromised child should be treated aggressively with oral or intravenous acyclovir, as severe disseminated disease can occur, including pneumonia, encephalitis, and hepatitis.

Influenza vaccine is indicated yearly, beginning at 6 months of age (CDC, 1993). Household contacts of the immunocompromised child should also be immunized. Pneumococcal vaccine is recommended for all HIV-infected children, asymptomatic and symptomatic alike. Immunization guidelines are summarized in Figure 7–5.

When should therapy be changed? Often, family members have strong opinions regarding therapeutic interventions. Previous experience with medications, information from the lay press, anecdotal reports from community members, and religious and health beliefs will all have an impact on treatment adherence. The decision to initiate any therapy should involve frank discussions with the family and should specifically address the circumstances of the particular child.

In 1992, the National Pediatric HIV Resource Center facilitated the formation of a working group of expert clinicians to address these questions directly and to develop guidelines. The results of these deliberations were published in the *Pediatric Infectious Disease Journal* (1993). A summary of the recommendations is presented in Figure 7–6.

### When to Treat

Clearly, HIV disease presents with a broad spectrum of clinical manifestations and immune function abnormalities. The group looked at children from two major perspectives: clinical symptomatology and immune compromise. The decision to treat must first address the issue of when the benefits of treatment outweigh the risk. The consensus opinion of the group was that those children with serious clinical manifestations, serious immune compromise, or both should be started on antiretroviral medication. The symptoms that carry high morbidity and mortality and that indicate antiretroviral intervention are as follows:

1. Neurodevelopmental abnormalities/progressive encephalopathy
2. Development of opportunistic infections
3. Severe wasting disease or failure to thrive
4. Pneumocystis carinii pneumonia

Severe immune compromise is also a recommendation for beginning antiretroviral therapy. Using CD4+ lymphocyte cell counts as markers for immune function, the following guidelines were recommended:

1. Children under 1 year: <1,500 cells/mm$^3$ and/or <30% lymphs
2. Children 1 to 2 years: <1,000 cells/mm$^3$ and/or <25% lymphs
3. Children 2 to 6 years: <750 cells/mm$^3$ and/or <20% lymphs
4. Children over 6 years: <500 cells/mm$^3$ and/or <20% CD4+

It is important to recognize that these consensus recommendations are guidelines, and the practitioner, in consultation with the infectious disease specialist, may change or modify the decision to treat on a case-by-case basis.

### What to Use

Zidovudine (ZDV, Retrovir) 180 mg/M$^2$ per dose every 6 hours is the recommended initial antiretroviral treatment. Children must be closely monitored for zidovudine toxicity, intolerance (specifically bone marrow

| Age | Immunizations/Antigens |
|---|---|
| Birth | HBV[a] |
| 1 month | HBV[a] |
| 2 months | DTP, IPV, HbCV |
| 4 months | DTP, IPV, HbCV |
| 6 months[b] | DTP, HbCV, HBV [a] |
| 12 months[c] | TB test (if HIV infected, anergy screen) |
| 15 months[d] | MMR HbCV |
| 18 months | DTP or DTaP, IPV[e] |
| 24 months | Pneumococcal vaccine[f] |
| 4–6 years | DTP or DTaP, IPV, MMR |
| 14–16 years | dT, measles |

[a] Alternate schedule for HBV immunization: 1–2 months, 4 months., 6–18 months.
[b] Seasonal influenza is indicated, starting at 6 months of age
[c] Every 6–12 months.
[d] May give earlier in areas of high prevalence/epidemic. Check with local health department
[e] May use OPV if child has seroreverted and there are no immunodeficient household members.
[f] For HIV-infected children only.

    dT = adult diphtheria and tetanus
    DTaP = diphtheria, tetanus, acellular pertussis
    DTP = diphtheria, tetanus, pertussis
    HbCV = hemophilus influenza b conjugate vaccine
    HBV = hepatitis B vaccine
    IPV = inactivated polio vaccine
    MMR = measles, mumps, rubella

*Note:* HIV-infected infants and children may lose vaccine-associated antibody titers over time.Therefore:

1. Serologic testing for protective measles titers is indicated at least yearly.
2. Immediate prophylaxis is recommended after exposure to
   * Measles:           human serum imune globulin
   * Varicella:          varicella zoster immune globulin (VZIG)
   * Pertussis:          erythromycin
   * Diphtheria:        diphtheria toxoid and penicillin
   * H. influenza type b:   rifampin

FIGURE 7–5    Immunization guidelines for HIV-exposed/infected children.

*Source:* Adapted with permission from Herman Mendez, "Primary Care Guidelines for H[ ]Exposed Children."

## Antiretroviral Therapy: More Questions Than Answers

The decision to begin antiretroviral therapy is a complex o[ ] The practitioner must consider a number of major and possibly conflicti[ ] concerns. It is clear that HIV is a progressive disease, and some interventi[ ] to slow viral growth is indicated. But when should therapy be starte[ ]

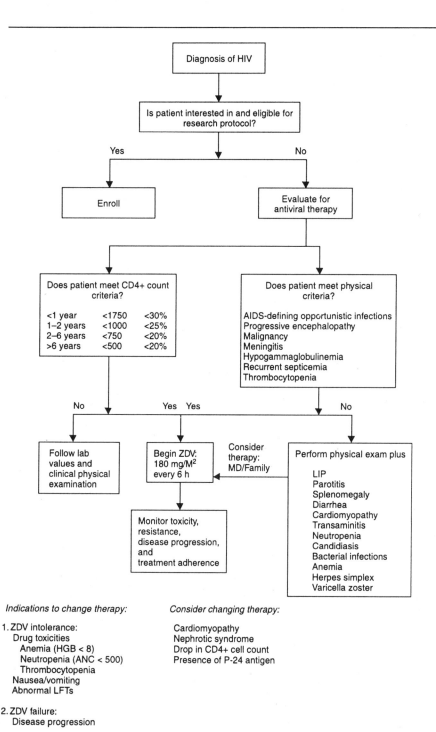

FIGURE 7–6   Algorithm for instituting antiretroviral therapy.

suppression), and evidence of disease progression. In the event of intolerance, toxicity, or disease progression, the practitioner should consult the infectious disease specialist regarding changes in therapy. Figure 7–7 presents guidelines for managing the HIV-infected child receiving zidovudine.

## Growth and Development

Supporting optimum growth and development of a child on his or her journey to adulthood is the foundation for providing primary care to children. Anticipatory guidance is akin to a signpost alerting parents to potential pitfalls and trouble spots. The child with HIV infection needs that same support and guidance, but like children with other chronic illnesses, the road may be steeper and shorter.

The HIV-infected child who appears to the practitioner as clinically stable cannot be assumed to be weathering the storm unscathed. Likely, the child, though growing, is smaller than classmates and may frequently miss school for medical care visits or hospitalizations. In addition to the expected disruptions of family life due to chronic illness, the HIV-infected child may also be struggling with multiple family losses, the burden of secrecy, social isolation, and the stigma of the disease.

The challenge to the primary care provider is to maximize the child's growth and development, provide support to the family during difficult times, and facilitate decision making when there seems to be no "right" answer.

## Nutrition

Nutrition is an ever-present concern for the child with HIV infection. Weight loss and the development of malnutrition may be one of the first clinical signs of HIV infection in adults (Kotler, Wang, & Pierson, 1985). Similarly, failure to gain weight may be the first sign of HIV in a child or may herald a change in the child's disease, and it indicates a need for immediate attention. The child's height, weight, and head circumference should be measured and recorded on standardized charts at every visit. The height and weight should also be plotted against each other. Any failure to gain weight, noted during a regularly scheduled visit, is cause for concern and should be closely monitored. Continued failure to gain weight or sustained weight loss may indicate a need for collaboration with the subspecialist.

Failure to thrive in the infected child may be caused by any one of a number of conditions, or a combination of them all, and can occur at any time during the child's life. These include decreased intake (anorexia, abdominal pain or distention, dysphagia), malabsorption (enteric infection, HIV-enteropathy), increased losses (diarrhea, GI blood loss, enteric protein loss), and increased requirements (fever, infection) (McLoughlin, 1992). The

| Week No. | 0 | 2 | 4 | 6 | 8 | 12 | 16 | 20 | 24 | 28 | 32 | 36 | 40 | 44 | 48 | 52 |
|---|---|---|---|---|---|---|---|---|---|---|---|---|---|---|---|---|
| **INITIAL & ONGOING CLINICAL EVALUATION** | | | | | | | | | | | | | | | | |
| Physical Exam every 1 month | * | | * | | * | * | * | * | * | * | * | * | * | * | * | * |
| NEURO Exam every 6 months | * | | | | | | | | * | | | | | | | * |
| Lumbar Puncture (HIV culture P24, chemistry, cell count, cryptococcal antigen) every 1 year[a] | * | | | | | | | | | | | | | | | * |
| Head CT (without contrast) every 6 months | * | | | | | | | | | * | | | | | | * |
| EKG every 1 year | * | | | | | | | | | | | | | | | * |
| ECHO Cardiogram every 1 year | * | | | | | | | | | | | | | | | * |
| Chest X-Ray every 6 months (if LIP, every 3 months) | * | | | | | | | | * | | | | | | | * |
| Neurodevelopment testing every 6 months | * | | | | | | | | * | | | | | | | * |
| **INITIAL & ONGOING LAB EVALUATION** | | | | | | | | | | | | | | | | |
| Hematology every 2 weeks for 2 months, then every 4 weeks | * | * | * | * | * | * | * | * | * | * | * | * | * | * | * | * |
| Chemistry every 2 weeks for 2 months, then every 3 months | * | * | * | * | * | | | * | | | * | | | | | * |
| T and B cells every 3 months | * | | | | | * | | | * | | | * | | | | * |
| Quantitative immunoglobins every 6 months | * | | | | | | | | * | | | | | | | * |
| HIV culture every 6 months | * | | | | | | | | * | | | | | | | * |
| P24 antigen every 6 months | * | | | | | | | | * | | | | | | | * |

FIGURE 7–7    Management of ZDV.

[a]Consider VDRL, AFB culture/smear, viral/fungal culture, India ink, or other clinically indicated studies.

following is a brief discussion of some of the possible factors and intervention strategies related to failure to gain weight.

Inadequate calories consumed may be due to poverty; there may be no consistent or adequate food supply in the home or no cooking facilities available in homeless shelters or motels. Sometimes, families are uncomfortable sharing with practitioners that they are in difficult situations, and an accepting, nonjudgmental attitude is necessary to build a trusting relationship. Asking families directly if there are times during the month when they are unable to provide adequate meals, whether food stamps are adequate, and what food bank they use may help to elicit this vital information.

Pain secondary to candida, herpetic lesions, gingivitis, stomatitis, dental caries, or esophagitis may interfere with sucking, chewing, or swallowing. This may be compounded by poor dental hygiene and limited concern over children's baby teeth. Frank explanations regarding caries as potential sites for infection can motivate parents or guardians to obtain the necessary dental care. Ideally, clinicians with expertise in oral and dental manifestations of HIV disease should be a part of the child's multidisciplinary health care team.

Abdominal pain, secondary to opportunistic infections like mycobacterium avium intracellularae or organomegaly, may also contribute to anorexia or "feeling full." Around-the-clock pain medication given as a trial for 1 to 2 weeks may have the effect of allowing the child to "feel better" with a subsequent increase in appetite.

Neurological disease, associated with HIV infection of the central nervous system, may cause dysphagia or uncoordinated suck and swallow. Evaluation by a feeding team or speech pathologist may lead to helpful suggestions and interventions (Pressman, 1992).

Diarrhea is often a major problem. Frequent loose stools not only impact on growth, but also can be an important quality-of-life concern. In many anecdotal reports, caregivers and children alike identify diarrhea as frustrating, annoying, and uncomfortable. One 12-year-old with symptomatic HIV infection was asked how she was doing, coping with her disease. She stated very clearly, "I can stand the blood tests, and I'm pretty good with my medicine, but can't you do anything so I don't have to go to the bathroom every minute? It's embarrassing!" The diarrhea may be related to HIV itself or may be secondary to opportunistic infection, medication, high-calorie food supplements, or possibly stress. For children receiving multiple oral medications, chronic intractable diarrhea may limit their usefulness. The challenge to the child, family, and care team is a formidable one and likely will require consultation and collaboration with subspecialists.

Interventions for the child with failure to thrive can be difficult to implement. The goal is to maintain enteral feeding whenever possible and should begin with a thorough assessment of the child's intake, using a 3-day diet recall and stool history, preferably written, or at least a day-to-day recall. Defining the terms the family uses for bowel movements and what they consider to be diarrhea is essential. Asking the school-age child direct, simple questions such as, "Do you ever have to run to the bathroom or feel that you will have a bowel movement [or whatever term the child uses] before you make it to the toilet?" may elicit a smile, but it also gives the child permission to talk about it. Follow-up questions about frequency, color, and quantity may be preceded with a statement that although embarrassing to talk about, diarrhea happens to a lot of kids, and knowing about it is important for the child's health.

Outpatient stool collection for ova and parasites, routine culture and sensitivity for enteric pathogens, Camphylobacter, C-difficile, and stools for acid fast bacilli (AFB) to identify atypical tuberculosis, such as Mycobacterium avian intracellularae (MAI), should be obtained on three separate occasions. An outpatient assessment for malabsorption can be achieved by giving a 0.5 g/kg oral dose of D-xylose and obtaining a serum D-xylose level 1 hour after ingestion; the child must have nothing by mouth after midnight.

The use of oral supplements can be successful if absorption is not impaired and there is no underlying treatable disease. Although literature addressing safety and efficacy is lacking, appetite stimulants, such as megasterol, have been used with spotty success in children.

Calorie counts, stool patterns and collections, and nutrition evaluations are noninvasive and may seem easy to obtain. The reality for many children living in families with ill caretakers and suboptimal living conditions is that medical concerns, if not an emergency, often take a backseat to daily survival. The successful implementation of any therapeutic plan requires total involvement with all family members involved. Asking the family directly, "How do you think we can do this?" is the first step. Assuming that prescriptions will be filled, refrigerators stocked, or supplements obtained is likely to result in mutual disappointment between family and practitioner.

## Neurological Abnormalities

Similar to HIV infection itself, the clinical spectrum of neurological abnormalities associated with HIV infection in children is a varied one. Symptoms can range from mild to severe, and it may be difficult to sort out prenatal and environmental factors from the direct effects of HIV. Early in the epidemic, neurological manifestations were frequently observed (Epstein et al., 1986; Mintz, Epstein, & Koenigsberger, 1989; Oleske, Minnefor, & Cooper, 1983) and in up to half of the children with perinatally acquired HIV infection, they may be the first sign of HIV disease. Studies have identified neurological manifestations in up to 50% of HIV-infected children under 1 year of age and possibly up to 90% of all children with HIV.

These central nervous system (CNS) abnormalities may be conceptualized as (1) primary neurological abnormalities resulting from HIV infection of the brain (HIV encephalopathy) or (2) secondary neurologic complications resulting from immunodeficiency causing opportunistic infections of the CNS (i.e., cytomegalovirus, cryptococcus, toxoplasmosis), CNS lesions (such as neoplasm or vascular lesions), or other organ involvement resulting in hypoxia or stroke (HIV-associated thrombocytopenia).

**Primary Neurological Abnormalities**    Mintz (1992) classifies HIV-infected infants and children into three clinical neurological categories: progressive encephalopathy, static encephalopathy, or neurologically normal. The clinical findings associated with progressive encephalopathy in children with HIV infection include (1) impaired brain growth, either acquired microcephaly (assessed by serial head circumferences) or brain atrophy on CT scans; (2) progressive motor dysfunction; or (3) loss of developmental milestones.

The child may evidence changes in muscle tone, spasticity, changes in gait, or inability to walk (Browers, Belman, & Epstein, 1993). Equally as devastating to families as the decline in motor and cognitive function are the accompanying behavioral changes. The child may become apathetic and withdrawn, losing interest in school, friends, and surroundings (Belman et al., 1988). Although children with progressive encephalopathy may have periods of prolonged plateaus or occasional signs of improvement, the prognosis is poor, with continual deterioration.

**Static Encephalopathy**    Children with HIV who evidence a static encephalopathy have fixed nonprogressive cognitive and motor deficits. They may have evidence of attention deficits and hyperactivity. These children may continue to acquire additional developmental skills, but often at a slower rate than noninfected children. Because of this, it is important to note that over time, a static encephalopathy may appear as a progressive one, as the gap in expected development widens (Browers et al., 1993).

**Secondary Neurological Complications**    Children with HIV are also susceptible to CNS infections due to immunodeficiency. Although opportunistic infections (such as toxoplasmosis or cytomegalovirus) are not as common in HIV-infected children as in adults with HIV, as life expectancy continues to improve, more opportunities for acquiring these infections are likely to occur. Primary CNS lymphoma, rarely seen in children, is the most common neurological lesion associated with HIV infection in adults. Neurological deterioration may be rapidly progressive, with seizures, changes in behavior, or other focal deficits (Browers, Belman, & Epstein, 1993). Strokes or other cerebral infarcts are rare, but they do occur. This may be related to intracerebral hemorrhaging (secondary to HIV-associated thrombocytopenia) or to disease of the blood vessels.

Confounding the initial neurological evaluation of children exposed to HIV in utero may be prenatal exposure to drugs, inadequate prenatal care, poor nutrition, or maternal illness. In addition, the practitioner needs to be aware that children with HIV may live in home situations where the caregivers are unable to provide a stable and nurturing home. This may be due to substance abuse, illness or disease progression in the parents or other family members, lack of social supports, stigma and isolation, the burden of secrecy, court-ordered changes in living situations, or homelessness.

At the Children's Hospital AIDS Program in Newark, New Jersey, a number of children with stable HIV disease who undergo sudden changes in living situation, such as placement in foster homes where the primary language may be unknown to the child, prolonged hospitalization, or death of a parent, have been observed to demonstrate dramatic drops in CD4+ lymphocyte cell counts or exhibit regressive or aggressive behavior, withdrawal, or apathy. Outwardly, the home situation may appear improved, but the impact on the child may initially be one of overwhelming loss. Like pain in children, it is conceivable that the failure of the child to protest or cry out does not indicate the absence of physical or psychological trauma. Depression in children may not be something the primary care provider is comfortable assessing, but it must be included in the differential diagnosis when assessing neurological changes.

In light of what may be a complex medical/psychosocial problem, the primary care provider has an essential role in assessing the impact of HIV on the child's growth and development. Directly questioning the parent or guardian about life changes or different or unusual behavior may give him or her permission to talk about things that may not have been considered important. The practitioner is encouraged to look for subtle changes and to act quickly if any are noted. Serial-based head circumferences, plotted on standard graphs, are absolutely essential. Red flags, such as acquired microcephaly, loss of milestones, or change in behavior, indicate the need for prompt referral to a subspecialist.

As important as recognizing that HIV infection is rapidly becoming the largest infectious etiology of mental retardation and developmental disability in children (Harvey & Decker, 1992) is the role the primary care provider may assume in helping families access the services they need to maximize the child's potential. Early intervention programs, preschool handicapped programs, and Head Start programs as well as regular day care, preschool, or public school may all be required to meet the varied needs of children with HIV.

In Table 7–2 and Figure 7–8, guidelines summarize comprehensive primary care for children with HIV infection. This information is organized within a framework of regular child care visits.

## ❖ HIV and Schools: Help or Hindrance

Many of the issues regarding access to care that challenge families affected by HIV may not appear to be at all related to primary health care. However, secrecy, disclosure of diagnosis, confidentiality, and freedom from discrimination are at least as important as monitoring immune function and modifying immunization.

TABLE 7-2   Primary Care Guidelines for HIV Exposed/Infected Infants

| Age | Immun/Screening | Additional Lab Testing | Anticipatory Guidance / Comments |
|---|---|---|---|
| 0–Nursery | Hepititis B 1 | HIV culture, PCR, or p24 | History (Hx) and physical examination (PE) to include growth parameters, HIV-associated symptoms, recurrent infections, and nutrition<br>Review home care instructions: signs and symptoms to seek medical attention<br>Reassure family members regarding transmission, and review universal precautions<br>Discuss reporting laws, disclosure, contact notification<br>Refer mother for appropriate medical follow-up<br>Identify other household members at risk, offer testing<br>HIV culture, PCR, or p24 positive: repeat to confirm. |
| 1 month | Hepititis B 2 | RPR/VDRL (if not available from mother)<br>CD4+ | Hx, PE to include growth parameters, HIV-associated symptoms, recurrent infections, and nutrition<br>Consider referral to special child health services for case management, early intervention programs, WIC, or other entitlements<br>PCP prophylaxis, depending on results of CD4 count: CD4 <1,500, begin prophylaxis<br>Explore family perceptions of lab results |
| 2 months | IPV 1<br>DPT 1<br>HbCV 1<br>Praxis—2, 4, 6, 15 months<br>Merck—2, 4, 12 months | | Hx, PE to include growth parameters, HIV-associated symptoms, recurrent infections, and nutrition<br>The child with confirmed HIV infection and symptoms early in life will likely have rapid progression of disease, and close monitoring is indicated<br>Caution family that negative test results do not rule out HIV infection |
| 4 months | IPV 2<br>DPT 2<br>HbCV 2 | HIV culture, PCR, or p24<br>Quantitative immunoglobulins (QIGS)<br>CD4+ | HIV culture positive (child is infected): Evaluate and stage disease; consider referral to infectious disease (ID) specialist; review treatment options, including access to clinical trials<br>HIV culture negative (does not rule out disease): Continue monitoring immune functions, growth parameters, and HIV-associated symptoms<br>Elevated QIGs increase suspicion of HIV<br>Decreased QIGs may need further evaluation to identify other underlying immune deficiencies, accurately interpret serological testing, monitor serious HIV-associated immune compromise, and consider for IVIG replacement therapy |

| Age | Immunizations/Tests | Culture– E & WB CD4+ | Culture+ CD4+ | Assessment/Plan |
|---|---|---|---|---|
| 6 months | DPT 3<br>HbCV 3 (Praxis)<br>HepititisB 3<br>Flu vaccine (seasonal) | Culture– E & WB CD4+ | Culture+ CD4+ | Hx, PE to include growth parameters, HIV-associated symptoms, recurrent infections, and nutrition<br>Red flags: the child who fails to gain weight, fails to attain or loses milestones, or has recurrent infections<br>May need referral to the appropriate subspecialty<br>Review family's understanding of test results: Infant with negative HIV culture, normal QIGs, normal CD4+, and negative Hx and PE likely (90%) is not infected, but follow-up is essential<br>Assess need for crisis counseling, other agency supports<br>Discuss procedure for emergencies or serious illnesses |
| 9 months | Lead | E&WB CD4+ | CD4+ | Hx, PE to include growth parameters, HIV-associated symptoms, recurrent infections, and nutrition<br>Review prophylaxis for exposure to communicable disease<br>Recognize family response to diagnosis may be varied: Anxiety may manifest as frequent calls and visits; anger or denial may manifest as poor adherence to treatment and follow-up plans |
| 12 months | CBC, diff<br>HbCV 3 (Merck)<br>TB | E&WB CD4+ | CD4+ | PCP prophylaxis; if CD4+ <750 for children 12-24 months<br>If child is HIV infected, PPD >5 mm induration indicates infection with MTb; evaluate for prophylaxis/ treatment in consultation with ID subspecialist; if PPD negative and child is not anergic, repeat yearly |
| 15 months | MMR[a]<br>HbCV 4 (Praxis) | E&WB CD4+ | CD4+ | Hx, PE to include growth parameters, HIV-associated symptoms, recurrent infections, and nutrition<br>Review with family relationship of antibody and virus: Serial HIV antibody negative >15 months—probably uninfected; repeat at 18 and 24 months. Serial HIV antibody positive > 15 months—infected; evaluate and stage disease |
| 18 months | IPV 3<br>DPT 4 | E&WB | CD4+ | Hx, PE to include growth parameters, HIV-associated symptoms, recurrent infections, and nutrition<br>Post MMR titers are useful for evaluating functional antibody<br>Obtain every 6-12 months if child is HIV infected. Reimmunize if titers are not protective |
| 24 months | Pneumococcal vaccine (if HIV+) | E&WB | CD4+ | Serial HIV antibody negative at 24 months: Reassure family that child is not and never was infected with the virus that causes AIDS (HIV)<br>Anticipate requests for retesting at signs of illness; reassure that no further testing is necessary<br>PCP prophylaxis if CD4 <500 for children 2-6 years old with HIV infection |

[a] In areas where there is epidemic measles, an MMR may be given at either 6 or 12 months of age. If the MMR is given at less than 12 months, a repeat at 15 months is necessary.

Note: Children with HIV who are exposed to measles should receive serum immune globulin within 4 days of exposure, regardless of antibody titers.

Children with difficulty fighting infections may get the same illnesses as other children. However, these illnesses may make the child sicker or may take longer to cure.

---

Call your doctor or nurse for any of these problems:

• If anyone in the house has chickenpox or measles
  Change in activity: is more tired, lays around, does not play, sleeps more, is irritable and cranky
• Fever: has temperature higher than 101 F. Keep a thermometer at home and learn to use it. Keep acetominophen (Tylenol or Tempra) to give if instructed by the doctor
• Breathing difficulty: breathing that is faster or more difficult, a new or worsening cough
• Pain and discomfort: irritability, pulling on ears, not using an arm or a leg, walking funny
• Change in appetite or feeding: not eating as much or not eating favorite foods
• Vomiting or diarrhea: throwing up or having bowel movements more than three times a day
• Skin problems: new sores, rashes, lumps, bumps, redness or swelling
• Loss of weight: looking thinner or not gaining weight
• Frequent nose bleeds or bruises
• Pale color
• Slow development: not walking or talking as quickly as brothers or sisters, not listening, poor grades at school, difficulty learning
• Loss of skills: not able to do things such as walking or talking, that the child used to do

---

FIGURE 7–8   What should I watch for?

Since the beginning of the HIV epidemic, feelings have clearly outpaced facts in society's response to the disease. Although children have escaped some of the scorn and blame that members of the gay and drug-using populations have endured, integrating HIV-infected children into schools has been, at best, controversial and, at worst, violent (Ray brothers enter new school, 1987; Ryan White, 1986).

A framework for helping families and day-care, preschool, and school providers make sense of what appear to be conflicting concerns addresses the issue of school attendance with two distinct questions:

1. Can the child with HIV attend day care, preschool, or school? This is a discussion of facts and includes law and school policy.
2. Should the child attend day care, preschool, school? This decision is based on the health care and educational needs of the individual child.

In an extensive review of the federal statutes affording children with HIV disease protection from discrimination, Feldsman, Tucker, Leifer, Fidell, and Bank (1992) came to the conclusion that, "Children with HIV disease are entitled to a public school education." Figure 7–9 includes a review of relevant legislation. The opening statement of "Education of Children with Human Immunodeficiency Virus Infection," a publication of the American Academy of Pediatrics Task Force on Pediatric AIDS (1991), states: "Children with human immunodeficiency virus infection can participate in all activities in school to the extent that their health permits."

Despite these assurances, the reality exists that school policy is far more likely to reflect the prevailing sentiment of the community than to reflect the law (Katsiyannis, 1992). Policy and practice have often overlooked the medical facts and the legal constraints and have excluded students and teachers with HIV infection from the school setting. Despite the evidence that transmission of HIV in casual settings does not occur, people remain fearful. The practitioner may play a pivotal community role in addressing some of those fears. Experience has shown that fear must be addressed calmly and rationally, or board meetings, community forums, and parent-teacher meetings will easily degenerate into name calling and hysteria. Often, it is the children who are most eloquent at addressing these fears. For example, Joey DePaolo and Ryan White, two children with HIV infection, went public with their disease to help educate a nation.

## ❖ Disclosure

Any discussion of school placement is likely to raise the issue of disclosure. Confidentiality requirements are regulated by individual state statutes and may differ from state to state. Practitioners must familiarize themselves with their state's legal obligations for health care providers regarding the maintenance of confidentiality. For example, in New Jersey, confidentiality law requires the written permission of the individual's legal guardian to disclose HIV status, and breaches of confidentiality are subject to fine. Several states, including Illinois and South Carolina, require health care providers to notify the school of the child's HIV status.

In matters of secrecy and disclosure, family situations change frequently. The health care provider must continually assess how the family is addressing disclosure and should broach the subject. Specific questions to ask include these: Is there anyone in your family or community with whom you have shared the diagnosis of HIV infection? Who are you able to talk to when you're worried? Is your child asking you any questions about his illness? How do you explain to your child why she comes for care? Are you wondering whether she knows? Do you need some help to talk about it?

At the Children's Hospital AIDS Program (CHAP) in Newark, New Jersey, families and care providers together determine whether notifying the school principal and the school nurse is helpful or hurtful. Benefits of disclosure (receiving medications at school, being apprised of communicable disease exposure, appropriate evaluation and referral should the child become ill at school) are weighed against the consequences (stigma, social isolation, discrimination, "letting the secret out"). This is done by school

No specific federal law expressly prohibits discrimination against HIV-infected people. However, through application of existing laws prohibiting discrimination against people with disabilities, the courts have determined that individuals with both symptomatic and asymptomatic HIV infection are included. The following is a brief chronologic review of some of the major legislation prohibiting discrimination on the basis of disability.

### Section 504 of the Rehabilitation Act of 1973 (Public Law 93-112)

This legislation prohibits discrimination of anyone with disabilities by federal government agencies and programs or agencies that receive federal funds. People with disabilities, or "handicapped" individuals, are defined as having impairments that limit a major life activity. Symptomatic HIV infection was always considered to be an impairment under Section 504, and recent amendments passed in 1987 clearly indicated asymptomatic HIV infection to be covered as well.

Activities covered under Section 504 include Medicaid, Head Start, Title I, Elementary and Secondary Education Act, and transportation grants. Section 504 discusses exclusion from a program as acceptable if there is a significant risk to others that cannot be eliminated by "reasonable accommodation." Although not specifically addressed, it is assumed that the implementation of universal precautions does reduce or eliminate the risk of transmission of HIV disease.

### Individuals with Disabilities Education Act, 1975 (Public Law 94-142)

This law ensures that "a free and appropriate public education in the least restrictive environment" be made available to all children with disabilities. The cornerstone of this legislation is the Individualized Education Plan. The plan is the result of a multidisciplinary assessment of the child's strengths and areas of disability (usually through a child study team evaluation). It includes the parent/guardian's participation in the decision-making process. The law also guarantees the right of parents to challenge a school's decisions in a hearing or in a court of law. Public Law 94-142 defines handicapping conditions; a disability must impair a child's ability to learn. The law does not necessarily apply to asymptomatic HIV-infected children, but it does have tremendous value for children as the disease progresses.

### Early Intervention Program for Infants and Toddlers with Handicaps (Public Law 99-457)

The purpose of this legislation is to provide early intervention to infants and toddlers up to the age of 2 years who are determined to be developmentally delayed. Through comprehensive, statewide interagency systems, children with developmental disabilities are provided with case management, family training, counseling, home visits, nutritional services, and speech, occupational, and physical therapy. Each state is able to decide whether high-risk or potentially handicapping conditions are covered under this legislation.

### Americans with Disabilities Act, 1990 (Public Law 101-336)

Building on the definition of disability in Section 505, this legislation prohibits discrimination on the basis of disability in the use of a wide variety of services and facilities, including private organizations. These facilities may include schools, hospitals, day-care centers, and state and local government activities.

FIGURE 7–9  Freedom from discrimination.

*Source:* Adapted from Feldsman et al.

district. The child's teacher is not necessarily informed, though some families do choose to disclose as it may relieve the burden of secrecy.

Each individual child and family must choose what is best for them. Four children in the program, all 13 to 14 years old, have made completely different choices. One girl feels very strongly: "I don't want anybody else to know my business. I don't want people feeling sorry for me, or asking me questions." She carefully protects her privacy, and her family has chosen not to disclose her diagnosis to the school. Another girl feels similarly about her privacy, but the family felt it important to disclose to the school so they could be notified if there were any threats to her health. One boy's family had chosen not to tell him, the school, or anyone else the diagnosis. However, as the child turned 13 and was eligible for certain treatment protocols, the issue of informed consent and the rights of the child were considered. The family and professional staff met to determine this child's right to know his diagnosis and be actively involved in his own care. The decision was made to disclose the diagnosis to the child. Another boy has disclosed his diagnosis publicly and is involved in peer AIDS education throughout the nation.

One of the greatest challenges that the practitioner may face is that of disclosing the diagnosis to the child. In a beautiful book about HIV disease and disclosure, *How Can I Tell You?*, Mary Tasker (1992) proposes a continuum of phases of disclosure, with secrecy at one end and full disclosure at the other. Like Elisabeth Kübler-Ross's stages of death and dying (1969), there is no "right" phase; Tasker describes the experiences that families affected by HIV are having.

Tasker's first stage is secrecy. At the time of the child's initial diagnosis, the parents may vow never to share this information with anyone. The parents may enter a state of extreme isolation and bear the burden alone. The professional needs to respect that secret and must reassure the family that this information will not be disclosed to anyone. The practitioner may explore with the family the stress of keeping the secret and should emphasize that there is help if the parents ever feel overwhelmed. In time, the family may choose to reveal the secret to another trusted adult.

This may be evidence of movement toward what Tasker describes as the second, or exploratory, phase. During this time, the family may continue to keep the secret, but with less intensity. There may be some ambivalence about keeping the secret from the child, and the parents may be ready to offer some explanation to the child, but not use the terms *HIV* or *AIDS*. This phase may include collaboration by the parents and the practitioner on strategies to help the child cope with medical treatments and procedures. The parents may now be ready to join a support group where no explanations are necessary and others are having similar experiences.

Gradually, the family may approach the third, or readiness, phase. At this time, the parents may move closer to sharing the diagnosis with the child. They may ask the practitioner for suggestions about talking with the child or may actively ask for assistance in preparing to talk things out. They may ask how other families have dealt with this issue and what the outcomes were. At this time, the parents may practice disclosing to other adults.

At this point, families enter the disclosure phase. Each family may tell the child in a different way, some with assistance from a professional, others as a direct response to a child's questions, others when the moment feels right. It may be the first time they casually use the words *HIV* or *AIDS* or have a very specific, serious conversation with the child.

Although much has been written about the stigma, social isolation, and secrecy surrounding HIV and AIDS, it is possible that nothing can prepare the practitioner for some realities. For example, one 8-year-old boy who had been receiving care at CHAP for years had never been told his diagnosis. The family believed very strongly that he would suffer if others knew and that the child himself was too young not to tell other people. The professional staff supported the family's decision and kept the secret. However, on the night that Magic Johnson announced his HIV infection on television, this young boy turned to his parents and said, "Can you believe that? Magic has the same thing as me!"

## ❖ HIV as a Family Disease

Children with HIV infection may live with their natural parents, grandparents, extended family, in kinship care, foster care, transitional group homes, or a combination of the above. The social context of family problems often overwhelms attempts to individualize health care interventions. Transportation, housing, school placement, poverty, and legal status require sustained multidisciplinary problem solving.

Women with HIV infection frequently take care of their children to the best of their ability but neglect their own health. Compliance with the medical regimen is complicated by parental poor health, substance abuse or other conflicting family needs. Well siblings may be "lost" in the family or may be expected to assume the responsibilities of homemaker, nurse, or breadwinner. In families in which HIV is secret, this additional burden can exact a heavy toll on the uninfected children.

In such difficult social contexts, how can the practitioner help promote adherence to the HIV treatment plan? In my opinion, there is no one right answer. Each child and family need to be the primary decision makers and must work with the practitioner to find a mutually satisfying plan. Every treatment recommendation must be tailored to the family. The 2-year-old child living with her blind grandmother will require very different strategies to maximize treatment adherence than the 4-year-old living in a transitional care facility staffed by registered nurses, even if the children's care plans are nearly identical. The concerns of foster families who do not have legal guardianship or authority to consent for treatment or to partake in important decisions regarding the child's care may be very different from those of aunts or uncles who have assumed unreimbursed care of their sibling's children in addition to their own.

It is not helpful to prescribe antiretroviral therapy for a child whose grandmother believes the drug to be poison or to have hastened her own child's death. In addition, the practitioner is not likely to know that unless he or she asks—honestly, directly, and with genuine interest in the response. Similarly, it may not be helpful to prescribe cases of dietary supplements to a mother with severe wasting syndrome, fatigue, and no transportation unless the practitioner is able to devise a mechanism for getting the supplement into the home.

Recognizing the complexity of problems facing families, some programs use a system of case management as the foundation for coordinating services (chapter 12). If case management is not available, referral to entitlement programs for children with special health care needs may assist families to access the necessary services.

The practitioner must recognize his or her own biases and prejudices. Caring for children can be difficult when families choose a course of treatment, or no treatment, that conflicts with the practitioner's judgment. Where is the line between a parent's right to choose treatment options and being labeled medical neglect? I believe the only course is to be direct. State concerns clearly. Try to differentiate what is true from what you believe to be true. Listen to what families tell you. Be accepting without imposing a judgment. If there are concerns about a parent's ability to provide adequate care, say so and state what those concerns are. Focus on the identified problems and potential solutions without fixing blame. Be willing to admit mistakes, and do not give up!

Providing care to HIV-infected children is a formidable task. There may be frantic phone calls, baffling diagnoses, missed appointments, and less than ideal treatment options. It requires continual collaboration with subspecialty providers, involvement with multidisciplinary care teams, and knowledge of entitlement programs. As Dr. James Oleske, medical director of the Children's Hospital AIDS Program, has observed, "HIV in children is like Alice in Wonderland. What's down is up, what's big is small, and the hurrieder we go, the behinder we get."

## ❖ References

American Academy of Pediatrics Task Force on Pediatric AIDS. (1991). Education of children with human immunodeficiency virus infection. *Pediatrics, 88*, 645–647.

Belman, A. L., Diamond, G., Dickson, D., Horoupian D., Llena, J., Lantos, G., & Rubinstein, A. (1988). Pediatric acquired immunodeficiency syndrome: Neurologic syndromes. *American Journal of Diseases of Children, 142*, 29–35.

Blanche, S., Tardieu, M., Dulieye, A. M., Rouzloux, C., LeDist, F., Fukunaga, K., Caniglia, M., Jacomet, C., Messian, A., & Griscelli, C. (1990). Longitudinal study of 94 symptomatic infants with perinatally acquired HIV infection. *American Journal of Diseases of Children, 144,* 1210–1215.

Borkowsky, W., Krasinski, K., Pollack, H., Hoover, W., Kaul, A., & Ilmet-Moore T. (1992). Early diagnosis of human immunodeficiency virus infection in children <6 months: Comparison of polymerase chain reaction, culture, and plasma antigen capture techniques. *Journal of Infectious Disease, 166,* 616–619.

Browers, P., Belman, A., & Epstein, L. G. (1993). Central nervous system involvement: Manifestations and evaluation. In P. A. Pizzo & C. A. Wilfert (Eds.), *Pediatric AIDS: The challenge of HIV infection in infants, children and adolescents.* Baltimore: Williams and Wilkins.

Burgard, M., Mayaux, M. J., Blanche, S., Feroni, A., Guihard-Moscato, M. L., Allemon, M. C., Ciraru-Vigneron, N., Firtion, G., Floch, C., & Guillot, F. (1992). The use of viral culture and p24 antigen testing to diagnose human immunodeficiency virus infection in neonates. *New England Journal of Medicine, 327,* 1192–1197.

Centers for Disease Control and Prevention. (1987). Classification system for human immunodeficiency virus (HIV) infection in children under 13 years of age. *Morbidity and Mortality Weekly Report, 36,* 225–230.

Centers for Disease Control and Prevention. (1991). Guidelines for prophylaxis against Pneumocystis carinii pneumonia for children infected with human immunodeficiency virus. *Morbidity and Mortality Weekly Report, 40(RR-Z),* 1–13.

Centers for Disease Control and Prevention. (1993). Recommendations of the Advisory Committee on Immunization Practices (ACIP): Use of vaccines and immune globulins for persons with altered immunocompetence. *Morbidity and Mortality Weekly Report, 42(RR-4),* 1–18.

Delfraisy, J. F., Blanche, S., Rouzloux, C., & Mayaux, M. J. (1992). Perinatal HIV transmission fads and controversies. *Immunodeficiency Reviews, 3,* 305–327.

Epstein L. G., Sharer, L. R., Oleske, J. M., Connor, E. M., Goudsmit, J., Bagden, L., Robert-Guroff, M., & Koenigsberger, M. R. (1986). Neurologic manifestations of human immunodeficiency virus infection in children. *Pediatrics, 78,* 678–687.

Feldsman, Tucker, Leifer, Fidell, & Bank. (1992). *Legal issues in pediatric HIV practice: A handbook for health care providers.* Newark, NJ: National Pediatric HIV Resource Center.

Harvey, D. C., & Decker, C. L. (1992). Legal overview: Rights and benefits. In A. C. Crocker, H. J. Cohen, & T. A. Kastner (Eds.), *HIV infection and developmental disabilities: A resource for service providers.* Baltimore: P. H. Brookes.

Katsiyannis, A. (1992). Policy issues in school attendance of children with AIDS: A national survey. *Journal of Special Education, 26,* 219–226.

Kotler, D. P., Wang, J., & Pierson, R. N. (1985). Studies of body composition studies in patients with acquired immunodeficiency syndrome. *American Journal of Clinical Nutrition, 42 ,* 1255–1265.

Kübler-Ross, E. (1969). *On death and dying.* New York: Macmillan.

McLoughlin, L. (1992). Gastrointestinal manifestations of pediatric HIV infection. In R. Yogev & E. Connor (Eds.), *Management of HIV infection in infants and children.* St. Louis: Mosby Year Book.

Miles, S. A., Balden, Z., Magprtay, L., Wei L., Leiblein, A., Hofheinz, D., Toedter, G., Stiehm, E. R., & Bryson, Y. (1993). Rapid serologic testing with immune-complex-associated HIV p-24 antigen for early detection of HIV infection in neonates. *New England Journal of Medicine, 328,* 297–302.

Mintz, M. (1992). Neurologic abnormalities. In R. Yogev & E. Connor (Eds.), *Management of HIV infection in infants and children.* St. Louis: Mosby Year Book.

Mintz, M., Epstein, L. G., & Koenigsberger, M. R. (1989). Neurological manifestations of acquired immunodeficiency syndrome in children. *International Pediatrics, 78,* 678–687.

National Pediatric HIV Resource Center. (1993). Antiretroviral therapy and medical management of the human immunodeficiency virus–infected child. *Pediatric Infectious Disease Journal, 12,* 513–522.

Oleske, J., Minnefor, A., Cooper, R., Thomas, K., delaCruz, A., Ahdieh, H., Guerrero, I., Joshi, V. V., & Desposito, F. (1983). Immunodeficiency syndrome in children. *Journal of American Medical Association, 249,* 2345–2349.

Palumbo, P., Hoyt, L., Demasio, K., Oleske, J., & Connor, E. (1992). Population-based study of measles and measles immunization in human immunodeficiency virus–infected children. *Pediatric Infectious Disease Journal, 11,* 1008–1014.

Pressman, H. (1992). *Communication disorders and dysphagia in pediatric AIDS.* American Speech-Language-Hearing Association.

Public Law 93-112. (1973). Rehabilitation Act of 1973. Section 504.

Public Law 94-142. (1975). Individuals with Disabilities Education Act. (Formerly the Education of All Handicapped Children Act).

Public Law 99-457. (1990). Amendments to the Education for the Handicapped Act. Part H, Early Intervention Program for Infants and Toddlers with Handicaps.

Public Law 101-336. (1990). Americans with Disabilities Act .

Ray brothers enter new school. (1987, October). *American Medical News,* p. 9.

Ryan White. (1986, February 14). *New York Times.*

Ryan White. (1986, February 22). *New York Times.*

Scott, G. B., Hutto, C., Makuch, R. W., Mastrucci, M. T., O'Connor, T., Mitchell, C. D., Trapido, E. J., & Parks, W. P. (1989). Survival in children with perinatally acquired human immunodeficiency virus type 1 infection. *New England Journal of Medicine, 321,* 1791–1796.

Simonds, R. J., Oxtoby, M. J., Caldwell, M. B., Gwinn, M. L., & Rogers, M. F. (1993). Pneumocystis carinii pneumonia among U.S. children with perinatally acquired HIV infection. *Journal of the American Medical Association, 270,* 470–473.

Tasker, M. (1992). *How Can I Tell You?: Secrecy and disclosure with children when a family member has AIDS.* Bethesda, MD: Association for the Care of Children's Health.

Working Group on Antiretroviral Therapy, National Pediatric HIV Resource Center. (1993). Antiretroviral therapy and medical management of the human immunodeficiency virus–infected child. *Pediatric Infectious Disease Journal, 12,* 513–522.

# ❖ Chapter 8

# Adolescents and HIV

JUDY COHN

DONNA FUTTERMAN

As of the beginning of 1993, adolescents aged 13 through 21 years accounted for 1% of the U. S. AIDS cases, or 3,058 cases out of 310,000 reported adult cases (Centers for Disease Control and Prevention [CDC], 1993). However, AIDS prevalence alone greatly underestimates the impact of HIV infection among adolescents. Approximately 20% of adults with AIDS are between 20 and 29 years, and given the average course of 10 years from viral infection to development of AIDS, many, if not most, of these adults were infected as teenagers. Indeed, the World Health Organization estimates that half of the world's 12 to 14 million AIDS cases were acquired between the ages of 15 and 24 years (Goldsmith, 1993). According to a report from the United Nations Development Program, female gender and youth are emerging as important variables in the acquisition of HIV infection. In the developing nations, the male-to-female AIDS case ratio is 1:1, and women are being infected at a significantly younger age than men, on average 5 to 10 years younger. Proportionately more girls and women in their teens and early twenties are becoming infected than women in any other age group (United Nations Development Program, 1992).

In the United States, AIDS cases among adolescents have disproportionately affected ethnic and racial minorities. In the CDC–defined age group of 13 to 19 years, African-Americans accounted for 37% of AIDS cases, Hispanics 19% and non-Hispanic whites 43%, while representing 14%, 8%, and 76% of the U.S. population, respectively, in that age group. AIDS has also had a relatively greater impact on adolescent females than on adult females. Among those aged 13 to 19 years, 37% are female; among those aged 20 to 24 years, 21% are female, whereas female adults older than 24 account for only 11% of reported AIDS cases (CDC, 1993).

HIV infection among adolescents should come as no surprise given that half the nation's high school students have had sexual intercourse and less than half of them had used condoms at last intercourse (CDC, 1992). Sexually active teenagers have the highest rate of sexually transmitted diseases (STDs) of any age group (Bell & Hein, 1984). In studies of selected populations of U.S. teenagers, widely varying HIV seroprevalence rates have been reported. The most recent study from the U.S. Job Corps found an overall seroprevalence rate of 3/1,000. Notably, the rate among females increased from 2.1/1,000 in 1988 to 4.2/1,000 through 1992 (Conway et al., 1993). HIV seroprevalence rates among adolescents under 20 years old attending STD clinics in Baltimore increased from 1.8/1,000 (1979–1983) to 21/1,000 (1987–1989) (Quinn, 1992).

## ❖ Counseling and Testing

HIV counseling and testing for adolescents has two goals: to bring adolescents with HIV infection into care and to raise awareness of risk behavior and stimulate behavioral change for uninfected youth.

### Developmental Issues

To work successfully with adolescents, it is important to recognize that the transition from childhood to adulthood is a time of emotional and cognitive change. Adolescents care a lot about what people think, and even those who may seem abrasive and rebellious are very sensitive to the way a clinician addresses them. Therefore, it is important that clinicians working with young people have experience with, interest in, and a genuine appreciation and respect for their issues.

Because the thought processes of adolescents are developing from concrete to abstract, an important element of communication is to speak in plain and explicit terms. It may be necessary to move at a slower pace and to schedule more than one counseling session prior to testing. The clinician may ask concrete questions about specific situations or may engage in role play to gain a sense of how an adolescent makes decisions.

### Risk Assessment

An important component of HIV counseling and testing of adolescents is an individualized risk assessment (Futterman & Hein, 1992). Adolescence is often characterized by risk taking and experimentation, which can put youth at risk for HIV infection. This section discusses some of the key ways in which adolescents are at risk.

During adolescence, boys and girls may experiment with same-sex and opposite-sex behaviors that may put them at risk for HIV transmission in the process of discovering their sexual identity. Adolescent boys may have sex with other boys in several contexts. They may be experimenting with same-sex behaviors, or they may be in the process of "coming out" but may not yet identify themselves as gay or bisexual. Either way, they may not believe they are at risk for HIV. Family and community prejudice against homosexuality may cause a gay adolescent to deny his sexual preference, and he may not incorporate the safer sex messages of the adult gay community or the general public. When a clinician asks specifically about male and female partners, he or she not only acquires important information, but also begins to create a more open and supportive communication.

A behavior that places most adolescent girls at risk is unprotected heterosexual intercourse. Adolescent girls may feel they are not at risk for HIV if they have only one sexual relationship at a time. In an adolescent HIV clinic in New York City, where 85% of the girls acquired HIV infection through heterosexual transmission, very few were aware of their partner's risk for HIV at the time of exposure (Futterman, Cohn, Monte, & Shaffer, 1992). For adolescent girls, a sexual relationship may be one of the first ways they move apart from their parents and develop an adult identity, and thus relationships may assume an exaggerated importance. They may feel unable to make demands of their partners, such as condom use, that might jeopardize their relationship. Gender inequality and a tendency for teenage girls to have older sexual partners also place them at increased vulnerability. As one adolescent stated, "If a guy doesn't want to wear a condom and he's giving you love and attention, it seems like a small sacrifice to get the love and affection you want."

Adolescents who have a history of sexual abuse are at particular risk for HIV due to direct infection at the time of the abuse or indirect infection due to the resultant earlier onset of coital activity or an increased number of sexual partners. Individuals who have been sexually abused begin intercourse at an earlier age and have more sexual partners (Cassesse, 1993; Harrison, Hoffman, & Edwall, 1989). The impact of sexual abuse can also interfere with self-esteem and the ability to practice safer sex or to communicate about sex (Cassesse, 1993).

A substance use history is also an important component of a risk assessment. Although fewer adolescents than adults with HIV infection report injection drug use, adolescents may use needles in a variety of other ways. In addition to injection of drugs, needles may be used for tattoos, skin piercing, and the administration of anabolic steroids by adolescents involved in sports. Substances like alcohol or marijuana pose an indirect risk by impairing judgment and sexual decision making. Crack cocaine use is strongly associated with high-risk sexual behavior, including the exchange of sex for drugs. Forty percent of HIV-infected adolescents seen in the same New York City clinic reported heavy crack use, and more than 80% of crack-using youth engaged in sex for drugs, food, money, or shelter (Futterman, Cohn, Monte, & Shaffer 1992; Futterman, Hein, Reuben, & Dell, 1993).

Perinatal infection is another transmission source for adolescents. As more effective treatments develop, children who have been infected at birth will live into puberty. Some children may not be diagnosed until they reach adolescence. It is important to question adolescents with HIV infection regarding the HIV status of family members. However, due to the social stigma of HIV, some families may not have disclosed HIV as the cause of a parent's illness or death.

Adolescents who have had blood transfusions or have received blood products prior to 1985 are also at risk for developing HIV disease. Although people with hemophilia account for only 1% of adult cases of AIDS, they constitute one third of AIDS cases among 13- to 19-year-olds (CDC, 1993). Additionally, the risk to teenagers with sickle-cell anemia or other conditions that required multiple blood transfusions prior to 1985 must be ascertained.

## Pretest and Posttest Counseling Issues

A key element of counseling and testing is to help the adolescent develop a strategy for coping with a positive or a negative test result (Kunins, Hein, Futterman, Tapley, & Elliot, 1993). A clinician can encourage an adolescent to think about how he or she handled a problem or difficult situation in the past. For example, one might ask, "What do you usually do when you get very upset or nervous?" For adolescents who need help in thinking abstractly about the future, a role play in which they receive a positive result may be helpful. The clinician must also assess each teen's potential for suicide, with particular attention to past ideation and attempts. An evaluation of the potential for initiation or return to alcohol or drug-using behaviors is also valuable.

It is important for adolescents to have a supportive adult involved in the testing process to provide ongoing emotional support and to decrease the sense of isolation. This individual could be a parent, teacher, youth agency counselor, or older friend or relative. Part of the assessment is to help the young person to identify this support.

## Risk Reduction

The challenges and difficulties of changing sexual behavior are magnified in adolescents. Unlike adults, who may have prior experience or skills in negotiating sexual relations, adolescents may not perceive themselves to be at risk for acquiring HIV infection and may lack the insight and skills necessary to change high-risk behaviors (Bowser & Wingood, 1992). Additionally, societal ambivalence and denial of adolescent sexuality and substance use send a contradictory message to youth.

Successful risk reduction programs for adolescents must incorporate the following elements: (1) increasing knowledge; (2) offering opportunities to explore attitudes regarding HIV transmission, including personal susceptibility to HIV; (3) building communication, problem-solving, and decision-making skills; (4) role playing and assertiveness training to facilitate condom use and decrease incidence of unprotected sex; (5) providing information about safer sex practices; and (6) providing a forum to identify and discuss barriers to implementing safer sex practices.

## Linkage to Care

HIV counseling and testing programs for adolescents must include linkage to care. Although anonymous testing may provide an adolescent with an increased sense of security that HIV information will not be released, confidential counseling and testing allow the provider an opportunity to develop an ongoing relationship with the adolescent that facilitates linkage to care. Ideally, HIV counseling and testing should take place in a setting in which an adolescent can also obtain HIV care. Adolescents who are HIV negative or of unknown serostatus should be linked to general adolescent or primary care sites for ongoing care.

If a provider plans to refer a young person to another site for care, that site should be comprehensive and sensitive to the needs of adolescents. A comprehensive site should offer medical care, ongoing counseling, help with concrete services like entitlements and housing, and clinicians who have experience working with the medical needs of adolescents.

In addition to identifying a referral site, the provider should take an active role in ensuring that the linkage is successful. Potential barriers, such as cost of services, payment mode, transportation, and confidentiality, should be addressed. Follow-up should continue at least until the adolescent has been to the first scheduled visit or has adjusted to the new service.

## Legal and Policy Issues

HIV counseling and testing for adolescents pose several legal and policy questions, specifically in the areas of consent, confidentiality, and mandatory testing (English, 1992). The National Center for Youth Law in San Francisco (114 Sansome St., Suite 900, San Francisco, CA 94104) is an important resource. It has recently documented laws and regulations regarding adolescents and HIV testing and treatment throughout the country.

### Consent

One major concern is whether adolescents can legally consent to HIV testing and treatment. Adolescents who are 18 years or older may give their own consent for medical care. Historically, minor adolescents have been able to provide their own consent for health care services pertaining to contraception and sexually transmitted diseases in recognition of the fact that requiring parental consent might drive them away from needed care. Additionally, in certain states, specific groups of adolescents, including emancipated minors, those living apart from their parents (the homeless, street youth, and married minors), have the right to consent for HIV testing. In 11 states, adolescents of any age are able to give consent for HIV counseling and testing under specific AIDS confidentiality laws (English, 1992). In New York state, the law allows minors, not restricted by age, to consent if they have the "capacity," as determined by their ability to process information and make an informed decision.

## Confidentiality

Confidentiality is an important concern for adolescents. For example, an adolescent girl who is having sex may decide not to be tested for HIV because she is afraid that her parents will learn that she is sexually active. Generally, an adolescent who can legally consent for HIV testing has the right to control the disclosure of related information in accordance with state laws (English, 1992). Clinicians should reassure adolescents that their wish for confidentiality will be respected but should also help them to understand the limits of confidentiality. In New York, for instance, clinicians or agencies are required to disclose an adolescent's HIV test result to foster care or correctional institutions upon request. Additionally, a physician has the right in some states to inform a minor's parent of a positive test result if the physician believes it is in the minor's best interest.

## Mandatory Testing

Adolescents already experience mandatory HIV testing in institutions like the military, the Peace Corps, and the Job Corps. Testing practices in these settings vary. For instance, young people who test HIV positive are not admitted into the military, but Job Corps applicants with HIV infection can be admitted and can receive medical care. Adolescents who attempt to join the military or the Job Corps as an opportunity for career advancement may not be aware that they will be tested for HIV. Those who test HIV positive can find themselves at risk for discrimination, psychological distress, and limited access to medical care (Hein, 1991).

## ❖ Natural History

Little research has been done to describe the course of HIV infection in adolescents. Because most adolescents are infected after their immune system has already developed, the course of HIV infection in adolescents is more similar to that of adults than of children.

A unique issue for adolescents appears to be the enhanced biological susceptibility to HIV infection for peripubertal females. To date, the biology of HIV transmission to women is not fully understood. It has not been established whether the majority of HIV transmission is through the vaginal wall or the cervix. To the degree that HIV is transmitted through the cervix, adolescents may be more vulnerable to infection than adults because the cervix is in the process of development. During puberty, the endocervical columnar cells, which extend onto the outer portion of the cervix, are being replaced by squamous epithelial cells. These "ectopic" endocervical cells are more vulnerable to infection with gonorrhea and presumably viral infection. Additionally, the cervical mucus of an adolescent is more permeable to sperm and infectious viral agents until several years after menarche and the establishment of progesterone-induced ovulatory cycles (Futterman & Hein, 1990). This biological susceptibility, coupled with social and political vulnerability, may help explain the high rates of HIV transmission among adolescent females.

## ❖ Clinical Evaluation and Care

The initial evaluation of an adolescent with HIV infection includes a medical, sexual, and substance use history, a psychosocial assessment, a physical examination, and laboratory evaluation (Futterman & Hein, 1990). This may be divided over one to three visits so as not to overwhelm the young person.

### Medical History

An initial medical history may begin with questions concerning HIV testing. It is important to learn why an adolescent decided to be HIV tested, when the test was done, how he or she is coping, and who knows of their HIV status.

In addition, the clinician should establish a history of prior illness, with particular attention to any evidence of seroconversion illness or infections that might be HIV related. The clinician must also inquire about tuberculosis. Adolescence is a time when tuberculosis can reactivate, and coinfection with HIV increases this risk. Hospitalizations, childhood illnesses like asthma or varicella, and history of blood transfusions, before 1985 should also be assessed. Adolescents should be questioned regarding previous immunizations because homeless, immigrant, or disadvantaged youth may not have had access to primary care and thus may not have received a tetanus booster or a measles, mumps, and rubella (MMR) booster, which should be administered at age 14 or 15.

History of sexually transmitted diseases (STDs) is another component of the medical history. An adolescent may not realize that he or she has had an STD; therefore, the clinician should not only name each STD, but also describe the symptoms. The site of infection and the treatment history should also be recorded. An STD history includes gonorrhea, chlamydia, syphilis, genital herpes, warts (condyloma), vaginal candida, and pelvic inflammatory disease. Adolescent females should also be asked if they have had a previous pelvic exam or Pap smear, with attention to a history of abnormal cytology.

A menstrual and pregnancy history should also be obtained. Women with HIV infection may present with changes in menstrual cycle, flow, or pain. These issues may be difficult to sort out in young adolescents, who may have less predictable ovulatory patterns. The date of the last menstrual period should be noted.

All adolescents need to be asked if they have borne or fathered children. If they have living children, the clinician should determine their ages, health, and HIV status and who is responsible for their care. Adolescents may need help in obtaining HIV testing or care for their children as well as assistance in making custody arrangements.

## Behavioral History

### Sexual History

A sexual history not only helps the clinician to plan care, but also signals to an adolescent that he or she can ask questions or talk about sexual behavior or orientation. Questions should include the adolescent's age at first intercourse and the number, age, and sex of subsequent partners. This can be asked, "How many partners have you had who are male? How many partners have you had who are female?" In this way, an adolescent is encouraged to speak about his or her same-sex and opposite-sex experiences. The clinician should ask explicitly if a teenager has had oral, anal, or vaginal intercourse. History of sexual abuse and survival sex (the exchange of sex for food, money, drugs, or shelter) should also be ascertained as part of ongoing care because a young person may initially be uncomfortable sharing this personal information.

### Substance Use History

A substance use history includes the use of cigarettes, alcohol, marijuana, crack cocaine, heroin, uppers, downers, hormones, steroids, and other substances that may impair judgment. A complete drug history should establish the adolescent's age at first use, past and current patterns of use, whether he or she shares needles or "works," and how drug use affects sexual decision making. Past drug treatment and family history of substance use should also be noted.

## Psychosocial History

A psychosocial history includes current living situation, education, work status, or other economic support and family and social supports. It is important to find out who an adolescent has told about the HIV infection and whether they are a source of support or hostility. The provider should also record any history of depression, anxiety, psychosis, suicidal thoughts or attempts, and psychiatric hospitalizations or treatments.

## Physical Evaluation

Adolescence is a time of physical and cognitive growth. The physical exam should be performed with attention to the failure of growth as well as physical pathology. In terms of the general exam, a clinician should note vital signs, pubertal changes like breast development, slowing of height and weight growth rates, and nutritional status.

A dermatologic exam should be done. Acne is a common skin problem of adolescence; it is important to reassure an adolescent that this is a normal development and to differentiate it from dermatologic signs of HIV progression. Lymph nodes should be examined and described, noting number, size, location, and consistency. A head, neck, ear, nose, and throat (HEENT) exam includes inspection of nasal passages and palpation for sinus tenderness. Recurrent sinusitis is a frequent problem among adolescents with HIV infection. The provider should check for thrush, oral lesions, dental decay, and periodontal disease. Visual acuity and fundoscopy should be performed to screen for evidence of cytomegalovirus (CMV) retinitis or toxoplasmosis, particularly in youth with CD4 cell counts of less than $200/mm^3$.

The genitalia exam should include sexual maturity staging using the Tanner and Whitehouse scale (Tables 8–1 and 8–2). This five-point scale describes the development of breasts, pubic hair, and male genitalia during puberty (Tanner, 1962). The external genitalia and anus of adolescents should be assessed for sores, lesions, and warts/condyloma. The anal area should always be examined because an adolescent may not be ready to discuss anal intercourse but may have anal warts or herpes. Condyloma are caused by the human papilloma virus (HPV), and certain serotypes of HPV may develop into genital, cervical, or anal neoplasia, particularly in immunocompromised patients.

All adolescent females who have had sexual intercourse, pelvic pain, or are over 18 should have a pelvic exam every 6 months. For some adolescent girls, this may be their first exam and thus their first opportunity to learn about their bodies. This can be done through diagrams, models, and the use of a mirror for adolescents to view their external genitalia and cervix.

TABLE 8–1    Classification of Sex Maturity Ratings in Boys

| Rating | Pubic Hair | Penis | Testes |
|---|---|---|---|
| 1 | None | Preadolescent | Preadolescent |
| 2 | Scanty, long, slighty pigmented | Slighty enlarged | Enlarged scrotum, pink, less smoth |
| 3 | Darker, curls, small amount | Longer | Larger |
| 4 | Adult-type but less; curly, coarse | Larger, breadth increases | Larger, scrotum is darker |
| 5 | Adult pattern; spreads to inner thighs | Adult | Adult |

*Source:* From Tanner, J. M. (1962). *Growth at adolescence.* The American Academy of Pediatrics. Oxford, England: Blackwell Scientific Publications, p. 53.

TABLE 8–2   Classification of Sex Maturity Ratings in Girls

| Rating | Pubic Hair | Breasts |
|--------|-----------|---------|
| 1 | Preadolescent | Preadolescent |
| 2 | Scanty, slighty pigmented, straight, on inner part of labia | Breast elevated as small mound |
| 3 | Darker, starts to curl, increased amount | Breast and aerola enlarged, no separation |
| 4 | Coarse, curly, more but less than in an adult | Areola and future nipple form a secondary mound |
| 5 | Adult feminine triangle: spreads to inner surface of thighs | Mature; nipple projects, and areola part of general breast shape |

*Source:* From Tanner, J. M. (1962). *Growth at adolescence.* The American Academy of Pediatrics. Oxford, England: Blackwell Scientific Publications, p. 53.

## Laboratory Evaluation

The laboratory evaluation for adolescents is similar to that of adults. The HIV test should be repeated for confirmation. CD4 counts are generally done every 3 months to monitor immune function and disease progression.

Laboratory tests, such as a complete blood count and chemistry and enzyme panel, can detect hematologic, renal, and hepatic involvement and can also monitor the effects of medications. Certain laboratory values are notable for differing from normal adult values. During puberty, boys experience a rise in hemoglobin due to the effect of increased androgens. Elevated alkaline phosphatase, whose levels may reach 104 U/L, compared with adult values of 13 to 39 U/L, may reflect bone growth during the adolescent growth spurt (Futterman & Hein, 1990).

All sexually active adolescents should be screened every 6 months for sexually transmitted diseases because infections may often be asymptomatic. The screen should include a syphilis serology, culture for gonorrhea at three sites (oral, genital, and anal), and a genital chlamydia test. For girls, microscopic examination of a slide prepared with potassium hydroxide (KOH), for candida, and a slide prepared with saline, for trichomonas or bacterial vaginosis, should be done. Ulcers should be cultured for herpes. A Pap smear should be done every 6 months to screen for cervical dysplasia, which, if present, should be followed up with colposcopy and a biopsy.

Laboratory evaluation also includes hepatitis B serology (antibody and antigen), toxoplasmosis titer, and urinalysis. Tuberculosis assessment consists of the administration of purified protein derivative (PPD) and an appropriate anergy panel (tetanus, mumps, or a multidose). Networking with community agencies for a reading of the PPD at 48 to 72 hours can facilitate the completion of this exam. If a patient has a positive PPD or is anergic, a chest radiograph should be done.

## Immunizations

All adolescents with HIV infection should receive a one-time pneumococcal vaccine and a yearly influenza vaccine. Additionally, age-appropriate immunizations such as tetanus and diphtheria (Td) and MMR should be given; pregnancy should be ruled out before giving rubella vaccine. Hepatitis B vaccine is also recommended for all nonexposed adolescents.

## Medication Dosing

To date, adolescents have been minimally included in AIDS clinical trials. The treatment of HIV infection for adolescents has thus been extrapolated from adults. However, the changes in body composition and metabolism, which occur during puberty, may alter drug distribution and dosing. As a general guideline, adolescents in Tanner Stage 1 should receive pediatric dose schedules, and adolescents in Tanner Stage 5 should receive adult dose schedules, regardless of chronological age. Appropriate dosing for adolescents in Tanner Stages 2, 3, and 4 have not been developed, so medications should be closely monitored (Futterman & Hein, 1992).

## Treatment Adherence

Adolescents and their providers face major challenges regarding adherence to medical treatment. The developmental level of a teenager may affect his or her ability to follow a treatment regimen. Adolescents who are facing complicated medical treatments may need a structured, supportive approach to care that can include simple explanations, telephone calls or reminders, and assistance in anticipating problems and devising solutions.

The clinician also needs to balance young people's need for direction with their desire for autonomy. The family of one adolescent developed a system in which her mother or older sister reminded her to take zidovudine every 4 hours. Although it was initially helpful, eventually it became difficult for the rebellious 17-year-old to accept continual advice and reminders.

Adolescents frequently have significant financial problems that prevent them from following a medical regimen. Young people who are impoverished or homeless may feel they have more immediate concerns, such as security, food, or shelter, that they must confront on a day-to-day basis. Practitioners also need to recognize payment issues that are unique to adolescents. Adolescents who make an insurance or Medicaid claim on their parents' policy may lose confidentiality.

## ❖ Psychosocial Issues

The social issues of living with HIV are of equal importance to the medical issues. By providing young people with emotional and social support while helping them to identify strengths and resources, providers can facilitate a process of coping and empowerment.

### Disclosure

One of the first major issues facing an adolescent who has HIV infection is disclosure. Disclosure offers potential benefit to a teenager by helping to build a system of support that can lessen isolation. However, some teenagers fear the rejection of family and friends, which they believe may come with disclosure. For some teenagers, the disclosure of HIV status may mean revealing stigmatizing behaviors, such as drug use or survival sex. Adolescents who come from families already affected by HIV may fear causing additional burden. Moreover, some teens may have realistic fears of abandonment or physical abuse. Disclosure to sexual partners is a particularly difficult issue for many adolescents, who may need time to acknowledge their own fears before they are able to think about notifying others.

### Developmental Issues

HIV can impact on the developmental tasks of adolescence. Because adolescence is a period of increased independence, a teenager may find it difficult to ask assistance of family and friends. For instance, a teenage boy with advanced disease may resist moving back into his mother's home although he needs extensive home-based services. Adolescence is also a time when future plans and goals are developed; teenagers with HIV may believe that these plans are now futile. Clinicians can help youth to continue their plans by helping them to understand what is realistic and hopeful about their lives.

### Women's Issues

Adolescent girls have much in common with adult women with HIV, but they also have their own unique experiences. Unlike male homosexuals, who may have a larger community, adolescent girls may appear isolated from family, friends, and peers. Through peer support groups, many teenage girls are able to meet others with similar issues and begin to build a support network.

Reproductive decision making poses many issues for young women. HIV infection does not destroy dreams and goals for the future, and many young women express a strong desire to bear children. Teens who experience an accelerated maturation due to this serious illness may feel they are more ready to become parents. Sometimes, a teenage girl who has already had a child that was raised by someone else may want to raise a child on her own. Others, facing a potentially shortened life, seek to hasten the accomplishment of developmental milestones. Teenagers may need a great deal of help in thinking ahead to the future needs of their child as well as the possible consequences for themselves and their families.

For teens who are already parents, clinicians should develop referrals for a range of services, including parenting classes, day care, and entitlements. Adolescents with advanced disease may need help in making custody arrangements for their children.

### Sexuality Issues

Because a developmental task of adolescence is to develop one's sexual identity, issues of sexuality are particularly intense. An adolescent with HIV infection may feel that the infection is a punishment for being sexually active or for being gay or lesbian. Clinicians need to reinforce the fact that HIV infection does not occur because of one's sexuality but because of unprotected intercourse (Kunins et al., 1993).

### Death and Dying

Providers may need to help teens and their families address and plan for dying. Completion of a health care proxy and living will can sometimes be helpful in providing a structure to begin to communicate about death and dying (see chapter 17). These documents may also help an adolescent to gain a sense of control over the dying process. It is important to begin to work on these documents when the immune system declines (CD4 ≤ 200) but before the development of a medical crisis.

### ❖ Program Issues

### Organization of Care

Any approach to the clinical care of adolescents with HIV infection must be comprehensive and adolescent specific. As described in chapter 2, this is best accomplished by a multidisciplinary staff, which may include physicians, nurse practitioners and physician assistants, nurses, social workers, psychologists, and case managers. Care plans are developed through case conferences in which staff members discuss each patient and coordinate the various facets of their care.

The role of a community liaison or case manager is also essential; the community liaison facilitates care by providing follow-up when teens miss appointments and by helping to obtain concrete services, such as housing, substance use treatment, and entitlements. Due to the complexity of the ethical and legal issues that emerge in caring for adolescents with HIV, linkage with a lawyer/ethicist is invaluable.

An important concept of care is "one-stop shopping." This is a system by which subspecialists come to one clinic site to provide care to adolescents. For instance, a gynecologist may come to the clinic on a regular basis to provide consultation and colposcopy.

## Aging Out: Adolescence to Adulthood

The process of "aging out," or transferring a young person to adult care, poses several issues for adolescent or pediatric programs. Adolescence is not a period that can be strictly defined by age, and the developmental process of adolescence often extends beyond the 22nd birthday. In addition, teens coping with HIV may develop close relationships with clinicians that they may perceive to be arbitrarily severed. However, adolescent or pediatric programs may be limited by hospital or clinic policies regarding age. One goal of adolescent care might be defined as assisting a young person to develop the responsibility and independence required by an adult program. These issues can be addressed in two ways. Patients with advanced disease can remain in the program because a transition to a new program in the final stage of their illness would be detrimental. Other patients, with less advanced disease, can be offered individualized referrals to adult programs when they reach 22 years. The aging-out process might include participation in a group that addresses this transition as well as follow-up to ensure that patients actually continue in adult care.

## Outreach

Although it can be assumed that thousands of adolescents are infected with HIV, relatively few are actually in care. Clinical programs must have active outreach strategies for identifying high-risk youth and bringing them into care. This involves networking with health care facilities, community-based organizations, government youth-serving agencies, and HIV counseling and testing sites. Outreach must also include training and working with community agencies to address their concerns regarding HIV testing for teenagers. Peer educators, who provide credibility and further access, may also be incorporated into an outreach plan.

## ❖ Summary

Adolescents who are HIV positive or at risk for HIV infection face many medical and social issues. Programs caring for these youth must address legal and policy issues and provide comprehensive care. As an increasing number of teenagers become infected with HIV, programs will also need to intensify outreach strategies to identify and bring teenagers into care. Major research challenges include developing a better understanding of viral transmission and progression in adolescents and developing effective approaches to care, prevention, and risk reduction.

In this chapter, the unique features of HIV infection in adolescents and the key issues in providing care for youth were discussed:

1. Current epidemiological trends among adolescents, highlighting variables of gender, age, and race
2. Behaviors that place adolescents at risk for HIV infection
3. How to elicit a sexual and substance use history
4. Counseling and testing, with attention to developmental issues and linkage of teens with HIV infection
5. Legal and policy issues, such as consent, confidentiality, and mandatory testing
6. Natural history and the possible enhanced biological susceptibility to HIV for prepubertal females
7. Key aspects of clinical evaluation for adolescents: growth dynamics, Tanner staging, and screening for sexually transmitted diseases
8. Medical treatment, with special consideration to medication dosing, immunizations, and treatment adherence
9. Psychosocial and prevention issues, such as disclosure, sexuality, and risk reduction
10. Unique experiences of adolescent females, including isolation, reproductive decision making, and the role of peer support groups
11. Programmatic issues, including multidisciplinary staff, legal/ethical consultation, and outreach
12. Challenges for the future, including medical and psychosocial research, case finding, and prevention

## ❖ References

Bell, T., & Hein, K. (1984). The adolescent and sexually transmitted diseases. In K. Holmes (Ed.), *Sexually transmitted diseases* (pp. 73–84). New York: McGraw-Hill.

Bowser, B., & Wingood, G. (1992). Community-based HIV prevention programs for adolescents. In R. J. DiClemente (Ed.), *Adolescents and AIDS: A generation in jeopardy* (pp. 194–211). Newburg Park, CA: Sage.

Cassesse, J. (1993, April/May). The invisible bridge: Child sexual abuse and the risk of HIV infection in adulthood. *SIECUS Report, 21,* 1–7.

Centers for Disease Control. (1992). Youth risk behavior survey 1990. *Morbidity and Mortality Weekly Report, 41,* 33–35.

Centers for Disease Control and Prevention. (1993). Acquired immunodeficiency syndrome—United States—1992. *Morbidity and Mortality Weekly Report, 42,* 547–557.

Conway, A. G., Epstein, R. M., Hayman, R. C., Miller, A. C., Wendell, A. D., Gwinn, M., Karon, M. J., & Petersen, R. L. (1993). Trends in HIV prevalence among disadvantaged youth: Survey results from a national job training program, 1988 through 1992. *Journal of the American Medical Association, 269,* 2887–2889.

English, A. (1992). Expanding access to HIV services for adolescents: Legal and ethical issues. In R. J. DiClemente (Ed.), *Adolescents and AIDS: A generation in jeopardy* (pp. 531–560). Newbury Park, CA: Sage.

Futterman, D. C., Cohn, J., Monte, D., & Shaffer, N. (1992, July). HIV infected adolescents: Risk behaviors and clinical status of a New York City cohort. Paper presented at the Eighth International Conference on AIDS, Amsterdam. (Abstract No.Th 1560)

Futterman, D. C., & Hein, K. (1990). Medical management of adolescents. In P. Pizzo & C. Wilfert (Eds.), *Pediatric AIDS: The challenge of HIV infection in infants, children and adolescents* (pp. 531–560). Baltimore: Williams and Wilkins.

Futterman, D. C., & Hein, K. (1992). Medical care of HIV infection in adolescents. *AIDS Clinical Care, 4,* 95–98.

Futterman, D., Hein, K., Reuben, N., & Dell, R. (1993). Establishing an adolescent AIDS program: The first 50 HIV positive patients. *Pediatrics, 91*(4),730–735.

Goldsmith, M. (1993). Invisible epidemic now becoming visible as HIV/AIDS pandemic reaches adolescents. *Journal of the American Medical Association, 270,* 16–19.

Harrison, P. A., Hoffman, N. A., & Edwall, G. E. (1989). Differential drug use patterns among sexually abused adolescent girls in treatment for chemical dependency. *International Journal of Addiction, 24,* 499–514.

Hein, K. (1991). Mandatory HIV testing of youth: A lose-lose proposition. *Journal of American Medical Association, 266,* 2430–2431.

Kunins, H., Hein, K., Futterman, D., Tapley, E., & Elliot, A. (1993). Guide to adolescent HIV/AIDS program development. *Journal of Adolescent Health, 14*(5), 55–56.

Quinn, T. C. (1992). Evolution of the HIV epidemic among patients attending STD clinics. *Journal of Infectious Diseases, 165,* 541–544.

Tanner, J. M. (1962). *Growth at adolescence.* The American Academy of Pediatrics. Oxford, England: Blackwell Scientific Publications.

United Nations Development Program. (1992). *Young women: Silence, susceptibility and the HIV epidemic.* New York: UN Development Program New York.

## ❖ Suggested Readings

DiClemente, R. J. (Ed.). (1992). *Adolescents and AIDS: A generation in jeopardy.* Newbury Park, CA: Sage.

Haymes, R., Karlson, K., Kunreuther, F., & Schnee, L. (1992). *HIV antibody counseling and testing for adolescents: Policy recommendations and practical guidelines.* New York: AIDS and Adolescent Network of New York.

Hoffman, N., & Futterman, D. (1993). Human immunodeficiency virus infection in adolescents. *Seminars in Pediatric Infectious Disease, 4,* 113–121.

Larkin Street Youth Center. (1990). *HIV and homeless youth: Meeting the challenge.* San Francisco: Larkin Street Youth Center.

NYS AIDS Advisory Council. (1991). *Illusions of immortality: The confrontation of adolescence and AIDS.* Albany: New York State Department of Health.

# ❖ Chapter 9

# HIV Counseling and Testing for Women

Susan Holman
Ann Kurth

It is now estimated that by the year 2000, more than 13 million women will have been infected with HIV, with as many females as males worldwide (World Health Organization [WHO], 1993). In the United States, AIDS is now the fourth leading cause of death for women in the reproductive-potential ages of 24 to 44 (Centers for Disease Control and Prevention [CDC], 1993). Given the increasing incidence of HIV disease in both women and men of reproductive age—and the goal of earlier interventions for those who are infected—HIV risk assessment, counseling, and testing will increasingly become a standard of care. Incorporating HIV counseling and testing within the context of women's health can serve several purposes: education, to provide specific information about the virus, its transmission, and the HIV antibody test; prevention, to discuss means of reducing the risk of acquiring or transmitting HIV; support, to provide a caring framework within which patients may make decisions about HIV testing, implement behavior changes to reduce risk, and cope with HIV test results; and treatment, to allow the initiation of appropriate clinical interventions to prolong the asymptomatic phase, to treat opportunistic infections, or possibly to reduce perinatal transmission risk. However, certain fundamental principles must be incorporated if these goals are to be met adequately. This chapter reviews some of these principles and their practical application for workers involved with HIV counseling and testing.

Testing is addressed from a policy perspective as well as a pragmatic one, including provider preparation and a pretest and posttest counseling model for HIV-negative and HIV-positive women. Long-term follow-up for some issues of particular significance to reproductive-age women will be discussed.

## ❖ Testing Policies: What Constitutes a Standard of Care?

National and international entities have called for the provision of HIV counseling and testing of women at risk, with the goals of education, prevention of transmission, and, more recently, treatment (WHO,

1990). From the outset, concern in the United States focused on prevention of vertical transmission. This led to a public health policy recommending HIV testing of reproductive-age women and anonymous newborn sero-prevalence screening, along with advice to HIV-positive women to refrain from childbearing until more was known (CDC, 1985).[1] Although the American College of Obstetricians and Gynecologists endorsed these early recommendations, by 1990 it was stating that "an individual woman's reproductive choices should be respected regardless of her HIV status" (Berer & Ray, 1993). In the fall of 1993 the American College of Obstetricians and Gynecologists (ACOG) endorsed the concept of universal (mandatory) counseling with the option of voluntary testing (ACOG, 1993).

The U.S. Public Health Service recommends that prenatal HIV testing be made routinely available to women (CDC, 1987). No similar policy or recommendations have yet been constructed for men of reproductive-potential age. Of the numerous seroprevalence studies of women of childbearing age, none have attempted to test male partners (Sherr, 1993). The logical fact that vertical transmission can involve both parents should be incorporated into research, policy, and service delivery.

Given the focus on perinatal transmission, it is perhaps not surprising that, over the years, calls have been raised for mandatory HIV antibody testing of women or newborns (Angell, 1991; Hunter, 1992). At present, the tenuous consensus about mandatory testing (see chapter 16) is that such testing is not ethically justified, cost-efficient, or beneficial as it would likely drive many women away from the health care system (Faden, Geller, & Powers, 1992; Naber & Johnson, 1993). However, there are legitimate concerns that as improvements in infant diagnosis and treatment accumulate, as with the evidence that perinatal HIV transmission may be reduced with the use of ZDV (ACTG 076 trial results described later), there will be increasing pressure for HIV testing of women. This could place women in the subordinate role of being important mainly in the context of their potential children (Amaro, 1993).

The benefits to knowing one's HIV status include the ability to seek appropriate emotional and clinical support and as a factor in life planning and other decisions. The expanding array of chemotherapeutic interventions, including antiretroviral treatment and prophylaxis, has increased the benefits of HIV testing, at least in settings where people have access to such care. Learning one's antibody status must involve informed consent; an understanding of the risks, benefits, and meaning of the test; and a plan of action following discussion of the results (reinforcement of safer behaviors

---

[1] The specific impact of this policy is not known. It is interesting to note that while the percentage of total AIDS cases occurring among women is increasing steadily, the pediatric AIDS incidence has remained almost unchanged throughout the epidemic, at less than 2% of total reported AIDS cases per year (data derived from CDC database, 1982–1992; see Kurth, 1993).

if negative; appropriate referrals, risk-reduction information, and services if positive).

This information should now include discussion of the results from the AIDS Clinical Trial Group 076 study (CDC, 1994). According to preliminary results released on February 21, 1994, zidovudine (ZDV/AZT) therapy reduced by two-thirds the risk of HIV transmission from mother to baby. The trial began in April 1991 and enrolled 477 women in their 14th to 34th week of pregnancy who did not need ZDV as part of their medical care through December 20, 1993 (all the women had CD4 counts >200 cells/mm$^3$). In this randomized, double-blind study, women received either a placebo or a standard dose of ZDV (1) during pregnancy (100 mg orally five times a day); and (2) intravenously administered during labor and delivery (loading dose 2 mg/kg followed by continuous infusion 1 mg/kg/hr until delivery). The infants received a syrup of placebo or of 2 mg/kg ZDV orally four times a day for six weeks. Of the 421 babies born, at least one HIV culture test was available for 364. Of the 263, 53 were HIV-infected: 13 of them born to mothers receiving ZDV (8.3% transmission) and 40 to mothers on placebo (25.5% transmission). There were no significant short-term side effects noted with the exception of mild, reversed anemia in the infants.

Because the long-term effects of this perinatal ZDV use are unknown (the infants will be followed for up to 20 years), no final recommendations regarding treatment during pregnancy and delivery have yet been made (NIAID/NIH Office of Communications, 1994). Several panels are being convened to address the clinical implications and other ramifications of these significant findings. The Public Health Service has provided the following interim recommendations: (1) all health-care workers providing care to pregnant women and women of childbearing potential should be informed of the ACTG 076 results; (2) HIV-infected pregnant women meeting the protocol eligibility criteria should be informed of the potential benefits but unknown long-term risks of ZDV therapy as administered in the trial; (3) women should be informed that this ZDV regimen substantially reduces but does not eliminate the risk for perinatal HIV transmission; and (4) ZDV therapy should not be instituted earlier than the 14th week of gestation until more is known about possible teratogenic effect (CDC, 1994). Knowledge of HIV status may help a women decide what kind of treatment to seek for herself and for her infant, and whether to forego breast feeding with its estimated 15% additional HIV transmission risk (HRSA Clinical Practice Committee draft statement, courtesy of Ann B. Williams).

Given the opportunity but also additional complexity of this information, it is particularly important that women receive comprehensive support in their pre- and posttest counseling.

Sherr (1993) pointed out that much of what passes for HIV testing (particularly in a reproductive health context) is not counseling in the fullest sense of the word, that is, with attendant psychological support. Others have stressed the fact that in the United States, there is unequal access to health care services, a history of the use of reproductive coercion—particularly for racial and other minorities—and the potential for discrimination if women are identified as HIV positive (Amaro, 1993).

Nonetheless, it is critical for women to protect themselves from, or have information and services for, HIV infection. For a number of years, much of the discussion about testing revolved around whether to offer testing to all women or to offer it selectively, that is, only to women who self-identified certain risk behaviors. Risk assessment has not always proved to be a sensitive tool in identifying at-risk women, either because of reluctance to admit to, or ignorance of, socially stigmatizing risk behaviors (Barbacci, Repke, & Chaisson, 1991; Minkoff et al., 1988). A comprehensive review of the many issues regarding prenatal testing approaches can be found in Faden and colleagues (1992). In an era in which HIV disease has become a leading killer of women in many U.S. cities, it can be argued that the time has come to move beyond the "targeted" versus "routine" testing debate (Minkoff et al., 1988). Universally offering *voluntary* HIV testing—with pretest and posttest counseling, confidentiality mechanisms, and referrals for needed care—to women and men who are sexually active or substance-using is a reasonable standard of care. In geographical areas where the seroprevalence of HIV is high (some suggest 2% or more as a risk factor in itself; Mitchell, Brown, Loftman, & Williams, 1990), it may be efficacious to recommend testing, with appropriate referrals (Institute of Medicine, 1990; Minkoff, 1992). As one researcher points out, "simply testing women does not result in behavior change; continuing education and counselling must also be provided"; assurances of legal protection for reproductive choice and from coercion are likewise needed (Amaro, 1993). Women must be empowered to understand both their risks for HIV acquisition and their options if they are HIV positive.

## Risk Screening

It has been documented in several settings that comprehensive risk assessment, particularly of sexual histories, is not usually conducted by health care providers, even among high-risk populations. Schoenbaum and Webber (1993) found that HIV infection in women was underrecognized in a cohort of patients attending a Bronx emergency room, with risk assessments being recorded less frequently for women (11.2%) than for men (15.9%). For 92.5% of those with any behavioral risk assessment, injection drug use was the only behavior assessed. A random sample of 1,000 internists and family and general practitioners in California revealed that only 10% of them asked new patients questions specific enough to identify those at high risk of HIV exposure (Lewis & Freeman, 1987). A survey of gynecologists in the Washington, DC, area showed that 20% of the obstetricians/gynecologists were not familiar with recommended HIV antibody screening and confirmation tests, only 40% regularly assessed the risk of new adult patients, and 30% did not recommend that women at risk use condoms. The study authors conclude that many obstetrician/gynecologists "do not perceive HIV as a major threat to their patients and are not prepared to address the problem" (Boekeloo, Rabin, Coughlin, Labbok, & Johnson, 1993). Other women's health providers, such as nurses and counselors, likewise need to become well informed about the risk and management of HIV disease in women (Hanley & Lincoln, 1992) as these workers often form the front line of care.

Providers may be hampered by personal bias and discomfort regarding frank discussion of sexual and substance use behavior more often than they realize. Testing recommendations also may arise from clinicians' personal motivations or fears, rather than patient-driven concerns, as one California study found (Partridge & Milliken, 1991). Wider use of the *harm reduction model*, which emphasizes health enhancement rather than total drug abstinence, may help clinicians and patients alike. In this model, open, nonjudgmental discussion of the client's drug use can be more productive "than the usual games we play which encourage clients to be dishonest with workers and workers to feel manipulated and incompetent" (Springer, 1991).

The lack of a consistent approach from health providers, coupled with AIDS prevention messages that tend to focus on nonmainstream behaviors like needle use and prostitution, may perpetuate myths of safety. Many women may believe that unprotected sex is not risky as long as it is heterosexual, and for women who have sex with women, a "powerful myth of lesbian invulnerability to HIV/AIDS" may be prevalent even among those who are at risk due to their injection drug use (Young, Weissman, & Cohen, 1992).

All people who are sexually active or who engage in behaviors that may put them at risk of HIV must be allowed an opportunity to explore the possible impact of their behaviors. A nonjudgmental, respectful attitude on the part of the health care worker can create a climate in which these sensitive topics can be explored. Questions regarding risk behaviors should avoid making assumptions. For example, asking "When you have sex, do you have sex with men, with women, or with both?" rather than "Do you use birth control?" allows the clinician to establish whether a female patient is celibate or lesbian or engages in a mix of behaviors. It also avoids placing labels or constraints on the ensuing conversation. If a written questionnaire detailing risk history is used, it should be culturally and literacy-appropriate to the patient population and should include "Don't know" in addition to "Yes" and "No" response choices. This allows the clinician and patient to review the answers together and to address any areas of concern or lack of information.[2]

It also must be acknowledged that many of the behaviors that put a woman at risk may not be amenable to change. Many women are economically or otherwise dependent on their partners and may have no control over the partner's behavior.

[2] This is the approach used at San Francisco's Bay Area Perinatal AIDS Center, for example (M. Shannon, personal communication, May 1993).

## ❖ Optimal Framework for Counseling and Support

In the sensitive discussion of pregnancy in HIV-positive women, reproductive autonomy must be balanced with harm reduction (Nolan, 1989). This topic can be difficult for some providers, who may have strong personal feelings about childbearing in the context of HIV, active substance abuse, or both. Nonetheless, providers must maintain a clear, factual, and emotionally supportive approach to HIV counseling. Insight can be gleaned from the experience of genetic counseling; both help a woman to negotiate a potentially difficult decision through the use of technical and often ambiguous information. Several authors have pointed out that there is a contextual nature to reproductive decision making for genetic disorders as well as with HIV (Hutchison & Kurth, 1991; Levine, 1979; Nolan, 1989), where "such diagnoses are interpreted in light of prior reproductive histories, community values and aspirations that particular women and their families hold for the pregnancy being examined" (Rapp, 1987). Others have documented that the ability to make use of health information depends primarily on such factors as socioeconomic status, educational level, sense of empowerment, and vocation. The unique psychological, sociocultural, and medical belief systems of African-Americans and other minorities need to be considered if effective AIDS prevention strategies and care are to reach that population (Flaskerud & Rush, 1989; Mays & Cochran, 1987).

As with genetic disorders, a nondirective model of counseling for HIV is essential. Staff must anticipate what to do when positive results occur and must ensure that necessary referrals to primary and reproductive care are available (therapeutic abortion, prenatal services with infectious disease consultation as needed, and ongoing HIV care). Support needs to be given to HIV-positive women outside of the reproductive cycle, including a need for grief work for the woman's own identified illness as well as other issues concerning impending or occurring loss (Hutchison & Kurth, 1991).

## ❖ Implications for Health Care Workers

HIV counseling and testing can and should occur in all settings where women's health care is provided. However, before routinely providing HIV counseling and testing, whether in an office or a clinic, several issues must be considered: staff preparation, documentation, confidentiality, consent, and referrals.

### Preparation for HIV Counseling and Testing

It is important to know which staff will be doing the counseling because it can be time intensive when done appropriately. As the volume of clients seeking testing increases, designated staff may need to change. All staff working in the clinical setting must be thoroughly educated about

HIV and about infection control procedures. Additionally, they will need to know the policies and procedures for HIV counseling and testing in a given setting. In some settings, patients will be counseled by the primary clinician; in others, it will be the responsibility of dedicated counselors or other staff who have received training. Emergency room and other staff who are likely to counsel at service entry points for women at risk should be trained. Regardless of who provides the counseling, it is important that they are thoroughly knowledgeable about HIV, have a caring attitude, and are able to communicate HIV information accurately and objectively (WHO, 1990). It is also important for clinicians to examine their own attitudes and the part that values play in discussing the HIV test and the behavioral aspects of HIV infection, such as sexual practices and preference, reproductive decisions, and drug use (Macks, 1988).

A list of appropriate local referrals should be developed before HIV counseling and testing are routinely provided. Referrals for ongoing medical care for HIV infection, social services, drug treatment, evaluation and care of partners and children, and psychological treatment may be necessary. In addition, HIV-positive women often need referrals to community-based AIDS organizations, support groups, and self-help groups. The availability of these resources may be dependent on the prevalence of HIV in the community. Resources that are relatively easy to locate in areas of higher seroprevalence may be scarce in areas of lower seroprevalence.

Two primary issues to be considered are documentation and confidentiality. Where the HIV test results will be recorded may be governed by law as well as by hospital or clinic policy. Additionally, there may be laws governing the subsequent disclosure of HIV test results, such as the mandatory reporting of HIV-positive tests to public health authorities. Twenty-six states now require HIV test-result reports by name. The limits of confidentiality are, in large measure, determined by such laws. It is incumbent on providers to be knowledgeable about the laws that govern this issue. They must also be aware of the penalties for disclosure and the legal resources for patients if breaches of confidentiality occur or if discrimination is encountered. It is also important to be clear with patients about both the safeguards and limits of confidentiality in a given system. Patients should be informed where HIV test results will be recorded and about procedures for the release of information during pretest counseling. The privacy of the counseling session itself should strive to ensure a sense of safety.

Another issue to be considered is consent and how informed consent will be obtained. Verbal consent should be documented, or a copy of the written consent should be placed in the patient's medical record. Clinicians should give serious consideration to the process of obtaining consent; women who have had the time and opportunity to give an informed consent are better prepared if their test results are positive. The HIV test should not be incorporated into a battery of "routine prenatal screens" because a positive HIV result is anything but routine in its implications.

## *Preparatory Information for Voluntary Testing*

Particularly in areas with low seroprevalence of HIV, routinely providing counseling and testing services to all women may not be feasible or appropriate. An alternative approach might be to provide a level of general HIV education to all patients and to allow them, in a nonthreatening way, to self-select for the test. A possible means of achieving this is to prepare an information sheet describing risk behaviors for HIV and to ask each patient to read it, consider her history, and decide whether to be tested without asking for her specific risk behavior. A one-to-one pretest counseling session would then be conducted before the test is taken to ensure that informed consent has been obtained (Holman et al., 1989; WHO, 1990). In addition, if any risk factors or signs suggestive of HIV are obtained on history or examination, the clinician should provide HIV counseling and offer HIV testing.

## ❖ Recommended HIV Counseling and Testing Protocols

### *Pretest Counseling*

The principal goals of pretest counseling involve education and informed consent. Pretest counseling includes both information giving and discussion so that the patient understands the concepts presented and an interactive discussion is encouraged. Only when and if the patient has an adequate comprehension of HIV, its transmission, and the antibody test can informed consent be given for the test. Pretest counseling should be provided regardless of a patient's decision to be tested; it is an opportunity to provide patients with information about this sexually transmitted disease and to discuss the adoption of behaviors that will reduce the risk of infection.

Basic information about HIV and the antibody test can be provided through the use of written educational materials, videotapes, group presentations, or some combination of these methods to augment the necessary counseling component. However, only through a patient-provider session can the clinician ensure that the patient has an adequate understanding of the information and has made an informed decision about testing. Additionally, the provider can evaluate the patient's coping skills and support system and can assist and support the patient in developing a plan for reducing risk of HIV infection.

The informational content of pretest counseling includes (1) an explanation of HIV infection and its relationship to AIDS; (2) modes of HIV transmission; (3) sexual and drug-related risk-reduction behaviors; (4) the purpose of HIV antibody testing; (5) the meaning of HIV antibody test results; (6) the importance of knowing one's HIV antibody status, particularly with regard to treatment, pregnancy, and perinatal transmission; and (7) documentation and reporting of test results.

A basic explanation about HIV disease and its transmission is critical to a patient's understanding. Many women may be unaware that HIV can be heterosexually transmitted or that early treatment of HIV infection (antiretrovirals and Pneumocystis carinii pneumonia [PCP] prophylaxis) is available. Patients may also hold misconceptions about the long asymptomatic phase of HIV infection or the risks of perinatal transmission. Sexual risk reduction should always be discussed in the pretest counseling session, with the woman's partner if possible, keeping in mind cultural and religious practices and norms as well as sexual preferences and constraints in effecting behavior change (Table 9–1). A woman may fear her partner's reaction, including abandonment, the withdrawal of economic support, or emotional or physical violence (Holman, et al., 1989; Macks, 1988). Clinicians can support women in introducing safer practices into their relationships by discussing possible partner reactions, by offering to counsel the couple together, and by exploring alternatives that may offer some protection, such as the use of a spermicidal agent with a diaphragm if condoms will not be used.

Risk reduction for injection drug users can be accomplished by eliminating needle use altogether; referrals for treatment should be offered to all drug users. If legal, sterile needles should be available for those who continue to inject drugs; injection paraphernalia should never be shared. If sterile needles are unavailable, equipment (needles, syringes, spoon) can be sterilized before and after reusing by boiling or by effectively decontaminating with a virucidal agent. Early studies indicated that HIV is inactivated by chlorine bleach (Martin, McDougal, & Loskoski, 1985), leading to recommendations that patients rinse needles and syringes twice with chlorine and then rinse them twice with water. However, more recent findings indicate that these widely recommended techniques may not be sufficient to remove HIV risk entirely (National Institute on Drug Abuse, 1993).

Finally, the HIV antibody test, its meaning, and its purpose should be reviewed, including the concept of the "window phase," the 3- to 6-month period from the time of exposure to the time of detectable antibody production. Women should be apprised of where HIV test results will be documented and who will have access to the results.

To give informed consent for HIV testing, women must first understand the numerous health and social implications that HIV testing incurs. The patient's coping skills and support systems may be assessed by ascertaining the following: (1) Who are the supportive people in her life? (2) If HIV positive, who can the patient confide in who will be supportive and will keep her confidence? (3) How has the patient generally reacted to stressful situations? (4) How does she think she might deal with a positive test result? In addition, suicide risk and history of psychiatric problems should be assessed (James, 1988). Women who believe that they cannot deal emotionally with positive test results should be allowed to decline the test.

TABLE 9-1  Risk Behaviors and Prevention of HIV Transmission

### Behaviors

| Safest | Low Risk | Possibly Unsafe | High Risk |
|---|---|---|---|
| Abstinence | Wet kissing | Cunnilingus | Unprotected receptive anal intercourse |
| Self-masturbation | Vaginal intercourse with latex condom | Fellatio | Unprotected vaginal intercourse |
| Monogamy (both partners uninfected and not engaged in risk activities) | Anal intercourse with condom and spermicide | | Unprotected anal penetration with hand |
| | | | Oral-anal contact |
| Hugging, massaging, touching, mutual masturbation (if no breaks in the skin) | | | Multiple sexual partners and unprotected sex |
| | | | Sharing sex toys or douches |
| Dry kissing | | | Sharing needles for any purpose |
| Drug abstinence | | | |

### Prevention Strategies

| Safest | Low Risk | Possibly Unsafe | High Risk |
|---|---|---|---|
| Avoid increased risk behaviors. | Avoid exposure to possibly infected body fluids. | Use dental dam or female condom with cunilingus. | Avoid exposure to possibly infected body fluids. |
| | Consistently use latex condoms and spermicide with vaginal intercourse. | Use condom with fellatio. | Consistently use condom and spermicide with vaginal intercourse. |
| | Avoid anal intercourse; if anal sex occurs, use latex condoms and spermicide. | | Avoid anal penetration (penile or hand); if anal penetration occurs, use condom with anal intercourse, latex glove with hand. |
| | | | Avoid anal-oral contact. |
| | | | Do not share sex toys or douching equipment. |
| | | | Do not share needles; if sharing occurs, clean with bleach before and after use. |

*Source:* Adapted from Cohen, 1990; De Ferrari, 1989. Reprinted with permission from Ann Kurth (Ed.), *Until the Cure: Caring for Women with AIDS.* New Haven: Yale University Press, 1993. Copyright © 1993, Yale University Press.

## Counseling during Pregnancy and
## Pregnancy Decisions

Obstetric and gynecologic care providers are those most likely to provide care to young, otherwise healthy women who may be at risk for or infected with HIV. For these reasons, providers of women's health care are faced with the need to incorporate HIV counseling and testing into their practices. Due in part to the emphasis on prenatal testing, many women have their HIV infection diagnosed only during pregnancy, often during the second trimester. The emotional repercussions of this vary but can be enormous. Many women experience pregnancy as a time of hopefulness and vulnerability. To receive what is often initially seen as a death sentence is more than some women can cope with during pregnancy. The psychological adaptation to an HIV diagnosis is thus compounded by the fact of already being pregnant. For many women who discover their HIV status late in the pregnancy, there is limited reproductive choice. Some women choose to terminate the index pregnancy but become pregnant again and, having adapted to living with HIV disease, choose to keep subsequent pregnancies.

HIV positivity may not be the major deciding factor in an HIV-positive woman's decision about whether to continue a pregnancy (Johnstone et al., 1990; Selwyn et al., 1989; Sunderland, Minkoff, Handte, Moroso, & Landesman, 1992). Prenatal testing policy in the United States appears to have been predicated on an assumption that cognitive fact giving ("You have HIV; here are the probable risks") will affect reproductive behavior. This assumption may not be accurate, and in any case, it ignores the affective or emotional component of reproductive decision making.

Several studies have pointed out that knowledge of HIV status does not appear to have been related to effective contraception use (Dattel et al., 1991) or pregnancy decisions (Selwyn et al., 1989; Sunderland et al., 1992). HIV-infected women, like their HIV-negative counterparts, experience pregnancy and parturition or face pregnancy decisions, such as whether to terminate.

Sunderland and colleagues (1992) followed 98 HIV-positive and 108 HIV-negative women in Brooklyn, New York, for a mean length of 18 months. Nineteen percent of the positive and 3% of the negative women terminated their index pregnancies. In subsequent pregnancies, 23% of the positive and 19% of the negative women carried their pregnancies to term, a finding of no statistical significance difference between the groups. In a study involving 28 HIV-positive and 36 HIV-negative women, Selwyn and coworkers (1989) found that termination rates were similar between the two groups. Decisions to terminate were associated with whether the pregnancy was unplanned, whether it induced negative or anxious feelings in the woman, and whether the pregnancy decision was difficult. Johnstone and colleagues (1990) found no difference in pregnancy decisions between HIV-positive and HIV-negative injection drug users, despite more directive counseling than is customary in the United States (Kelly, 1992).

In a cohort of HIV-infected sexual partners of hemophiliac men, 280 out of 2,276 couples reported pregnancies, a fertility rate comparable to the U.S. average. Nine out of 24 completed pregnancies of HIV-positive women were planned; 15 were unplanned. The reasons given for the planned pregnancies included a denial of risk, a willingness to "take chances," a sense of invincibility, and a desire for a child despite HIV disease (Jason et al., 1990).

Much of the difficulty in making a pregnancy decision—and in counseling at this time—has to do with the number of unknowns. Although there is increasing documentation that certain factors may statistically increase the chance of perinatal transmission, these may not be clearly predictable for a given individual. As one clinician put it, women "have no absolutes with which to guide their thinking. There is no way to know how much of a chance a woman takes in continuing a pregnancy or how likely it is that an abortion would have been unnecessary" (Williams, 1990). The indications from ACTG trial 076 that perinatal HIV transmission can be reduced are very encouraging (CDC, 1994); still, there is no guarantee that all women can tolerate the ZDV regimen equally, or that all infants will be protected from transmission. Nonetheless, the benefits and risks of ZDV use as a viable option need to be discussed with HIV-positive women.

Reproduction is a complex issue with profound personal and cultural meanings for women, and childbearing and child rearing may be a woman's most significant life task. The impact of asking women not to reproduce because they have an infection that carries a limited chance of transmission must be considered within this context.

## Posttest Counseling

After a woman has been tested, there may be a waiting period before results are available. This may be an anxious time for the patient, and it is advisable that she be informed of the average time lag between testing and the availability of test results to help reduce concern. Posttest counseling should occur as soon as possible after the results are received. The counseling should be conducted in person, regardless of test results. Some women may feel that they are not ready to hear the results immediately but will agree to learning them after a period of time. The clinician must decide together with the patient as to how this will be handled in a way that is respectful of the woman's wishes, yet does not impede appropriate treatment.

### HIV-Negative Results

In almost any clinical setting, the majority of patients will test HIV-negative. The posttest counseling session, the content of which is summarized in Table 9–2, represents another opportunity to provide education and support risk-reduction behaviors while informing a patient that she is HIV negative. If a woman has engaged in risk behaviors in the past 6 months, she should be advised to be retested. Women who are identified as having an ongoing risk of acquiring HIV infection should be engaged in ongoing follow-up (see the following section on long-term follow-up). Occasionally, clinicians may encounter patients who are known as the "worried well." These patients may be convinced that they are actually HIV infected despite a negative test result and may ask to be tested repeatedly without reason. They may have emotional problems or underlying depression and may need to be referred for more extensive counseling (Brotman & Forstein, 1988).

## Inconclusive Results

Occasionally, the results of a woman's HIV antibody test are inconclusive, reported as neither positive nor negative. *Indeterminate* and *equivocal* are other terms that laboratories use to describe the test results in this situation. An inconclusive HIV antibody result is due to insufficient criteria for serologic diagnosis, the presence of a nonspecific Western Blot banding pattern, or both (Sandler, Dodd, & Fang, 1988). The usual practice in this situation is to redraw the patient's blood and repeat the HIV antibody test. The patient should be informed that this occurs occasionally and does not necessarily indicate that the test result will be positive, except in the case of seroconversion. In most cases, the repeat test will be negative. Understandably, however, the patient may need reassurance during this additional period of waiting for results.

## HIV-Positive Results

The purposes of posttest counseling for HIV-positive women are to provide accurate information about the meaning of HIV infection and to provide support as they cope with their test results. It is helpful to prepare for the session by reviewing the patient's support network and developing an initial medical and psychosocial follow-up plan before an HIV-positive woman arrives for her posttest counseling appointment. A second staff person may sit in on the counseling session to act as a support person and to assess gaps in understanding.

At a minimum, the following issues should be covered in the initial session: (1) the patient's positive test results and the reliability of the test; (2) the meaning of a positive test result and a review of how HIV is transmitted and how the infection affects the immune system; (3) maintenance of health issues, including the availability of early treatments, such as zidovudine; (4) a review of safer sex practices and safer needle use, if appropriate; (5) where the test results will be recorded and who has access to the record; (6) issues relating to perinatal transmission if the woman is pregnant or planning pregnancy; and (7) identification of a support person for the patient.

Table 9–2   Posttest HIV Counseling Protocol

| Negative Result | Indeterminate Result |
| --- | --- |
| • Patient informed that HIV antibody result is negative<br>• Reliability of test result (ELISA and blot > 99%, sensitive/specific) discussed<br>• Meaning of negative test result: probable nonexposure to HIV<br>• If exposed to HIV in past 6 months, antibody may not have developed, and retesting is recommended<br>• Review of HIV transmission modes: sexual contact, blood/blood product injection, perinatal transmission<br>• Ways to avoid exposure to HIV reviewed<br>   "Safer" sex guidelines:<br>     -Decreasing number of sexual partners decreases chance of exposure<br>     -If sexual partner has engaged or is engaging in past/present risk, patient may be at risk of HIV exposure<br>     -Use of latex condoms and spermicide<br>     -HIV counseling and testing of partner<br>   "Safer" use guidelines, if appropriate:<br>     -If using needles, do not share; instruct to use sterile needles, if available, or to decontaminate them (chlorine/rinse)<br>• Patient informed blood supply is HIV tested and safe<br>• Discuss partner testing<br>• Literature for HIV-negative results given<br>• Other patient questions/concerns discussed | • Patient given result<br>• Test technology discussed<br>• Reasons can include "window period"<br>• Retesting required |

*Source:* Adapted with permission from the Perinatal HIV Transmission Study Team, SUNY Health Science Center, Brooklyn, New York, 1990.

TABLE 9–2   *(Continued)*

Positive Result

- Patient informed that HIV antibody test result is positive
- Reliability of test result discussed (ELISA is confirmed with Western Blot; false positives rarely occur)
- Meaning of a positive test result: indicates infection with HIV; duration of infection is considered lifelong; patient at risk for developing AIDS-related conditions
- Explanation/review of HIV infection:
    CD4 cell depletion, opportunistic infections
    Spectrum of disease (asymptomatic to AIDS)
    Asymptomatic stage lasts years; individual rate of disease development
- Maintenance of health:
    Treatment options: ZDV and PCP prophylaxis as appropriate, based on CD4
    Nutrition
    Avoidance of drug use
    Importance of close medical follow-up
- Modes of transmission reviewed:
    Sexual contact, blood/blood product injection, perinatal transmission
    Casual, household contact not a mode.
- Prevention of HIV transmission:
        "Safer" sex guidelines:
                - Use of latex condoms and spermicide
                - Informing current/future sexual partner(s)
        "Safer" needle use guidelines, if appropriate:
                - If using needles, do not share; instruct to decontaminate
                  needles with chlorine/water rinse
    Do not donate blood or organs
    Inform health care personnel of HIV status
    Perinatal transmission averted if no pregnancy
- Confidentiality:
    Discuss where HIV status is noted and who has access to record, discuss who to share HIV test results with, why, and in what circumstances
- Perinatal/reproduction issues (as appropriate):
    Probabilities of perinatal transmission (based on current data & woman's disease status)
    Spectrum of disease if child infected
    Option for pregnancy termination p.r.n.
    Breast feeding discouraged if infant formula a suitable alternative
    Risks of infant to other children or caregivers (HIV not casually transmitted)
- Support systems: patient identified support network; option of attending support group discussed
- Referred for HIV evaluation and ongoing medical care: patient; other family members at risk for HIV (e.g., sexual partner, young children)
- Literature for HIV-positive results given to patient
- Other patient questions/concerns discussed

Patients should be informed of their positive test results as soon as the session begins. Women's initial reactions to learning that they are HIV positive vary from stoicism to shouting and crying (Holman et al., 1989). Lack of comprehension and denial are commonly seen as patients first begin to assimilate this information. Occasionally, a woman may want to leave the counseling session while still in crisis, but it is important to allow her enough time during the session to work through some of her initial reactions. This initial session may last between 45 and 75 minutes.

Usually, a woman's first concerns are about the implications of HIV infection for her health and for her children's health. A realistic review of HIV infection can be combined with an outline of the available treatment options. If the woman is asymptomatic, this should be stressed. It is not uncommon for patients to believe that they have AIDS when they learn of a positive test result. The use of "realistic optimism" and practical support, such as referrals to community-based support systems, is more useful than quoting statistics about HIV disease at this stage (Volberding, 1990). If the woman has young children, she may be concerned that they are infected, and arrangements should be made to have them evaluated for HIV. Patients may also worry about the possibility of household transmission. Numerous studies have shown no evidence of household transmission (Gershon, Vlahov, & Nelson, 1990), and the improbability of this type of transmission should be stressed.

A review and discussion of "safer" needle use should occur if there is a history of intravenous needle use. Referrals for drug treatment should be made available. For drug users, substance abuse is a means of attempting to reduce stress, and it is not uncommon for drug users to react to the stress of learning that they are HIV positive by increasing their drug use for a period of time (Cancellieri et al., 1988).

Safer sexual practices and the issue of partner notification should be discussed at the initial counseling session. Some women may choose not to inform their partners immediately, preferring to wait until they have adjusted somewhat and feel the time is appropriate. Others may tell their partners right away and may want to bring the partner in for counseling and testing. Intense emotions may be at play with respect to partner notification: guilt about past behaviors, anger toward the partner, fear that the partner may have been infected, a sense of loss of "normal" sexuality. It is important to be sensitive to these intense, possibly conflicting feelings and to remain nonjudgmental and accepting.

Perinatal and reproductive concerns must be addressed at the initial session if the patient is pregnant or is planning a pregnancy. Transmission of HIV from infected mother to child occurs approximately 25% of the time (see chapter 6 for an in-depth discussion of perinatal transmission), and at this time, there is no standard method to detect which pregnancies will result in an infected child. As more information accrues about particular factors associated with an increased risk of perinatal transmission, there may be a need to tailor what is known about transmission to help the patient assess her individual health status and risks. However, staff should bear in mind that—as occurs with HIV-negative women—much of the reasoning about whether to keep or terminate a pregnancy may have to do with nonclinical issues, such as whether the pregnancy was planned.

If a woman is pregnant, the discussion about perinatal transmission and the possibility of disease in the infant is particularly salient to her current situation. The option of abortion, if legal and appropriate to the circumstances, should be discussed in a neutral, noncoercive manner. If a woman is considering abortion, her general feelings about abortion and the baby as well as her partner's feelings should be explored. The issue of who will take care of the children if she becomes ill or dies is a difficult but necessary one to explore. The patient should be encouraged to involve any appropriate significant others in the decision about an abortion. Mechanisms for obtaining an abortion should be discussed, and the patient's decision, regardless of whether she opts to continue the pregnancy or to terminate it, should be supported.

It is helpful to have the patient identify a support person before they leave the initial session, if possible. This person must be able to keep the patient's confidence and be supportive of her and her situation. Some women choose to disclose to their partners, some to their mothers or sisters, and some, more rarely, to a friend. Occasionally, a woman may not feel she is able to tell anyone in her family or network of friends. In these cases, it is especially important to offer ongoing counseling, participation in a support group, or both.

There are other issues to discuss, but not necessarily at the initial counseling session: the need to maintain a good nutritional intake and to avoid drugs and alcohol, the avoidance of donating blood or organs, the importance of informing other health care providers so they are able to provide appropriate care, and referrals for other family members for evaluation of HIV status and care.

Arrangements should be made for an evaluation and ongoing HIV-related medical care. A follow-up appointment for another counseling session is usually necessary and should be made before the patient leaves the initial session. Significant others, especially the sexual partner, should be encouraged to attend the follow-up session. At the follow-up session, which should ideally be scheduled a short time after the initial one, the patient's emotional status and gaps in knowledge can be assessed. The counseling of any significant others can occur, and additional information can be provided to the patient. It is important to stress the health care provider's continued availability to discuss HIV-related issues. HIV literature should be provided to reinforce and clarify information for both the patient and her support network. All posttest counseling of HIV-positive women should be documented in the patient's record, including referrals that were provided and arrangements for ongoing care. Table 9–2 summarizes the information to be covered in the posttest session.

## Long-Term Follow-Up

HIV-negative women who continue behaviors that put them at risk of acquiring HIV should be counseled periodically. This follow-up counseling should focus on the reduction of risk: the initiation and mainte-nance of safer sexual behaviors. To promote a shared responsibility for risk reduction, sexual partners should be included whenever possible. Retesting should be offered every 6 months, and again, sexual partners should be encouraged to be tested as well. Women who continue to use intravenous drugs should receive additional counseling on safe needle use. Some women may also benefit from peer support groups to help them initiate and main-tain risk-reduction behaviors. Another essential element in long-term fol-low-up of at-risk HIV-negative women is the supportive attitudes of health care providers toward their patients, especially with regard to sexual be-havior.

HIV-positive women require ongoing care for multiple needs, including clinical and psychosocial care, access to research as appropriate, support with material needs such as housing and temporary child care, and contra-ception/safer sex options (Figure 9–1). It has been pointed out that many women of reproductive age, especially those with a history of drug addic-tion, have undergone surgical contraception/tubal ligation but also need health prevention messages and reproductive services (Armstrong, Samost, & Smith, 1991).

The importance of preventing HIV transmission to partners must be discussed, often over a period of time. Many women experience sexual dysfunction and depression on learning of their HIV diagnosis. They may react with feelings of shame, guilt, worthlessness, or denial because of the inordinate stigma still placed on this disease and the fact that they face an uncertain future with a high likelihood of fatal outcome. Many women become abstinent and may need psychological and/or psychiatric services in learning to cope with their diagnosis. Establishing a trusting relationship with health care workers can prove an invaluable source of support for dealing with the diagnosis of HIV, its impact on one's physical, sexual, and emotional health, and the discussion of one's status with existing, past, or potential sexual partners (Denenberg, 1993).

HIV-positive women require long term follow-up of their chronic dis-ease, both medically and psychosocially. Women with advanced HIV dis-ease have additional needs that may be addressed through counseling. These include concerns about physical well-being and loss of functioning,

- Ongoing counseling and support for safer sex, contraception, interconceptual planning
- Clinical care
- Access to research trials (adult, pediatric)
- Social services (case management, housing, health coverage, income entitlement programs)
- Legal resources (life planning, child-care issues such as temporary custody and aftercare)

FIGURE 9–1   Ongoing needs of HIV-positive women—Long-term follow-up.

death and dying issues, both short- and long-term child care and custody arrangements, and other legal issues, such as wills. (For a more detailed discusssion of these issues, see chapters 10 and 17.)

## ❖ Summary

HIV poses unique concerns for women of reproductive age. Most current public health strategies recommend that HIV testing and counseling be offered to all women of reproductive age. Some recommend routine testing, with counseling, in areas of high seroprevalence. With a proper system in place, it is clear that knowledge of HIV status can provide benefits by ensuring that a woman's health and pregnancy can be better monitored and supported (Williams, 1990).

As discussed in detail in chapter 2, the ideal HIV-disease caregiving system has several components. Counseling is essential and should include information sharing and assistance in grief processing. For some, emotional support may be found in groups comprised of seropositive women. The social service needs of women with HIV must be addressed. They include the treatment of addiction, housing and financial concerns, and child care. Clinical care specific to HIV disease presentation in women, such as early detection of gynecologic markers and the availability for enrollment in clinical treatment trials, is essential.

As the HIV pandemic has evolved over the past decade, the number of women affected by this virus has swelled. HIV counseling and testing is increasingly becoming a standard of primary care practice, and providers need to incorporate the appropriate knowledge and skills in order to provide these services. It is up to these providers not only to develop but also to safeguard a standard of care for counseling and testing that ensures confidentiality and referral for a comprehensive array of needed services. Public policy should stress a multifactorial approach to preventing further HIV transmission, including appropriate addiction treatment strategies, outreach to men to prevent transmission to female partners and to children, and clinical and psychosocial support for HIV-positive women and their families.

## ❖ References

Amaro, H. (1993). Reproductive choice in the age of AIDS: Policy and counselling issues. In C. Squire (Ed.), *Women and AIDS—Psychological perspectives*. London: Sage.

Angell, M. (1991). A dual approach to the AIDS epidemic. *New England Journal of Medicine, 324,*(21) 1498–1500.

Armstrong, K., Samost, L., & Smith, H. (1991, June). HIV related risks of sterilized and non-sterilized drug abusing women. Paper presented at the Seventh International Conference on AIDS, Florence.

Barbacci, M., Repke, J. T., & Chaisson, R. (1991). Routine prenatal screening for HIV infection. *Lancet, 337* (8743), 709–711.

Berer, M., & Ray, S. (1993). *Women and HIV/AIDS: An international sourcebook.* London: Pandora Press.

Boekeloo, B. O., Rabin, D., Coughlin, S., Labbok, M., & Johnson, J. (1993). Knowledge, attitudes, and practices of obstetrician-gynecologists regarding the prevention of human immunodeficiency virus infection. *Obstetrics and Gynecology, 81*(1), 131–136.

Brotman, A. W., & Forstein, M. (1988). AIDS obsessions in depressed heterosexuals. *Psychosomatics, 29*(4), 428–432.

Cancellieri, F. R., Fine, J., Holman, S., Sunderland, A., Landesman, S., & Bihari, B. (1988). Psychological reactions to human immunodeficiency virus infection in drug using pregnant women. In R. E. Schinazi & A. J. Nahmias (Eds.), *AIDS in children, adolescents and heterosexual adults: An interdisciplinary approach to prevention* (pp. 207–209). New York: Elsevier.

Centers for Disease Control. (1985). Recommendations for assisting in the prevention of perinatal transmission of human T-lymphotrophic virus type III/lymphadenopathy-associated virus and acquired immunodeficiency syndrome. *Morbidity and Mortality Weekly Report, 34,* 721–732.

Centers for Disease Control. (1987). Public health service guidelines for counseling and antibody testing to prevent HIV infection and AIDS. *Morbidity and Mortality Weekly Report, 36,* 509–515.

Centers for Disease Control and Prevention. (1993). Update: Mortality attributable to HIV infection among persons aged 25–44 years—United States, 1991 and 1992. *Morbidity and Mortality Weekly Report, 42*(45), 869–872.

Centers for Disease Control and Prevention. (1994). Zidovudine for the prevention of HIV transmission from mother to infant. *Morbidity and Mortality Weekly Report, 43*(16), 285–287.

Dattel, B. J., Padian, N., Shannon, M., Miller, J., Cromblehome, W. R., & Sweet, R. L. (1991, June). *HIV serostatus and risk unrelated to pregnancy planning or contraceptive use*. Paper presented at the Seventh International Conference on AIDS, Florence.

Denenberg, R. (1993). Gynecological considerations in the primary care setting. In A. Kurth (Ed.), *Until the cure: Caring for women with HIV* (pp. 35–46). New Haven: Yale University Press.

Faden, R., Geller, G., & Powers, M. (1992). *AIDS, women and the next generation.* New York: Oxford University Press.

Flaskerud, J. H., & Rush, C. E. (1989). AIDS and traditional health beliefs and practices of black women. *Nursing Research, 38*(4), 210–215.

Gershon, R. R. M., Vlahov, D., & Nelson, K. E. (1990). The risk of transmission of HIV-1 through non-percutaneous, non-sexual modes—A review. *AIDS, 4*(7), 645–650.

Hanley, E., & Lincoln, P. (1992). HIV infection in women: Implications for nursing practice. *Nursing Clinics of North America, 27*(4), 925–936.

Holman, S., Berthaud, M., Sunderland, A., Moroso, G., Cancellieri, F., Mendez, H., Beller, E., & Marcel, A. (1989). Women infected with human immunodeficiency virus: Counseling and testing during pregnancy. *Seminars in Perinatology, 13*(1), 7–15.

Hunter, N. D. (1992). Complications of gender: Women and HIV disease. In N. D. Hunter & W. Rubenstein (Eds.), *AIDS agenda: Emerging issues in civil rights.* New York: New Press.

Hutchison, M., & Kurth, A. (1991). "I need to know that I have a choice": A study of women, HIV, and reproductive decision-making. *AIDS Patient Care, 5*(1), 17–25.

Institute of Medicine. (1990). *Prenatal and newborn screening for HIV.* Washington, DC: National Academy Press.

James, M. E. (1988). HIV seropositivity diagnosed during pregnancy: Psychosocial characterization of patients and their adaptation. *General Hospital Psychiatry, 10*(5), 309–316.

Jason, J., Evatt, B. L., & the Hemophilia-AIDS Collaborative Study Group. (1990). Pregnancies in human immunodeficiency virus–infected sex partners of hemophilic men. *American Journal of the Diseases of Children, 144*(4), 485–490.

Johnstone, F. D., Brettle, R., MacCallum, L., Mok, J., Peuthever, J. F., & Burns, S. (1990). Women's knowledge of their HIV antibody state; Its effect on their decision whether to continue the pregnancy. *British Medical Journal, 300*(6716), 23–24.

Kelly, P. (1992). Fertility, menstruation, and birth control in HIV. *Treatment Issues* (Gay Men's Health Crisis [GMHC]), *6*(7), 10–14.

Kurth, A. (1993). An overview of women and HIV. In A. Kurth (Ed.), *Until the cure: Caring for women with HIV* (pp. 1–18). New Haven: Yale University Press.

Levine, C. (1979). Genetic counseling: The client's viewpoint. In A. M. Capron, M. Lappe, R. F. Murray, T. M. Powledge, S. B. Twiss, & D. Bergsma (Eds.), *Genetic counseling: Facts, values and norms.* New York: Allen R. Liss.

Lewis, C., & Freeman, H. (1987). The sexual history-taking and counseling practices of primary care physicians. *Western Journal of Medicine, 147*(2), 165–167.

Macks, J. (1988). Women and AIDS: Countertransference issues. *Social Casework, 69,* 340–347.

Martin, L. S., McDougal, J. S., & Loskoski, S. L. (1985). Disinfection and inactivation of human T lymphotropic virus III/lymphadenopathy-associated virus. *Journal of Infectious Diseases, 152*(2), 400–404.

Mays, V. M., & Cochran, S. D. (1987). Acquired immune deficiency syndrome and black Americans: Special psychosocial issues. *Public Health Reports, 102*(2), 225–231.

Minkoff, H. L. (1992). *American Journal of Women's Health, 1,* 137–140, 193–196.

Minkoff, H. L., Holman, S., Beller, E., Delke, I., Fishbone, A., & Landesman, S. (1988). Routinely offered prenatal HIV testing. *New England Journal of Medicine, 319*(15), 1018.

Mitchell, J., Brown, G., Loftman, P., & Williams, S. (1990). HIV infection in pregnancy: Detection, counseling, and care. *Pediatric AIDS and HIV Infection: Fetus to Adolescent, 1* (5), 78–82.

Naber, J., & Johnson, D. (1993). Mandatory HIV testing issues in state newborn screening programs. *Journal of Law and Health, 7,* 55–68.

National Institute on Drug Abuse (NIDA). (1993, March 25). Proposed recommendations to prevent HIV transmission by sharing drug injection equipment. *Community Alert Bulletin.*

Nolan, K. (1989). Ethical issues in caring for pregnant women and newborns at risk for human immunodeficiency virus infection. *Seminars in Perinatology, 13*(1), 55–65.

Partridge, J., & Milliken, N. (1991, June). *HIV antibody tests in women: Physicians and informed consent.* Paper presented at the Seventh International Conference on AIDS, Florence.

Rapp, R. (1987). Counseling women at risk: Models, myths, ambiguities. Speech presented at The Hastings Center, New York, December.

Sandler, G. S., Dodd, R. Y., & Fang, C. T. (1988). Diagnostic tests for HIV infection: Serology. In V. T. DeVita, S. Hellman, & S. A. Rosenburg (Eds.), *AIDS: Etiology, diagnosis, treatment and prevention* (pp. 121–136). Philadelphia: J. B. Lippincott.

Schoenbaum, E., & Webber, M. (1993). The underrecognition of HIV infection in women in an inner-city emergency room. *American Journal of Public Health, 83*(3), 363–368.

Selwyn, P. A., Carter, R. J., Schoenbaum, E. E., Robertson, V. J., Klein, R. S., & Rogers, M. F. (1989). Knowledge of HIV antibody status and decisions to continue or terminate pregnancy among intravenous drug users. *Journal of the American Medical Association, 261*(24), 3567–3571.

Sherr, L. (1993). HIV testing in pregnancy. In C. Squires (Ed.), *Women and AIDS: Psychological perspectives.* London: Sage.

Springer, E. (1991). Effective AIDS prevention with active drug users: The harm reduction model. In M. Shernoff (Ed.), *Counseling chemically dependent people with HIV illness.* New York: Haworth Press.

Sunderland, A., Minkoff, H. L., Handte, J., Moroso, G., & Landesman, S. (1992). The influence of serostatus on women's reproductive decisions. *Obstetrics and Gynecology, 7*(6), 1027–1031.

Volberding, P. (1990, May). How to tell patients they have HIV disease. *AIDS Clinical Care, 2*(2).

Williams, A. (1990). Reproductive concerns of women at risk for HIV infection. *Journal of Nurse-Midwifery, 35*(5), 292–298.

World Health Organization. (1990). *AIDS prevention: Guidelines for MCH/FP programme managers, II. AIDS and maternal health.* Geneva: Author.

World Health Organization. (1993, September). *13 million HIV positive women by 2000*. Press release at the Second International Conference on HIV in Children and Mothers, Edinburgh.

Young, R., Weissman, G., & Cohen, J. (1992). Assessing risk in the absence of information: HIV risk among women injection-drug users who have sex with women. *AIDS and Public Policy Journal, 7*(3), 175–182.

# ❖ Chapter 10

# Women and Their Families: Psychosocial Stages of HIV Infection

JUDY WEAVER MASON

JOYCE E. PREISINGER

SISTER MARY DONOHUE

Intimately woven into all phases of debilitating, progressive, and fatal diseases like HIV infection are the emotional, social, and environmental variables that influence treatment, health-seeking behaviors, disease course, and outcome. The changing psychosocial needs of women with HIV infection are closely linked to the progressive course of the disease. Some needs are constant throughout the course of the illness, whereas others dominate during a particular phase. After diagnosis, patients and their families must begin the difficult task of reorganizing their lives (Becker & Becker, 1986; Rehr, Berkman, & Rosenberg, 1980; Sands, 1983). The strain of the prolonged and unpredictable disease course creates problems for those with whom the patient has personal or occupational ties and may precipitate a breakdown of the family unit (Christ, Weiner, & Moynihan, 1986). As changes in body functions and physical appearance begin to manifest, the woman may experience significant psychosocial changes.

We have delineated four psychosocial stages that occur during the progression of HIV disease: (1) confrontation, (2) adjustment, (3) spiraling, and (4) end of life. Confrontation with mortality becomes very real when first learning about a seropositive status. This frightening experience is often viewed as an immediate death sentence. During the asymptomatic stages, inconsistencies between the deadly internal processes at work and an external healthy appearance bring a need for adjustments and adaptations. One day a woman feels normal, and the next, she remembers she is seropositive. Her priorities and life-style begin to change, and it becomes increasingly evident that life will never be the same. As the spiraling effects of single or multiple symptoms are seen, the infected woman and her family must deal with reminders of disease progression: the episodic course of HIV disease, alternating between stable periods and sudden flare-ups, frequent clinic visits and hospitalizations, and body changes. Moving from the crisis of diagnosis to end-stage AIDS intensifies the need for social and spiritual supports. Dependency needs then are based not solely on functional problems, but also on the realization that the end of life is nearing. Patients grieve for themselves while grieving for their loved ones. Conceptualizing the psychosocial stages of HIV disease can contribute to the development of more effective treatment planning for women and their families as they confront lives irrevocably altered by illness.

## ❖ Confrontation

The patient's initial response to learning that she has tested HIV seropositive is often grief, shock, or terror. Reactions can cover the gamut of feelings from stunned disbelief to anger, shame, guilt, fear, anxiety, and loss. It is not uncommon to equate HIV with death and to feel condemned by the disease, society, and even family and friends. Common reactions include these: "Does this mean I'm going to die?" "How long do I have to live?" "This must be a mistake." When told that she is infected with the virus that causes AIDS, a woman may sit, disbelieving, in stunned silence or may sob uncontrollably. Sadness and depression frequently follow the initial shock of diagnosis.

Many who are faced with the diagnosis of HIV infection react with the psychological defense of denial, which is used to keep unconscious thoughts and feelings from the conscious mind. Denial is an important and natural reaction to trauma, and it can serve to cushion the impact of receiving devastating news. However, if used for an extended period of time, the result can be maladaptive. A patient in denial may refuse treatment or related services or may continue high-risk and self-destructive behaviors, such as substance abuse or unhealthy sexual practices. Assessment of the degree of denial and how it affects the functioning of the client and family will provide direction for interventions. For some patients, denial can be supported, whereas for others, confrontation can allow them to move on with the remainder of life.

Denial at this time may also impede the early grief process, which is needed to anticipate and prepare for losses, deal with unfinished business, and eventually say good-bye. Acknowledgment of loss, facilitated by clear information and open communication, is crucial at this time because it is the sharing of experiences of loss that prepares for the next phase, adaptation or adjustment (Walsh & McGoldrick, 1991).

Anger is another emotion of this psychosocial stage that may become manifest in a number of ways internally or externally directed. Anger at oneself may be shown by an inability to cooperate or conform with the medical or social plan of care or by self-destructive behaviors related to alcohol and other substance abuse. Depression is another manifestation of anger. Anger may also be directed toward the person who is held responsible for transmission of HIV infection or someone not related to the illness. Domestic violence may be exhibited, including failure to take precautions to prevent HIV infection in others.

Issues introduced during the confrontation stage with HIV include coping with the woman's own illness and prospective death as well as the possible death of a child or partner; notification of family members, friends, and present and past partners; coping with feelings of guilt and failure related to dying before her children are grown; informing children about the illness and dealing with their grief about the loss or anticipated loss of a parent; and planning for the time when the patient will be physically unable to care for her children. Many issues relate to changes in the roles women play and which have an impact on their sense of self and on their families.

⌐The largest number of women infected with HIV are poor and from racial or ethnic minority groups seriously disenfranchised and medically disadvantaged (Minkoff & DeHovitz, 1991). For some women, HIV disease is one more blow in a life already seriously compromised by limited resources through substance use, violence, hopelessness, psychological problems, encounters with the criminal justice system, homelessness, and other manifestations of poverty. There are often few resources for these families to use in dealing with the overwhelming demands of a chronic, life-threatening illness. Even these infected women who are able to meet their basic needs wrestle with fears of becoming not only stigmatized, but also economically and physically dependent should they become ill (Benson & Maier, 1990). ⌐

Families with HIV infection may also experience numerous uncertainties related to the unpredictable course of HIV illness, the reactions of other people, the possibility that children or significant others may also be infected, and the impact on work, relationships, finances, sex life, reproduction, and parenting. These uncertainties can generate feelings of anxiety, a major component of which is guilt. Because HIV transmission has been primarily associated with sexual promiscuity and drug use, AIDS is viewed by some as a punishment for these behaviors (Krieger, 1988).

Many women infected with HIV are young, in their 20s and 30s (Levine & Dubler, 1990). During these peak childbearing years, the issues of child and reproductive health are of prime concern. To be identified as HIV-positive during pregnancy can be overwhelming, and the woman may be incapable of logically assessing the full impact of her serostatus on her pregnancy or of anticipating what effect decisions could have on her life. Some motivations considered by women in decision making are their reproductive capability and the meaning they place on being a mother. Motherhood may be an important source of pride and identity to them, a reason to go on living, or an attempt to right the wrongs of the past (Hutchison & Kurth, 1991).

With the inherent uncertainty of perinatal HIV transmission, many women are willing to take the risks of pregnancy because the alternatives—including rejection by their partner or disclosure of their HIV status to their family—may seem worse (Levine & Dubler, 1990). A value-neutral approach to counseling women, with a clear delineation of their range of reproductive choices, is essential (see chapter 9). Women need information about the impact of HIV infection on pregnancy, the effect of pregnancy on HIV infection, perinatal transmission, and pediatric AIDS. When dealing with decision making early in pregnancy, the pressures of time must be clearly stated in a supportive and nonjudgmental manner.

The patient's psychosocial needs should be assessed at the first contact and throughout the course of the therapeutic relationship. The patient's level of crisis must be assessed. This is done by evaluating her affective response, coping ability, history of trauma and loss, and her plans and wishes. General areas to be addressed include prediagnosis functioning, coping skills, current strengths and vulnerabilities, and present or past family dysfunction, such as drug or alcohol use, psychiatric problems, and family violence. The woman's perception of her support network must be carefully evaluated and should include extended family, house of worship, and neighborhood as well as the mechanics of mobilizing the support. A present-oriented, problem-solving approach is indicated in which information is provided, options presented, skills assessed, and the patient's decisions supported.

## Interventions

Care delivered to women in the confrontation stage should extend over several sessions. The kind of support, crisis intervention, and education needed for people dealing with HIV disease can best be provided through a multidisciplinary team approach (Cohen, 1990). Assistance may be required to help the patient balance use of defense mechanisms, such as denial, avoidance, projection, and intellectualization, with productive coping strategies in order to foster optimum involvement with others, health-promoting and life-enhancing activities, responsibilities toward others, and a sense of hope.

During the confrontation phase, the woman may want help to identify her own complex emotions and to make some sense of her overwhelming situation. For this to happen, a safe environment must be provided, free of judgment and guilt, where trust in caregivers can be established. Clinicians need to normalize the experience for the patient in order to develop a context into which the trauma of HIV can fit (Bidgood, 1991). This can be accomplished by promoting an atmosphere in which feelings are shared and validated. In doing so, the patient is helped to feel that she is not alone and that someone else understands. When someone else verbalizes the patient's responses, her feelings are acknowledged. The stage can then be set for the sharing of such life-sustaining feelings as hope and expectation, a starting point for adjustment.

Information and education about HIV disease help the woman to regain a sense of control over her life. Discussions should include how to stay healthy, reducing the risk of transmission, the need for medical evaluation and treatment to contain the illness, enhancing the quality of life, legitimate fears of rejection and discrimination, and issues relating to disclosure. Information helps to reduce stress as the client begins to move toward a more positive view of living. Consideration of the range of options available, prioritizing tasks, and delineating ways to take direct action are other skills that promote mastery.

When face to face with the life-threatening implications of HIV positivity, catastrophic fears can trigger thoughts of suicide, which must be carefully evaluated. Sharing suicidal feelings with an empathic listener is not only relieving, but may provide a different perspective. It is essential that a comprehensive multidisciplinary team approach be used that includes a component for psychiatric evaluation and follow-up. In settings where this is not available on site, familiarity with community mental health resources and good linkage systems is needed to ensure that referrals have a successful outcome. To resolve a suicidal crisis, the patient's bonds with a supportive network of family, friends, and caregivers should be reestablished.

Assisting the patient to articulate a concrete plan can serve to provide a structure at a time when the internal foundation is unsteady. Prioritizing on the basis of a patient's individual situation, taking into account her strengths and weaknesses, can help her feel less overwhelmed as permission is given not to deal with everything at once. (See Case 1 Vignette.)

## ❖ Case 1 Vignette ❖

In the case vignette that follows, one woman is confronted with news of an HIV-positive test result.

Ms. B was a 30-year-old unmarried mother of seven children who earned her living as a security guard. The patient presented with a 12-week unplanned pregnancy. Initially, she expressed ambivalence about the pregnancy and was considering adoption, though her partner of 6 months favored termination. Although Ms. B denied any risk behaviors and agreed to voluntary HIV-antibody testing, she became angry and hostile when efforts were initiated to schedule a meeting to review the test result. The patient appeared in the clinic a few days later and was informed that she had tested HIV positive. At that time she was firm about her intention to keep her baby. For the duration of her pregnancy, this patient exhibited a range of ambivalent behaviors. For example, she vowed she would not return to clinic, then appeared unexpectedly. Ms. B refused to keep scheduled appointments, refused specialized medical care services, and refused to have any of her children tested. The patient also impulsively contacted an attorney to arrange permanent and immediate custody for her children.

**Analysis**    This patient's style of coping was proactive, heading off her losses in advance. This was exemplified by her efforts to make arrangements to have her children permanently placed in the custody of others, even before her medical status was evaluated. For Ms. B, the idea of dying was so present and unbearable that it was preferable to give her children up than to be a helpless, passive victim. This was a maladaptive response, but it was the patient's way of symbolically taking control of her life.

### Interventions

1. Assess coping skills, mental functioning (i.e., level of cognitive functioning, judgment, suicidal ideation), and support network.
2. Educate the patient about the characteristics of HIV disease, notification, safe sex, and medical treatment.
3. Introduce decision-making imperatives and strategies in the areas of medical care, disclosure, reproductive choices, child custody arrangements, and prevention.

## ❖ Adjustment

Moving from learning the diagnosis to living with HIV disease is a major transition. Feeling healthy, yet aware of her infection with HIV, the patient moves between hope and hopelessness, depression and escapism, fear and courage. Emotional responses can fluctuate moment to moment, day to day. There is the ever-present fear of waking up with some sign of deteriorating health or of being perceived differently by family, children, or friends. Consoled to see that the reflection in the mirror still looks the same, the fear may again submerge temporarily and precariously below the surface.

As the infected woman and the affected family members struggle to make sense of their lives with HIV infection, they often try to forget the seropositivity and return to normal patterns of interaction. Long-term personal and familial goals may be adjusted to short-term goals. As one woman indicated, "I no longer plan for a year. I plan for 3 months at a time." Family members may also make life readjustments, such as emphasizing quality moments spent with the infected individual. Still others seek refuge in defensive strategies like denial and violence.

When substance use is part of the patient's history, preexisting unresolved personal and social dysfunctions, such as poor self-esteem, feelings of alienation from family, or poor interpersonal and work histories, may also be present. Compounded by ill health, these stressors may precipitate relapse or increased risky behaviors associated with drug addiction (Stein, 1991).

Even before the onset of any symptoms, the continuing threat of illness and eventual death make loss an ever-present theme for women with HIV infection. For most women, not fulfilling their image of the mothering role generates grief, as evidenced in uncertainty about her own and her children's health, fear of not living to see children grow up, or disappointment in not having the number of children that the woman and her partner desire. Another threat to the mothering role is the actual or potential transmission of HIV infection to her children. For many women, concern for who will care for the children after their death is paramount. They may have to begin to let go of many aspects of the mother role to secure a safe place for their children to live well before they die.

The adjustment stage may usher in a renewed sense of spirituality. Women and affected family members may bargain for prolonged life or to have a child's life spared.

Disclosure is a major issue throughout the course of HIV disease. Women with HIV infection wonder who to inform, when, and under what circumstances. Most women choose to tell one or two intimates, those in need of testing and medical care, and those whom the woman feels can offer nonjudgmental support. Dilemmas of disclosure are further complicated when other family members are infected. Although secrecy may be perceived by the woman as her best defense, it threatens the integrity of the family, strains relations between members, and can mean exposing the woman and her family to rejection and discrimination. Family disorganization and instability often erupt because only selected relatives are allowed to know of the patient's status. These "chosen" members may become polarized from others in the familial support network. Considerations involving disclosure to children are especially difficult, given the unpredictable nature of entrusting youngsters with a family secret (see chapter 7). When preparing to inform an infected or uninfected child, women must confront their own anger and fears.

Perhaps the most troublesome adjustment during this phase is linked to sex and intimacy. The emergence of conflicting feelings of wanting to be desired or touched and feeling guilty, dirty, and at risk for reexposure is often frustrating or demoralizing for women with HIV infection and their partners. Feelings of anger and betrayal about transmission can destroy a relationship. Stress can also occur because relationships are ending early in life. For some women, physical violence may be a reality when they attempt to exercise control over their own health and sexuality, such as insisting on condom use. Fears and concerns of losing a close friend or partner are heightened when the patient learns she is infected with the disease, or she may withdraw from family and friends when she perceives their shame and embarrassment. There may also be worries of transmitting the infection to uninfected family members.

Until women with HIV infection experience their first or multiple signs of ill health, preventive care is often ignored. Historically, women assumed the role of primary family caregiver, often seeing to the needs of others while neglecting themselves (Rosen & Blank, 1991). In the case of indigent families, this problem is often compounded by limited access to services and mistrust of the health care delivery system. Familial conflict may surface if family members who are aware of the patient'a seropositivity realize she is not actively pursuing medical treatment. Health care neglect and lack of compliance represent a form of maladaptive denial.

A woman's sense of identity is closely linked to her career choices, her employment, and the other financial means by which she provides for herself and her family. In the case of the impoverished woman, financial resources may have always been scant and marginally sufficient for the family. The career-oriented woman may not have previously had financial concerns, but these may emerge for the first time, threatening long-held goals. Adjustment to HIV disease will likely require negotiating financial assistance, health insurance coverage, and other social service systems.

Caregiving functions and needs change throughout the course of HIV disease. They are also contingent on the number of other family members infected and the severity of ill health at any given time. In the absence of physical symptoms, caregiving during the adjustment stage largely centers around increased emotional availability from members of the disclosure circle. Tangible demonstration of willingness to listen, compassion, and acceptance of the infected individual are the primary functions of the caregiver.

### Interventions

During the adjustment stage, the mental health provider's treatment goals should be geared to helping the patient find a balance in the emotional upheaval and make a series of important decisions that will affect the overall functioning of the patient and her family. Specific interventions should include exploring and normalizing expressed emotions, monitoring and evaluating coping capacity, and helping the patient to develop problem-solving strategies. Counseling sessions must incorporate assistance with anticipating possible outcomes and consequences of disclosure, overcoming resistance to psychosocial support from health providers and support networks when evident, obtaining timely access to medical care, modifying unhealthy behavior, and preparing for financial or other needed services when the patient becomes ill. (See Case 2 Vignette.)

### ❖ Case 2 Vignette ❖

The following case vignette illustrates some of the psychosocial dilemmas encountered by people adjusting to living with HIV.

Ms. S, age 45, was an employed African-American mother of a teenage son. She was infected through heterosexual transmission and was asymptomatic. Her husband of the past 6 years, a former intravenous drug user, had end-stage AIDS. Ms. S was actively involved in her spouse's medical care and regularly accompanied him to his clinic visits. She was not compliant with her own medical care because she did not feel sick. She had disclosed her illness to immediate family members, except her son. The family members discussed among themselves their feelings of shame about the illness and anger at the source of infection. The family had also encouraged Ms. S to tell her son of her serostatus. They frequently inquired about her health and encouraged her to seek needed medical care. This was met with dismissal and denial by Ms. S, whose maladaptive health-seeking behavior continued. In addition, Ms. S constantly refused invitations to traditional family gatherings.

**Analysis** This woman was unable to work through her denial and conflicted feelings of shame and fear of rejection in order to achieve acceptance of her illness. These immobilizing emotions were manifested through avoidance and denial of medical care, interaction with her family, disclosure to her son, and assistance from caregiving agencies.

### Interventions
1. Attempt outreach efforts to engage the patient in needed medical and counseling services.
2. Explore and normalize expressed emotions. Evaluate coping capacities, problem solving strategies, and barriers to medical care and familial interactions.
3. Assist the patient in anticipating possible consequences and outcome of disclosure to her son.
4. Educate the patient about caregiving resources, and assist in securing service for her spouse.

## ❖ Spiraling

The onset of symptoms, which for women may present as vaginal thrush that is unresponsive to treatment, cervical diseases or decreased appetite and wasting, brings a foreshadowing of disability, disfigurement, and eventual death to a previously asymptomatic woman. Alternatively, the patient's first hospitalization may force a realization of the physical, emotional, and social impact of HIV infection. At this time, the protective structures of denial typically begin to break down. Psychosocial reactions may be extreme and may include unbridled anxiety, depression, rage, and escape into drug use and risky sexual practices.

The progression of HIV disease brings intermittent illnesses of sudden onset and unpredictable duration and severity. The constant waxing and waning of physical vitality, deteriorating bodily functions, and changes in appearance can initiate a growing sense of powerlessness, loss, and grief in the HIV-infected person and her loved ones. As symptoms become more severe, repeated hospitalizations are common, each time exacerbating the feelings of loss of control and powerlessness. The unpredictable roller coaster of multiple relapses, followed by periods of relative plateau, create an enormous strain for the woman and her familiy.

The ability to function independently and to carry out prescribed roles decreases as established patterns of life become disrupted. Relationships with others undergo significant changes. There may be a scaling down of work capacity or the loss of a job, which affects the woman's feelings of self-worth and can precipitate a financial crisis. In some cases, family members and friends may find the situation too stressful and may depart.

Family roles begin to be renegotiated and reassigned. The normal life cycle of the family is disrupted. Older children are asked to assume the care of parents and younger siblings, often beyond age-appropriate expectations. Older adults may need to step in to parent their grown children and their children's children. The needs of uninfected family members may be postponed or completely neglected. Family members must also give up or make alterations in their future plans, dreams, and expectations. A long-term future orientation now focuses on the ordinary day-to-day aspects of life. Relationships with family and close friends take on great value. It is important to encourage women to build and maintain these relationships.

Many women with HIV infection are single-parent heads of household with primary responsibility for children and perhaps also for younger siblings or dependent parents. In our culture, women often assume the tasks of caregiving and bereavement for the terminally ill and surviving family members (Walsh & McGoldrick, 1991). Often, multiple members of the same family are infected with HIV and are at various points along the disease continuum. The woman with HIV infection thus frequently finds herself in the overwhelming position of being not only the patient, but also the primary caregiver to others, with the latter role exerting pressures to put her own care and needs aside.

Of all human experiences, death poses the most painful adaptational challenge for families (Walsh & McGoldrick, 1991). The sense of mortality experienced when there is an HIV-related death of someone close is especially acute for those family members who are themselves infected. They question who will be next. The death of a child can be the most tragic of losses for a family, disrupting the expected order of life. For a parent who has provided day-to-day care, this can mean the loss of a sense of purpose. The death of a child may trigger relationship changes, such as divorce, precipitous marriage, or the conception of another child. Although some changes bring a sense of renewal, hope, and joy, they also create new conflicts and can block mourning, which is essential for adjustment and resolution (Walsh & McGoldrick, 1991).

Multiple losses also diminish the support system and limit the number of remaining caregivers. Multiple or concurrent losses produce an accumulation of stress that is capable of overwhelming the most stable of families. The anxiety generated by facing the reality of death may lead to high-risk behaviors as anger and rage are acted out (Bidgood, 1991).

## Interventions

Families with AIDS need assistance in coping with the stress of these complicated situations. They require a supportive environment where members feel safe to express their hurt, anger, and fear. As they begin to make sense of the situation, an equilibrium can be established. Individual counseling works best in some instances, whereas in others, family sessions are of greatest benefit. Support groups and peer counselors are also valuable resources and should be considered. Stability can be provided to patients through supportive listening techniques, creating an environment where the patient's pain and grief can be heard and validated without judgment. The thoughts and feelings of surviving family members must be acknowledged and handled. When they are avoided, experiences of hopelessness, helplessness, and anxiety are promoted and can lead to dysfunctional behaviors and even psychiatric disorders.

## ❖ Case 3 Vignette ❖

This case vignette illustrates the effects of the spiraling phase of HIV disease that one woman experienced.

Ms. D was a 37-year-old Hispanic woman who was diagnosed with AIDS when she was admitted to the hospital in the first trimester of pregnancy with pneumocystis carinii pneumonia. She had three children, ages 14, 16, and 20. Ms. D had a history of intravenous drug use and for the past several years was successfully participating in a methadone maintenance program. The patient was happily married to her new husband of 2 years and was eager to cement this relationship with a child they had planned together. Her commitment to the pregnancy remained strong, even after her HIV status was confirmed. Despite her hospitalization and declining health, Ms. D could not immediately bring herself to share her diagnosis with her husband. For his part, the husband conspired with Ms. D to deny the obvious. The patient did, however, share her HIV-positivity one by one with her children, with the enlisted assistance of her social worker. After the birth of the baby, Ms. D was finally able to inform her husband, also. Although he was initially supportive, as Ms. D's health deteriorated, family conflict increased. After the son identified himself as a homosexual, the husband left the home, leaving the infant in the custody of the oldest daughter. As the family crisis escalated, caregiving needs were reevaluated, and professional home-care services were put into place.

**Analysis**  This patient needed to experience her control in the timing and manner of disclosure to family members. This, along with the child custody and other legal arrangements with which she was assisted following the birth of her child, was an important source of empowerment and helped to facilitate the family grieving process. For some time, this patient resisted home-care assistance. However, as the family began to disintegrate with her son's disclosure and her husband's leaving, she gradually became more amenable to home health supports, which were critical in this case.

### Interventions
1. Enlist and coordinate formal and informal caregivers.
2. Provide on-going assessment of coping ability, mental functioning, expanding financial and entitlement needs as medical condition escalates, and emerging home-care needs.
3. Offer supportive counseling in areas of grieving, custody planning, diminished capacity, and changing role function.
4. Plan for end-of-life, including attention to living will, health care proxy, and property and funeral arrangements.

## ❖ End of Life

The care of people who are dying with AIDS remains surrounded by such issues as fear, rejection, and isolation. The health care provider must often "walk with" the woman and her family as they travel the often lonely road to death (Donohue, 1993). In the last stage, psychosocial responses and family issues relate to the process of dying. The patient who has reached this stage of illness may experience emotions ranging from denial, guilt, bargaining, and depression to peace and acceptance. Both patient and family experience these emotions in varying intensity, length, or sequence.

Some women and families facing HIV/AIDS are acquiescent about death, considering the infection a death sentence from the beginning. Although treatments for other illnesses, such as cancer, allow some hope for survival, current morbidity and mortality evidence about HIV disease suggests to the infected woman that she cannot conquer the illness. Health care providers should try to foster realistic hope, even when there seems to be no alternative to death. Realistic hope is honest and supports the relationship of trust between the woman and her care provider.

Feelings of guilt may relate to the behaviors that led to the HIV infection or to broken relationships with oneself, significant others, families, or God or a higher power. The patient's awareness that she is dying may intensify these feelings because there may not be time to correct these broken relationships. She may have a sense that she is failing her children because she is dying, and she may be concerned that she will not leave positive memories with her children.

For some people, their relationship with God or a higher power takes on special importance during illness. People from formal or structured religions may want to participate in specific healing rituals or prayers and may put a great deal of emphasis on these, as well as on attention from the chaplain or other religious representative. In most cases, these activities seem to reflect the patient's desire to mend her relationship with God in the face of death.

Although some conservative religious beliefs have done much to make people dying of AIDS feel unworthy of forgiveness (Francis, 1989; Johnson, 1989), others make a strong distinction between the acts that led to the illness and the beauty and value of the patient, with the concomitant obligation to support her in whatever way possible.

## *Interventions*

Women and their families can be enabled to cope with this last phase of HIV disease when they know clearly what is happening and what to expect. Honest conversations with the woman and her family about medical decision making will allow them to feel some sense of control and will assure them that they will not be abandoned medically, socially, emotionally, or spiritually. Assisting the patient in personal care and providing extra attention (combing her hair, encouraging her to wear daytime clothes, getting an extra cup of tea, spending time listening to whatever she wants to talk about, discussing the realities of her situation) can give her a sense of continued respect. These actions may also allow family members to feel as if they can provide concrete assistance and may enable them to remain close to the dying person. Identifying reasonable, limited goals for family support may make staying with the dying person more bearable. Many families may feel unable to remain physically or emotionally with the dying person for any number of reasons. Group support for family members offers a safe outlet for emotions and a sense of not being alone. Figure 10–1 provides many concrete suggestions to assist family members in supporting a dying loved one.

Providers can assist patients in meeting spiritual needs during the terminal stage. With the ultimate goal of helping the patient to have a peaceful death, it is paramount to encourage and assist her with the resolution of any unfinished business, such as the reassessment of her life, the evaluation of its positive and unpleasant aspects, and the search for forgiveness or reconciliations.

At the moment of death, religious services or rituals and the spiritual assistance of clergy can be very comforting to the woman and the members of her support system. This is especially true if the chaplain has been a part of the journey all along, assisting the woman to have a peaceful death.

Care providers can assist the woman in achieving a peaceful death by being present and providing care in a way that reflects human dignity and respect.

- Be sensitive to your own fear of death, your resistance to letting the person go, and your grief from previous losses.
- Do not do it all alone! You need support, also. Learn the lessons for *you*.
- Take time to readjust your perspective before and after visits, avoiding abrupt changes of focus.
- Do not take it personally if the person does not want to see you or does not recognize you. Calling just before a visit and identifying yourself on arrival minimizes this possibility.
- Be sensitive to the discomforts of the illness and the medical interventions, such as IVs and catheters.
- Do not be offended if the person economizes on politeness and seems abrupt or irritable.
- Be aware of the side effects of medications on the personality (drowsiness, hallucination, disorientation).
- Be sensitive to the person's right to physical, emotional, and spiritual privacy. Support his or her attempts to be honest with you about your relationship.
- Encourage the person to make decisions, no matter how small, and to do what they can for themselves.
- Feel free to share humor; it is healing.
- A new level of honest communication may reveal previously hidden prejudices, old resentments, and suppressed emotions.
- Allow the dying person to reciprocate, to be there for *you*.
- Be patient. The timing is not ours.
- Be willing to listen, and be present to the person in the process. Allow his or her feelings of denial, anger, fear, depression, and acceptance.
- Communication is not always verbal. It is fine just to be present silently.
- As death nears, you may find yourself wanting to be with the person more often. Pace yourself. You are not essential to the process. A dying person may express a desire to have you present at the moment of death but then choose to die in your absence.

FIGURE 10–1   Suggestions for supporting a family member who is dying.

*Source*: Adapted with permission from B. Hermes (1993), *Together We Care: Kairos: Support for Caregivers*, 114 Douglass St., San Francisco, CA 94114-1921, tel. 415-861-0877.

## ❖ Summary

Women living with HIV face psychological and social adaptive tasks that are unique to their gender. Their access to health care, health-seeking behaviors, reproductive health choices, child-rearing responsibilities, and substance use have direct bearing on prognosis. The clinical manifestations and emotional and social factors engendered by HIV transmission are all distinguishing characteristics of a woman's vulnerability.

For proposed interventions to have optimal relevance and benefit, early crisis and supportive counseling is essential. Each stage of infection has its own set of psychosocial stressors that may emerge and recede sporadically along the disease continuum and intensify with progression. This model of distinguishing need by stage allows the affected women, families, and the providers to anticipate need and engage in strategic problem solving and advanced planning.

## ❖ References

Becker, N. E., & Becker, F. W. (1986). Early identification of high social risk. *Health and Social Work, 11,* 26–35.

Benson, D., & Maier, C. (1990). Challenges facing women with HIV. *Focus: A Guide to AIDS Research and Counseling, 6,* (6).

Bidgood, R. (1992). Coping with the trauma of AIDS losses. In H. Land (Ed.), *AIDS: A complete guide to psychosocial intervention* (pp. 239–251). Milwaukee: Family Service America.

Christ, G. H., Weiner, L. S., & Moynihan, R. T. (1986). Psychosocial issues in AIDS. *Psychiatric Annals, 16,* 173–179.

Cohen, M. (1990). Biopsychosocial approach to human immunodeficiency virus epidemic: A clinicians' primer. In I. Lopez (Ed.), *General Hospital Psychiatry* (pp. 98–123). New York: Elsevier.

Donohue, M. (1993). A special kind of ministry. *Focus: A Guide to AIDS Research and Counseling, 9,* 6.

Francis, R. A. (1989). Moral beliefs of physicians, medical students, clergy, and lay public concerning AIDS. *Journal of the National Medical Association, 81,* 1141–1147.

Hutchison, M., & Kurth, A. (1991). "I need to know that I have a choice": A study of women, HIV, and reproduction decision-making. *AIDS Patient Care, 5* (1), 17–25.

Johnson, S. D. (1989). Discrimination against AIDS victims. *Psychological Reports, 64*(3, Pt. 2), 1261–1262.

Krieger, I. (1988). An approach to coping with anxiety about AIDS. *Social Work, 33*(3), 263–264.

Levine, C., & Dubler, N. (1990). HIV and childbearing: Uncertain risks and bitter realities: The reproductive choices of HIV-infected women. *Milbank Quarterly, 68*(3), 321–351.

Minkoff, H., & DeHovitz, J. (1991). Care of women infected with the human immunodeficiency virus. *Journal of the American Medical Association, 266*(16), 2253–2258.

Rehr, H., Berkman, B., & Rosenberg, G. (1980). Screening for high social risk: Principles and problems. *Social Work, 25,* 403–406.

Rosen, D., & Blank, W. (1991). Women and HIV. In H. Land (Ed.), *AIDS: A complete guide to psychosocial intervention* (pp. 141–151). Milwaukee: Family Service America.

Sands, R. G. (1983). Crisis intervention and social work practice in hospitals. *Health and Social Work, 8,* 253–260.

Stein, J. B. (1991). HIV disease and substance abuse. Twin epidemics. Multiple needs. In H. Land (Ed.), *AIDS: A complete guide to psychosocial intervention* (pp. 107–115). Milwaukee: Family Service America.

Walsh, F., & McGoldrick, M. (1991). Loss and the family: A systemic perspective. In F. Walsh & M. McGoldrick (Eds.), *Living beyond loss: death in the family* (pp. 1–29). New York: Norton.

# ❖ Chapter 11
# Cultural Sensitivity

JOANNE BRADLEY

Values, beliefs, and ways of interpreting and finding meaning in the world are specific to each culture. No single scale of values applies to all cultures; beliefs and practices must be judged relative to where they appear. Health beliefs are similarly diverse, with customs and practices relative to wellness and illness strongly tied to a particular racial or ethnic group. The concept of cultural sensitivity has emerged as an important variable in providing primary care services to the culturally heterogeneous population of women and children with HIV infection. Primary care physicians, nurses, and social workers will enhance care if they integrate culturally sensitive intervention strategies into their clinical practices.

## ❖ Patients in Context

In addition to family and community, many factors influence patients' attitudes about health and their responses to illness. These include but are not limited to the following:

❖ Race
❖ Ethnicity
❖ Understanding of illness and death
❖ Language
❖ Socioeconomic status
❖ Religion
❖ Family structure and supports

### *Race*

*Race* is a biological term that refers to population-specific and genetically determined distinguishing physical characteristics. Blacks represent the largest racial minority in the United States and are disproportionately represented among AIDS cases. They are a heterogeneous group whose health beliefs are determined by the various cultures in which they were raised. African-Americans from southern rural communities make extensive use of both prayer and folk medicines as healing modalities. These practices contrast with those of some Haitians, who may use candles and oils to prevent illness or may ascribe specific types of illnesses to supernatural etiology (Leavitt & Lutz, 1989).

## Ethnicity

An ethnic group has a sense of collective distinctiveness as a result of shared characteristics, such as geographic boundaries, diet, dialect, and daily customs. Many health beliefs and practices have their roots in a patient's ethnic community. In traditional Chinese homes, illness is viewed as an imbalance between yin and yang foods. This is similar to the beliefs of some Hispanics who view the proper quantities and timing of prescribed amounts of "hot" and "cold" foods as important in maintaining health. The evil eye, or the infliction of physical illness by directly staring at someone, is a belief held by many ethnic groups. Protection, especially for babies, is offered by the wearing of amulets.

In the concept of machismo, which is common in Latin cultures, men are in-control, dominant decision makers. In many cultures, women may be unable to implement health education instructions, especially those about sexual behavior, unless their male partners are taken into account.

## Understanding of Illness and Disease

Some injection drug users feel that AIDS is a just punishment for the sins they have committed ("I played and now I pay"). Mexican-Americans often believe that health is either a result of good luck or a reward from God for good behavior. Mexicans also believe in *susto*, an illness in which the soul leaves the body as a result of a fright and which can only be treated by a *curandero*'s healing rituals (Spector, 1991). Western Europeans and North Americans believe in a Cartesian duality in which mind and body are thought to operate independently of each other.

## Language

Patients from different cultures and classes vary in their use and understanding of English language. A patient may show agreement but not truly understand a health education message if it is not conveyed in her native tongue. Interpreters may give a less precise meaning to the questions and instructions of the provider whom they are translating. The use of family members as interpreters is problematic when gathering sexual or gynecologic histories. Topics relevant to HIV transmission, such as sex and drugs, are taboo subjects for discussion in many cultures, further complicating clear communication with women.

Both patients and providers use words and sentences that represent what is meaningful in their culture but are often misinterpreted by a listener with a different cultural or social class perspective. For example, patients who express a belief in voodoo or who describe emotional states in terms of the supernatural have been described as pathologic by providers who are not sensitive to the client's cultural beliefs.

## Socioeconomic Status

Poverty is often used as a proxy for or compounder of other social divisions, such as race. Poor families may lack access to the health care services and supports that are available to middle-class families. Poverty or its resultant limitations and demands may be reasons for the seeming non-compliance with medical treatment plans. For example, pride can prevent a woman from explaining that the reason for missing a clinic appointment was a lack of carfare. Although perhaps a trivial amount to a middle-class provider, the $2 transportation cost may be critical to feeding a patient's family. Because a large number of families with HIV infection live below the poverty level, it is important to be sensitive to the hidden costs of many health care services; these include time, distance, and stress as well as money.

## Religion

Religion provides a meaningful support for many families with HIV infection and is also an important determinant of belief systems. However, the tenets of some religions may be at odds with the teachings of HIV workers. For instance, some religious organizations forbid the use of condoms or any form of mechanical contraception. As a result, some women often feel a conflict between the advice of the health system and that of the Church. Some fundamentalist religions advocate healing by salvation and a belief in God, to the exclusion of regular medical care. A woman's church may view HIV disease as punishment for sins. Providers who are sensitive to the significance of religion in the lives of their patients can help negotiate disparities between church teachings and appropriate health practices.

## Family Structure and Supports

The nuclear family has been the norm in Western culture, and it is the structure with which most middle-class providers are familiar. Early in the AIDS epidemic, gay men and their network of friends and community forced many providers to expand their definition of family. The "buddy system," in which friends and volunteers from the gay community provided day-to-day housekeeping, nutrition, and social support services for people with AIDS, provided essential social support. In African-American and Latino families, kinship solidarity and mutual help are not confined to the immediate family, and different patterns of cooperation exist. African-American families often have a pivotal person available within the extended family who operates as a filter between the larger society and the individual. Puerto Ricans expect family members, especially those in stable positions, to assist when a relative is having a crisis or problem. They will access social systems only when all else has failed (Badillo-Ghali, 1974). It is important for the provider to learn to respect and work with the family structures of patients, however different they may be from the provider's expectations and experience.

### ❖ Providers and Patients

These factors form part of a larger cultural gulf that exists between providers and the women and children with HIV disease for whom they care. Most women and children with HIV disease receive health care from providers who do not share their racial, ethnic, or cultural background. Differences exist between the culture of the health care professional and that of the patient. In the patient-provider relationship, the provider is the dominant partner, with the knowledge, technology, and resources needed to treat the patient. The provider is comfortable in the health care setting and has some control over the immediate environment. Patients are often discomforted by these differences and are ill at ease in the physical setting. This is exacerbated by the reluctance of many patients to question the authority of the health provider or to ask for clarifications. The patient's resultant anxiety often results in misunderstandings about illnesses and treatments.

Bridging this patient-provider gap through effective cross-cultural communication is the responsibility of the health care provider. The following specific suggestions are designed to help providers with this task:

- ❖ Adopt a work style that is congruent with the expectations of your population and is generally unhurried, sensitive yet persistent, and respectful of the patient.
- ❖ Spend time listening.
- ❖ Elicit information from patients about their health beliefs, family roles, and healing practices.
- ❖ Avoid the use of familiar terms such as *Mother* or *Honey*.
- ❖ Be aware of your body language and the message it may be conveying.
- ❖ Avoid any assumptions about groups that are different from your own. This includes conjecture about sexual or drug using behavior of women who are HIV positive. Do not assume heterosexuality.
- ❖ Negotiate treatment plans that are acceptable to both patient and provider. These might include plans that preserve helpful cultural beliefs and practices, accommodate neutral practices, and repattern harmful practices (Jackson, 1993).
- ❖ Try to have appropriate health education materials available in the native language of your patients.
- ❖ Check the physical environment of your clinic: Are signs only in English? Do wall posters and health education materials depict only white, middle-class people?
- ❖ Seek out articles, books, and educational seminars about the different groups with whom you are working.

❖ Make contact with individuals, groups, and communities with different values, life-styles, and religious and ethnic backgrounds in order to appreciate and accept differences.

❖ Develop an understanding of your own culture and the degree to which you are conditioned by it. Remember that even providers are culture bound and have been influenced by the healing systems of Western, industrialized societies.

## ❖ Summary

Considerable satisfaction can be gained from taking the initiative to bridge this cultural gap by working with patients from different backgrounds. The basis of trust on which a primary care relationship is built must include acceptance and respect—of differences as well as similarities, of the familiar as well as the strange.

Patients' view of and response to illness and disease are directly relative to the cultural context in which they appear. Understanding the client's own perception of illness and her use of language to convey meaning is important in delivering primary care. Caregivers have an obligation to remove any obstacles to care that lie within their control. Cultural understanding and sensitive behaviors are integral to primary care.

## ❖ References

Badillo-Ghali, S. (1974). Cultural sensitivity and the Puerto Rican client. *Social Casework, 55*(1), 100–110.

Jackson, L. A. (1993). Understanding, eliciting and negotiating clients' multicultural health beliefs. *Nurse Practitioner, 18*(4), 30–43.

Leavitt, R., & Lutz, M. E. (1989). *Three new immigrant groups in New York City and the human services: Dominicans, Haitians, Cambodians.* New York: Community Council of Greater New York.

Spector, R. E. (1991). *Cultural diversity in health and illness.* East Norwalk, CT: Appleton-Century-Crofts.

# ❖ Chapter 12
# Continuity of Care

Stephen Paul Holzemer
Rosalie Rothenberg
Carolyn A. Fish

The course of HIV disease is so extended, varied in intensity, and unpredictable that providing continuity of care for patients can be a challenge for primary care providers. Long asymptomatic periods, when the monitoring of immune status and health maintenance are the only health care priorities, are interspersed with severe life-threatening opportunistic infections that interfere with sustaining activities, such as child rearing and employment. The HIV disease process generally concludes with an overwhelming illness during which the patient may need all the supports available from the health care community. During the course of an HIV disease, patient and family needs change along with functional abilities and the modalities and settings for delivering care (Afzal & Wyatt, 1989; Beresford, 1989; Boland & Klug, 1986; Special Treatment and Research Clinic, 1992). The special needs of women (Cohen & Durham, 1993; Kelly & Holman, 1993) surface as a complex set of physical, emotional, and social needs (Hurley & Ungvarski, 1993; Rose, 1993).

This chapter reviews some of the services women may need throughout the trajectory of HIV disease in order to provide continuity of care. Special attention is given to home care because of its potential to keep women and their children together as a family (Center for the Future of Children, 1993). The role of the case manager is explored as one way in which primary care professionals can offer continuity of care (Mor, Piette, & Fleishman, 1989; Piette, Fleishman, Stein, Mor, & Mayer, 1993; Schmidt, 1992).

The concept of continuity of care can be valuable in designing programs for women and children with HIV disease. Evashwick defines such a program as "an integrated, client oriented system of care composed of both services and integrating mechanisms that guides and tracks clients over time through a comprehensive array of health, mental health and social services spanning all levels of intensity of care" (1987). The goal of a continuity-of-care program is to predict, prevent, or minimize problems through the use of early interventions and anticipatory preparation. With the proper use of resources (Callahan, 1990; Wilensky, 1991), continuity of care can result in improved quality of life, independence, and maintenance of family integrity for those affected by HIV disease (Clark, 1991; Davis, Ferguson, &

195

Stapleton, 1992; Harris, Nyquist, Avery, Hahn, & Reichgott, 1989; Ryndes, 1989; Smits, Mansfield, & Singh, 1990; Sonsel, 1989).

The context for continuity of care for women and children with HIV infection may be understood as it relates to the location of care, such as within a home, day clinic, hospital, or nursing home. The context of care is also a reflection of care provided within the patient's family, community, and ethnocultural group. For women, obtaining continuous care for themselves and their dependents—at any location—depends on coordination (Ickovics & Epel, 1993; Rogers, 1992; Rosenthal, 1993).

The idea of continuity of care is not meaningful unless services are available, acceptable, financially realistic, and delivered in a manner that women can use. Figure 12–1 identifies some of the questions primary care providers need to consider to address plans for continuity of care. Primary

---

**Availability of Services**

• Are the medical and social services needed for the patient and family members available at the same time and location?
• Are services offered in the evening and on weekends?
• Can home visits be scheduled for physical assessment and specimen collection as well as emotional support?
• Are services accessible by affordable public transportation?

**Acceptability of Services**

• Are services culturally appropriate for women in the community?
• Were women involved in the development and planning of services?
• Are interpreters available?
• Is privacy provided for interviewing and interactions?

**Financial Resources**

• Is the patient the sole generator of income?
• Are there savings accounts, life insurance policies, or other assets?
• Is the patient taking advantage of unemployment or disability benefits?
• Is she eligible for Medicaid, food coupons, or Aid to Families with Dependent Children (AFDC)?

**Ability to Ask for Help**

• Is the patient able to ask for assistance in obtaining self-care or care for others?
• What are the past patterns of caregiving behavior?
• Does the patient have care commitments (sick relatives or friends)?
• Are friends or family members willing to plan respite periods for the patient who is sick and/or caring for others?

---

FIGURE 12–1   Questions that assess ability to access health care services.

care providers must work with women to identify the appropriate lay or professional caregivers who provide the needed services (Schmidt, 1992).

To develop an individual plan for continuity of care, the primary provider must consider what the woman with HIV infection and her family might need over the course of the disease. The provider must attempt to balance, with the patient, her potentially infinite needs with finite resources (Callahan, 1990). Comprehensive care during the course of HIV illness includes outpatient, inpatient, and emergency medical and psychiatric services; financial assistance; psychological and emotional supports; family services; child care; legal services; and home care. The primary care provider and the patient must identify which resources will best meet her multiple needs.

Because the health care needs of women with HIV disease may change abruptly, plans should be developed and systems of access designed so that the services are available when needed. To enhance access to and participation in health care services, women should be involved in developing their own individual plans. Figure 12–2 outlines the types of support services that women may need during their illness. These services must be user-friendly, particularly for the poor or for women with specific cultural beliefs different from the care system.

Women can explore services by contacting a number of resources, including the following:

- ❖ AIDS Clinical Trial Information Service, 800-874-2572
- ❖ Centers for Disease Control and Prevention National AIDS Clearinghouse, 800-458-5231
- ❖ National AIDS Hotline, 800-342-AIDS
  (Spanish-speaking callers) 800-344-SIDA
  (Deaf or hearing-impaired callers) 800-AIDS-TTY
- ❖ National Pediatric HIV Resource Center
  (outside New Jersey) 800-362-0071
  (in New Jersey) 201-268-8251

## ❖ Systems of Communication

The patient should keep summary records of all health care visits (primary care, emergency room care, and specialty care) in a folder and should take them to all health care visits. A list of current prescribed medications, with dosages and the patient's responses, should be included. Contributing to this health record should be the caregiver's responsibility, but the patient should keep the records for the entire family and bring them to health care visits. Health-related information will then be available when it is needed.

Women with HIV infection can meet in small groups to share similar problems, validate their responses, and prevent isolation. Support groups have served as an outlet to reduce stress and help patients resolve problems. Although a professional person may be present as a resource, support

**Providing Emotional Support**

- Weekly phone contacts
- Monthly group meetings
- Hospital/home visits as necessary
- Peer support networks, "buddies"

**Tracking Clients**

- Home visits to monitor general health status and environmental support
- Periodic self-assessment reports mailed to case manager
- Phone contacts

**Holding Educational Meetings**

- Provide information about specific OB/GYN needs and services.
- Conduct classes on health promotion topics like stress, nutrition, sleep, and exercise.
- Discuss available research protocols and treatment options.
- Provide written or taped materials for women unable to attend meetings.

**Providing Written Information About Resources**

- Provide lists of counselors, care providers, therapists, and support groups; offer referrals for medical, psychological, and spiritual resources.
- Compile resources that relate to "unfinished business," such as wills, power of attorney, health care proxy, and funeral arrangements.
- Dedicate an area for written materials about health care, legal, financial, and social service resources; inform patients of these materials.
- Improve access to resources; facilitate resources.
- Provide an opportunity for clarification and discussion of written materials.

**Support Groups**

- Develop groups based on needs of women with HIV/AIDS.
- Conduct groups in a private, comfortable setting.
- Enhance attendance through the use of refreshments and child care.
- Remind staff and patients to practice confidentiality at all times.

FIGURE 12–2  Systems of support.

groups may be most helpful when co-directed by participants and a professional. Co-leadership may allow women to guide group work in a way that makes them most comfortable. Special groups can be designed for families or partners of people with AIDS, mothers of infected children, or women in drug treatment. Support groups should be available to women at different stages of HIV disease.

Regular telephone calls made by volunteers, other patients, or professionals can reduce isolation, provide support, and monitor health status, especially between scheduled visits and when the woman's health begins to deteriorate. Some women may benefit from telephone or informal drop-in services if they are unable or unwilling to participate in structured group activities.

Simple instructions about what to do and whom to call in an emergency should be given to patients in anticipation of problems. Lists and reminders may help women to use resources properly and to reduce the chance of manageable problems escalating into disasters.

## ❖ Financial Services

People with HIV infection and AIDS may be impoverished, often from the inability to work or from the costs of illness. Basic information about currently available benefits and entitlements for which women diagnosed with HIV infection are eligible should be reviewed with patients early in their health care. Many entitlements take weeks or months to initiate, so early processing is important, and correct documentation is essential.

Entitlements change from state to state and can vary from year to year. Some entitlements available throughout the United States are Social Security disability insurance, supplemental security income, food coupons, Medicaid, and Medicare. Other local and more variable entitlements include housing, income maintenance, and state disability insurance. Questions about entitlements should be directed to the local Social Security office, a volunteer financial advocacy agency, or a hospital social service department. Local financial resources and services are usually listed in the telephone book.

Planning for the use of entitlements is important. The following are some key suggestions from the Gay Men's Health Crisis (1989) for helping patients to organize the process:

- ❖ Keep a log of *all* phone calls made to an agency, the instructions received, and the name of the person who provided the information.
- ❖ Keep personal documents in one place, including birth certificates, passports, immigration documents, Social Security card, lease or rent receipts, and W-2 forms or income tax records.
- ❖ Keep a photocopy of everything mailed to a benefit agency or service. If original documents are requested, verify that they are actually necessary. Send important documents and applications by registered mail to obtain a receipt of delivery.
- ❖ Notify all relevant agencies immediately if a change of address is anticipated.

Those who use entitlements should work with a knowledgeable social worker or counselor to access all appropriate benefits. A family member or friend should be aware of how the patient is progressing with applications, to provide assistance and encouragement.

The legal concerns that often accompany financial services are discussed in chapter 17. Problems of child care, housing, finances, discrimination, and immigration often assume priority over health care and cause severe stress. Resolution of these problems is often prerequisite to the comprehensive planning of health care for women.

## ❖ Family and Child-Care Services

Reducing the use of foster care and group housing for HIV-infected children and women may be possible through the use of services aimed at keeping the family intact. These services may include substance abuse treatment for women, protected shelters for abused women, respite services, homemakers, parenting classes, and day care for children. Although all services may not be available in all areas of the country, advocacy for essential family services should be a goal of primary care providers.

Respite services can provide short-term relief for caregivers of women and children with HIV disease. Professional counseling related to the family's response to illness and to death and dying (chapter 10) may strengthen the ability of family members to cope with their experiences. Tangible supports from volunteer, religious, or community-based organizations, such as money, transportation, clothing, medication, and equipment, may be necessary to supplement other benefits.

Children with HIV infection who need day care can be integrated into regular day-care settings (chapter 7). General instructions for child-care providers should focus on reducing physical hazards related to the spread of HIV and other infections and on the care of all children who experience a tendency to bruise or bleed, who have frequent infections, or both. Health screening of caregivers, meticulous personal cleanliness, and strict hand-washing procedures must be established. Child-care staff should separate feeding and diapering areas, provide basic health screening of children, and follow the child-to-caretaker ratios established by licensing agencies.

Special child development day-care services can offer an environment that is supportive of the child's level of function and can assist in monitoring changes in neurological development. Early intervention programs provide the special supports needed to maintain the optimal functioning of children living with a debilitating illness (Center for the Future of Children, 1993). Mothers and other caregivers can be incorporated in the care process to improve their ability to parent successfully.

## ❖ Home Care Services

Advances in the treatment of HIV-related symptoms and con-comitant infections have made the management of HIV disease at home possible for many. Many health care needs can be treated as well or better at home as in a hospital. Hospitalization may be reserved for treatment of the most severe opportunistic infections and for women and children whose homes are not suitable for care. If home care is considered to be appropriate, a professional will make an assessment home visit to identify and explore needed resources and initial care strategies. A variety of personnel and a range of durable medical equipment resources are available for home care across the country. The goals and advantages of home care include promoting normal developmental activities of individuals, maintaining family relationships and routines, and allowing women and their families more control in setting priorities. Although each person may need a different program of services, home care needs should be identified by the patient and her home care provider, who will develop a written plan of care.

Information about home care services should be discussed with the patient so she can contract for the services that best meet her needs. Medicare-certified agencies, for example, provide comprehensive services that meet basic national government standards. In addition to certification, accreditation of home care agencies provides assurance of excellence beyond minimal state or federal regulations (Community Health Accreditation Program, 1994). The local department of health will verify Medicare certification, and the National League for Nursing (1-800-669-1656) or the state hospital association will verify the accreditation of agencies.

## *Nonprofessional Workers*

Both professional and nonprofessional workers provide health-related service in the home. Entitlement and insurance companies have referred to professional and nonprofessional home care workers differently.

Women living with HIV disease often need help to care for themselves and their children. Many in-home services are provided by paraprofessionals called home attendants or personal care workers. They have had limited education in health care matters and should not be expected to provide skilled care. These workers, hired privately or as part of an insurance or disability package, are supervised by a registered professional nurse (RN) who provides a list of expected duties.

Semiskilled home workers provided under Medicare benefits are called home health aides (HHAs). The HHA can assist with personal care, help with cooking and light housework, and escort patients to their health care appointments. The HHA is specifically trained to work with a family and can implement a written plan of basic care under the supervision of an RN.

Volunteers, sometimes called buddies, can assist with limited homemaking, shopping, and personal care activities. Lay religious workers, for example, may bring companionship and prayer to a person living with HIV while helping with household chores or errands. Individual organizations providing volunteer services have orientations and ongoing education about the role of the volunteer and his or her work with patients and their families.

## Professional Workers

Nurses educated to meet the health care needs of people at home are called visiting nurses, public health nurses, or home care nurses. They have special expertise in working within the health care team and can monitor the health status of women and their families at home. In many home care agencies, visiting nurses provide high-technology services in the home that until recently were restricted to the hospital environment. These services include administering oxygen therapy, intravenous medications, and fluid and nutritional supports. Phlebotomy can be performed in the home in order to update the patient's plan of care as it relates to blood work. In this situation, the woman or child would not need to leave the home for the monitoring of laboratory results.

Physical, occupational, nutritional, speech, and social service therapists are often available to implement care regimens in the home. Regardless of whether these therapists are self-employed or work for an agency, their services will be coordinated by the primary care provider and the patient's case manager. Patients need to be instructed on which therapy services are appropriate and how much service is reimbursable by the entitlement or insurance program.

## Hospice Care

As HIV illness progresses, hospice care may be needed to allow patients and their families to approach death honestly and with less fear. A central hospice principle is pain management. Care in a hospice program can help women to die with the least pain while remaining alert and oriented. Hospice care also strives to ensure that patients will not die alone, and it enables families and friends to be present for psychological support. Primary care providers should encourage dying women to consider hospice services and to initiate them if appropriate (Holzemer, 1986). The idea of considering the need for hospice care should be introduced to patients while they can still make informed decisions.

## ❖ Case Manager

Someone is often needed to coordinate service delivery and to escort women with HIV infection through the often crisis-driven health care delivery system. In some settings, the primary care provider assumes this role. In other settings, these responsibilities are designated to a provider called a case manager. Early in HIV disease, when acute health care needs are few, caregivers and case managers can work with patients to outline the range of available services that might be needed in the future. Planning services in advance makes their implementation less difficult and allows women more control over health care decisions.

Ideally, each family affected by HIV disease should have one person or a team of people to assume continuous responsibility and accountability for the coordination of health care services through all the phases of HIV disease. In addition to expertise in HIV disease assessment and management and knowledge of the expected disease course, the case manager should know how to use HIV-specific health care resources effectively. The case manager coordinates the use of community and family resources for the delivery of care. Women are usually assigned a case manager after a hospitalization or AIDS-defining diagnosis.

The case manager often facilitates access to services from a variety of agencies and vendors and acts as the liaison or patient advocate between agencies in the management of care. The case manager may be responsible for evaluation of care as it relates to patient satisfaction with service and perception of the quality of care. The case manager should assist the patient to access and participate in all physical, mental health, and social services that she needs and can use effectively.

Communications, both verbal and written, between health care settings are needed to clarify the client's needs, family resources, and division of responsibilities. Networking and establishing communication and service linkages are necessary to minimize care delivery problems while maximizing access to specialized services. The case manager acts as an information resource for community agencies, other providers, and especially women and their families. In addition, the case manager may also be a direct care provider. In this role, the case manager teaches the family about caring for the person with HIV infection in the home while managing a cluster of patients with other needs.

## ❖ Adapting to Change

Any change can bring psychological and physiological stress, anxiety, and fear of the unknown. Predictable points of change-related stress during the course of HIV disease include learning the HIV diagnosis and prognosis, the first lab report of falling CD4 cells, the first opportunistic infection, weight loss, loss of a child's developmental skills, and hospitalization. While recognizing the stress inherent in these changes, the caregiver can offer appropriate supports, such as providing care or making a referral to a support group or to a member of the clergy. Providing counseling, positive reinforcement, and additional resources may be needed until the patient adjusts to the change. Changes in the woman's disease intensity or the location where she receives care may alter her need for services, information, and skill training. With each transition, a fresh look at the patient's entire health picture may identify the need for new resources and changes in care priorities.

Home visits and telephone contact in the early days after any change will provide support. A return visit to the clinic or doctor's office should be scheduled within a short time. The frequency of follow-up visits should be planned with consideration for the client's needs, not the system's. The opportunity to learn and practice additional skills and patterns of behavior should be arranged as early as possible. Community-based nurses, family caretakers, and homemakers need orientation and practice with any new care skills.

## ❖ Summary

As caregivers ensure continuity of care to women who are HIV infected, they must address the unique issues that women experience. These issues range from advocacy for women who are homeless or injection drug users to coordination of care when many family members are ill. The different needs of women and their children must be planned in such a way to ensure that the woman is able to care for both herself and her family. This is particularly true when HIV cuts across generations or affects family members in the same generation.

The primary care provider and case manager, working with the woman with HIV infection, can create a plan that may include day treatment, social support services, hospitalization, skilled home care, and hospice care. Care providers can assist women in learning about resources and in creating systems of support that will improve their ability to get the services they need. Including family members in an understanding of the plan of care increases the support available to women living with HIV disease and fosters the continuity of their care.

## ❖ References

Afzal, N., & Wyatt, A. (1989). Long term care of AIDS patients. *Quality Review Bulletin, 15*(1), 20–25.

Beresford, T. (1989). Alternative, outpatient settings of care for people with AIDS. *Quality Review Bulletin, 15*(1), 9–16.

Boland, M. G., & Klug, R. M. (1986). AIDS: The implications for home care. *MCN, 11*(6), 404–411.

Callahan, D. (1990). *What kind of life?* New York: Simon & Schuster.

Center for the Future of Children. (1993). Home visiting: Analysis and recommendations. *Future of Children, 3*(3), 6–22.

Clark, J. (1991). HIV nursing management in the home health care setting. *Journal of Home Health Care Practice, 3*(2), 1–9.

Cohen, F. L., & Durham, J. D. (1993). *Women, children, and HIV/AIDS.* New York: Springer.

Community Health Accreditation Program. (1994). *Quality through accreditation.* New York: National League for Nursing Press.

Davis, K. A., Ferguson, K. J., & Stapleton, J. T. (1992). Moving home to live: Migration of HIV-infected persons to rural states. *Journal of the Association of Nurses in AIDS Care, 3*(4), 42–47.

Evashwick, C. J. (1987). Definition of the continuum of care. In C. J. Evashwick & L. J. Weiss (Eds.), *Managing the continuum of care* (pp. 23–43). Rockville, MD: Aspen.

Gay Men's Health Crisis. (1989). *You're entitled: A guide to government entitlement programs in New York City.* New York: Author.

Harris, C., Nyquist, R. P., Jr., Avery, S. J., Hahn, S., & Reichgott, M. J. (1989). Quality assurance for HIV-related care. *Quality Review Bulletin, 15*(1), 25–30.

Holzemer, S. P. (1986). The lodging of patients with AIDS as your guests. *American Journal of Hospice Care, 3*(2), 28–31.

Hurley, P. M., & Ungvarski, P. J. (1993). *Nursing care needs of adults with HIV disease/AIDS in homecare.* New York: Author.

Ickovics, J. R., & Epel, E. S. (1993). Women's health research: Policy and practice. *IRB: A Review of Human Subjects Research, 15*(4), 1–7.

Kelly, P. J., & Holman, S. (1993). The new face of AIDS. *American Journal of Nursing, 93*(3), 26–32, 34.

Mor, V., Piette, J., & Fleishman, J. (1989). Community-based case management for persons with AIDS. *Health Affairs, 8*(4), 139–153.

Piette, J. D., Fleishman, J. A., Stein, M. D., Mor, V., & Mayer, K. (1993). Perceived needs and unmet needs for formal services among people with HIV disease. *Journal of Community Health, 18*(1), 11–23.

Rogers, D. E. (1992). Report card on our national response to the AIDS epidemic—Some A's, too many D's. *American Journal of Public Health, 82*(4), 522–524.

Rose, M. A. (1993). Health concerns of women with HIV/AIDS. *Journal of the Association of Nurses in AIDS Care, 4*(3), 39–45.

Rosenthal, E. (1993, October 13). Is women's health harmed by medical specialization? *New York Times,* pp. A1, C14.

Ryndes, T. (1989). The coalition model of case management for care of HIV-infected persons. *Quality Review Bulletin, 15*(1), 4–8.

Schmidt, J. (1992). Case management problems and home care. *Journal of the Association of Nurses in AIDS Care, 3*(3), 37–44.

Smits, A., Mansfield, S., & Singh, S. (1990). Facilitating care of patients with HIV infection by hospital and primary care teams. *British Medical Journal, 300*(6719), 241–242.

Sonsel, G. E. (1989). Case management in a community-based AIDS agency. *Quality Review Bulletin, 15*(1), 31–36.

Special Treatment and Research Clinic. (1992). *Living with HIV.* Brooklyn: State University of New York at Brooklyn Health Science Center.

Wilensky, G. R. (1991). From the health care financing administration. *Journal of the American Medical Association, 266*(24), 3404.

# ❖ Chapter 13

# Complementary Therapies

Ana L. Oliveira
Rae L. Crowe

The use of complementary therapies, which emphasize the body's ability to heal itself, allows women with HIV disease to share the responsibility for their own health care. By maximizing the mind-body connection and the relationship between the physical, emotional, mental, spiritual, and environmental realms, an individual's overall satisfaction and quality of life can be improved. The wide range of available complementary therapies includes those with complex bodies of knowledge such as acupuncture, herbs, and homeopathy, that have been used for centuries and newer practices, such as exercise, massage, nutrition and vitamin supplements, meditation and imagery, and therapeutic touch.

Complementary therapies have been used since early in the AIDS epidemic, and their use has grown as the limitations of Western medicine have become more evident. Many women with HIV disease seek out therapies that permit them to have some control over their health and are culturally familiar and affordable. Learning how to control symptoms with the use of relaxation techniques or dietary modifications can be very empowering. Primary care providers are encouraged to become familiar with the complementary therapies used by the women and children for whom they care and to encourage their safe and rational use.

Women in particular are familiar with and open to the use of alternative medicines. As caretakers, they have long used herbal remedies or home remedies for their families. As healers, *curanderas*, or witches, they have exploited locally available resources for treatments. Many complementary therapies are rooted in indigenous peoples' medicines and are easily recognized and used by the communities most affected by the AIDS epidemic (Diaz, 1993).

## ❖ Mind-Body Therapies

Whereas some alternative therapies are derived primarily from Eastern philosophies and traditions, the mind-body strategies such as prayer, religious reading, meditation, imagery and visualization, and reaching out to others, are rooted in the Judeo-Christian tradition. Spirituality, or the faith that one is connected in some way to a transcendental entity, is a common denominator for many holistic therapies. Although spirituality is not necessarily connected to religious practices, it does encompass one's search for meaning in life and is often intensified when losses, grief, and one's own mortality are at issue.

Reed (1987) reported that terminally ill, hospitalized adults had a significantly greater spiritual perspective than both other hospitalized adults and healthy adults. Generally, terminally ill patients with high levels of spirituality reported a greater feeling of well-being. Reed (1991) suggested the use of journal writing, prayer, contemplation, tracking spiritual life history, and meditation and imagery as part of the patient's health care.

Mindful meditation, the intentional focusing of attention on one's breathing or senses, changes one's awareness and brings about a feeling of relaxation. Relaxation reduces distress by improving mood and decreasing anxiety and pain. Regular deep relaxation is an important health maintenance practice for patients with HIV infection. Deep relaxation can be done in a comfortable, relaxed position for at least 20 minutes while listening to meditation tapes or focusing the mind inward on one's breathing patterns. Many patients experience increased energy levels, improved digestion and sleep patterns, and, as the mind becomes quieter, a more balanced emotional state.

Imagery, or creating pictures in the mind, has been seen to affect both body and mind. The imagining of running elicits measurable amounts of muscle contraction in the muscles used in running (Jacobson, 1942). Imagery has been effective in relieving painful symptoms associated with cancer (Simonton, Simonton, & Creighton, 1978). It can help solve current dilemmas, transport the individual to a place associated with pleasant memories, or create a framework for the future use of imagery. The practice of visualization has potential for augmenting traditional therapies prescribed for those with HIV infection.

Meditation and visualization are essential components of therapeutic touch, which has been described as a moving meditation. Therapeutic touch, derived from the ancient art of the laying on of hands, is the intentional transfer of a universal energy by a helping person to an ill person (Krieger, 1979). Inherent in therapeutic touch is the premise that humans and the environment are energy fields coextensive with one other (Rogers, 1970). Illness is an imbalance in the human energy field. The intent is to stimulate the ill person's self-healing abilities by promoting the rhythmic flow of energy waves. The helping person becomes still within, focuses intention on healing, and uses the hands, thoughts, and visualization to balance the ill person's fields. This elicits relaxation.

Healing or wholeness may be a relief of symptoms, an absence of symptoms, a sense of well-being, or a peaceful death. Neushan (1989) describes treating people with AIDS with therapeutic touch. The cough and dyspnea of respiratory infection decreased. The fluctuating temperature patterns of an imbalanced immune system were steadied. Pain was relieved with a sense of peacefulness in a patient with Kaposi's sarcoma.

Therapeutic touch is an innate human potential that can be learned by family members, significant others, and friends of the HIV-infected person. These people can become active participants in caring for the person with AIDS in a way that can open communication and enhance intimacy (Heidt, 1990).

## ❖ Acupuncture

Acupuncture is an ancient form of medicine practiced throughout the world with other therapies or as an independent approach. The most widely practiced form is traditional Chinese medicine, which is based on the concept of the duality of and balance between yin and yang. Acupuncture is particularly effective in treating imbalances early in an illness when "things are not quite right" and symptoms are not specific. Based on a belief that disease can only take place when the host environment is vulnerable and the "pernicious influence" (traditional Chinese medicine's term for a pathogen) is not warded off, acupuncture aims to strengthen the individual as opposed to combating pathogens.

Acupuncture treatment involves the insertion of very fine presterilized disposable needles into different areas of the body, according to points specifically selected for each condition. Acupuncture practitioners also use other methods, including cupping, in which small suction cups are placed on different areas of the body to aid in the circulation of blood and *chi*, or "life force"; the use of *moxa* or artemisia vulgaris, a natural herb that provides a warming effect when placed on needles or near acupuncture points; and electrical stimulation, which is used to open pathways blocked by neuropathy, stroke, or pain. Acupuncture has been reported to provide effective relief for a great number of HIV-associated problems. These are listed in Figure 13–1.

## ❖ Homeopathy

Homeopathy is a scientific approach founded by Samuel Hahnemann in the 18th century. The basic principles of homeopathy are the following:

❖ The law of similarities, or "like cures like"—using a medicine that causes similar symptoms to the ones that an individual experiences during sickness

❖ The law of potentization, or "small amounts resonate powerfully"— allowing the body to heal naturally by creating resonance between the pattern of a substance and the pattern of the essence of a person (Ullman, 1989)

❖ Constantine Hering's principles of the healing process—last first (the last symptoms to appear will be the first to disappear) and externalization of disease (symptoms progress from more internal levels to more

**Symptom Relief**

- Night sweats
- Diarrhea
- Fatigue
- Weight loss
- Shortness of breath
- Nausea and headache from chemotherapy

**Detoxification of Addictive Substances**

- Alcohol
- Cocaine/crack
- Marijuana

**Increased Ability to Cope With Disease Process**

- Reduction of anxiety
- Promotion of relaxation
- Renewed vitality

**Health Maintenance in Presymptomatic HIV Infection**

- Boosting immune system
- Stress reduction

FIGURE 13–1   Uses of acupuncture in HIV management.

superficial ones, and healing occurs first at the top portion of the body, then progresses to lower areas)

Homeopathic interventions in HIV care are thought to be most effective as prophylaxes. Homeopathy strengthens the person to better resist and ward off infection by delaying or slowing down the breakdown of immunity that occurs as HIV disease progresses. Homeopathic treatments are believed to aid in the relief of specific symptoms, such as skin rashes, pain, shortness of breath associated with Pneumocystis carinii pneumonia (PCP), and asthma. Grief, sadness, fear, and hopelessness are also aided through homeopathic treatment (Ullman, 1989).

## ❖ Nutrition

For women and children, nutrition is a readily available intervention. Nutrition education is essential to assist the patient to make successful diet changes when they are necessary. Because the best nutrition plan is one that can be followed, planning a diet should involve the patient in order to increase the likelihood of informed choices. Reading labels, combining different kinds of foods properly, eating regularly, chewing thoroughly, abstaining from drinking water with meals, selecting less processed foods, using fresh vegetables, and budgeting to afford wholesome foods are practical issues to be taken into consideration when discussing changes in diet. A healthy diet includes foods that are natural or processed as little as possible and foods that are rich in minerals, vitamins, amino acids, proteins, and calories. The following simple rules will help patients achieve proper nutrition:

❖ Eat whole grains (brown rice, oats, cracked wheat, rye, millet, barley).
❖ Eat at least three servings of lightly cooked vegetables a day.
❖ Eat at least two servings of washed fresh fruits a day.
❖ Make up nutritious soups that can be served to the whole family and frozen in small containers for lunches and snacks.
❖ Eat a hearty breakfast every day.
❖ Avoid coffee, soda, sugar, alcohol, and raw fish.
❖ Store food properly to avoid spoilage and contamination.

## ❖ Vitamins and Nutritional Supplements

Nutritional supplements, including vitamins, amino acids, minerals, enzymes, coenzymes and fatty acids, are used in the prevention and treatment of HIV infection. Their use is intended to replenish depleted or absent nutrients that result from poor dietary habits or clinical conditions like wasting. In HIV disease, food digestion and absorption can be impaired and the capacity to sustain a nutritious diet reduced, so the consistent use of supplements that are appropriate to each medical condition and each person can enhance the functioning of the immune system (Kaiser, 1993). The cost of vitamin and mineral supplements can be minimized by buying the generic brands available from large drugstore chains or by joining a buyers' club and purchasing at bulk or wholesale prices. The use of different vitamins and minerals is discussed in this section.

Vitamin C has been used to treat viral diseases. In the treatment of AIDS and HIV infection, large dosages of Vitamin C have produced antioxidant effects, and increased numbers of T cells, interferon levels, and the phagocytic function of white blood cells. The effective dosage necessary to produce such effects is under debate and may range from 2 to 6 g to 20 g per day (Kaiser, 1993). Vitamin C is used for the prevention and treatment of colds and is associated with a lower risk of cancer. It is also used in the prevention of cervical dysplasia and in the treatment and prevention of urinary tract infections and vaginitis. Because of its rapid elimination in the urine, doses of this vitamin are taken several times a day. Large doses can cause diarrhea.

Vitamin E is used as a regenerator of mucous membranes and as an antioxidant. In large dosages, vitamin E is thought to neutralize the toxicity and increase the effectiveness of zidovudine (Kaiser, 1993). Vitamin E is also helpful in preventing some types of breast cysts, in preventing exacerbations of herpes outbreaks, and in facilitating the absorption of vitamin A.

Vitamin A and beta carotene are considered to be cancer-preventing agents. Beta carotene, a precursor of vitamin A, is safer for consumption in large dosages than vitamin A, which can be toxic in doses exceeding 10 mg per day.

B complex and brewer's yeast are supplements for the nervous system, facilitating the absorption of other substances (such as l-lysine). B-12, in particular, is effective in the prevention of herpes outbreaks. B complex can help to prevent urinary tract infections.

Zinc is used to speed up the healing of injured tissues and to treat vaginitis, herpes outbreaks, and other skin conditions.

Calcium is often used as a natural tranquilizer, soothing the nervous system and the musculature. Calcium deficiencies are associated with osteoporosis, insomnia, and menstrual cramps.

Magnesium is crucial for the absorption of other minerals including calcium and vitamins C, B complex, and E. It is effective for menstrual cramps and insomnia and is used for cancer prevention.

L-lysine is an amino acid used for prevention and suppression of herpes symptoms.

## ❖ Herbal Therapies

The pharmacology of traditional Chinese herbal medicines employs animal, vegetable, and mineral substances in formulas that are balanced to minimize specific physical problems and to counter side effects. There are usually between 8 and 12 herbs in a formula (Zhang & Hsu, 1990), which can be taken raw or cooked as a tea or in capsules or pills. These herbal formulas can often be found at low cost in natural pharmacies. Many patients with HIV infection have effectively integrated the use of Chinese herbal medicines in conjunction with Western therapies.

The American oral tradition has transmitted the healing beliefs of local cultures from one generation to the next. A large pharmacopoeia of herbal medicine practiced in the Americas has been collected and is available for the treatment of patients with HIV infection. These remedies include the following:

- ❖ Detoxing herbs, such as red clover, alfalfa, passion flower, dandelion, and catnip
- ❖ Digestive tonics, such as licorice, peppermint, ginger, slippery elm, and chamomile
- ❖ Natural antibiotics, such as goldenseal, echinacea, myrrh, and garlic
- ❖ Antifungals, such as pau d'arco, aloe vera, and tea tree oil
- ❖ Nervines, such as valerium, skullcap, hops, and passion flower

Although occasional toxic reactions can occur from the use of herbal remedies, in general they and the rest of the armamentarium of complementary therapies offer patients a safe opportunity to share in the treatment of their HIV disease.

## ❖ Exercise and Relaxation

Many practitioners consider exercise to be beneficial to the immune systems of both women and children. Exercises that require more energy expenditure are recommended for individuals who are stronger, whereas milder exercises are more appropriate for those who have constitutional symptoms. Aerobic exercises that maintain a pulse rate double the body's resting rate for at least 20 minutes promote circulation. Exercises of particular benefit for people living with HIV infection are walking, arm swings, and exercising as if bicycling upside down (Gregory, 1989).

Chi gong and t'ai chi ch'uan, moving meditations, are gentler exercises recommended for persons who have more severe immune deficiency. Chi gong, a widely practiced form of breathing exercise in China, is known for its powerful effects on well-being, longevity, and disease prevention and treatment. T'ai chi ch'uan develops the life force and centers it in the lower part of the abdomen through daily exercises (Man-ching, 1982).

## ❖ Massage

Therapeutic massage for emotional and physical healing comes from Japanese, Chinese, European, and North American schools of medical practice. Techniques that have been used in holistic clinics in the treatment of HIV infection and disease are shiatsu, acupressure, tui na, Swedish massage, rolfing, and polarity therapy. These therapies aim to unblock energy, relieve pain, alleviate stress, improve circulation, stimulate the release of toxicity from the lymph system, and enhance the immune capacity of the body (Rabinowitz, 1987; Wilson, 1991).

Chiropractic medicine is used in the United States to improve immune function of people living with HIV infection. Both osteopathy and chiropractic medicine are concerned with postural and skeletal problems and seek to stimulate the body's own resources to heal, by providing and maintaining alignment and optimal functioning of the organs.

## ❖ Summary

Women with HIV infection can assume some measure of responsibility for their own care by using complementary therapies. These modalities are compatible with the concurrent use of antiretroviral and PCP prophylaxis drugs prescribed by primary care providers educated in the biomedical model. Many women make use of these treatments, which are consistent with the health practices of their families and communities. These practices provide comfort and hope to women with a long-term, chronic illness for which Western medicine has limited alternatives.

## ❖ References

Diaz, M. D. (1993). Acupuncturist meets curandera: Responding to similarities in traditional medicines as a means for developing cultural and clinical sensitivity. *American Journal of Acupuncture, 21,* 1–6.

Gregory, S. J. (1989). *A holistic protocol for the immune system.* Joshua Tree, CA: Tree of Life Publications.

Heidt, P. (1990). Openness: A qualitative analysis of nurses' and patients' experiences of therapeutic touch. *Image, 22*(3), 180–186.

Jacobson, E. (1942). *Progressive relaxation.* Chicago: University of Chicago Press.

Kaiser, J. D. (1993). *Immune power: A comprehensive healing program for HIV.* New York: St. Martin's Press.

Krieger, D. (1979). *Therapeutic touch: How to use your hands to help and heal.* Englewood Cliffs, NJ: Prentice-Hall.

Man-ching, C. (1982). *Master Cheng's thirteen chapters on tai-chi chuan.* Brooklyn: Sweet Ch'I Press.

Newshan, G. (1989). Therapeutic touch for symptom control in persons with AIDS. *Holistic Nursing Practice, 3*(4), 45–51.

Rabinowitz, N. (1987). Acupuncture and the AIDS epidemic. *American Journal of Acupuncture, 15*(1), 3–6.

Reed, P. (1987). Spirituality and well-being in terminally ill hospitalized adults. *Research in Nursing and Health, 10,* 335–344.

Reed, P. (1991). Spiritual and mental health in older adults: Extant knowledge for nursing. *Family and Community Health, 14*(2), 14–25.

Rogers, M. (1970). *An introduction to the theoretical basis of nursing.* Philadelphia: F. A. Davis.

Simonton, O., Simonton, S. & Creighton, J. (1978). *Getting well again.* Los Angeles: J. P. Tarcher.

Ullman, D. (1989). *Discovering homeopathy: Medicine for the 21st century.* Berkeley, CA: North Atlantic Books.

Wilson, C. (1991). *AIDS treatment at Austin Immune Clinic.* Paper presented at the NADA Conference, Austin, TX.

Zhang, Q., & Hsu, H. (1990). *AIDS and Chinese medicine.* Long Beach, CA: Oriental Healing Arts Institute.

## ❖ Suggested Readings

Academy of Traditional Medicine. (1981). *Essentials of Chinese acupuncture.* Peking: Foreign Languages Press.

Balch, J. F. & Balch, P. *Prescription for nutritional healing.* Garden City, NY: Avery.

Bing-shan, Huang. (1991). *AIDS and its treatment by traditional Chinese medicine.* Boulder, CO: Blue Poppy Press.

Firebrace, P. (1989). *Acupuncture: Restoring the body's natural healing energy.* New York: Harmony Books.

Hemphill, C. (1988, March 3). Focus on AIDS: Turning to acupuncture. *New York Newsday.*

Maisel, E. (1963). *Tai Chi for health.* New York: Dell.

Mitchell, E. R. (1987). *Plain talk about acupuncture.* New York: Whalehall.

O'Connor, J. & Bensky, D. (1981). *Acupuncture—A comprehensive text.* Seattle: Eastland Press.

Oliveira, A. L. (1990, March). *Acupuncture and treatment of addictions.* Paper presented at Harvard University Medical School, Boston.

Oriental Healing Arts Institute. (1989). *AIDS, immunity and Chinese medicine.* Long Beach, CA: Author.

O'Sullivan, S. & Thomson, K. (1992). *Positively women.* London: Sheba Feminist Press.

Reuben, C., & Priestley, J. (1988). *Essential supplements for women.* New York: Perigee Books.

Siegel, L. (1986). AIDS: Relationship to alcohol and other drugs. *Journal of Substance Abuse Treatment, 3,* 271–274.

Smith, R. & Dharmanada, S. (1981). AIDS prevention: Preliminary consideration in the management of prodrome symptoms using the concept of traditional Chinese medicine. *Journal of the American College of Traditional Chinese Medicine, 20*–29.

## ❖ Resources

AIDS and Adolescents Network of New York (offering seminars, workshops, and referral services), 121 Sixth Ave., 6th Fl., New York, NY 10013, tel. 212-925-6675

AIDS Treatment Data Network, 259 W. 30th St., New York, NY 10001, tel. 212-268-4196

Asian and Pacific Islander Coalition on HIV/AIDS (APICHA), 41 John St., 3rd Fl., New York, NY 10038, tel. 212-349-3293

Caribbean Women's Health Association, Inc., 1600 Central Ave., Far Rockaway, NY 11691, tel. 718-868-4746

Hispanic AIDS Forum, 121 Avenue of the Americas, Room. 505, New York, NY 10013, tel. 212-966-6336

Homeopathic Educational Service, 2124 Kittredge St., Berkeley, CA 92704, tel. 510-649-0294

National Commission for the Certification of Acupuncturists, tel. 202-232-1404

National Directory of Holistic Practitioners and Services, American Holistic Medical Association, 4101 Lake Boone Trail, Suite 201, Raleigh, NC 27607, tel. 919-787-5146

National Homeopathy Referral Center, 801 North Fairfax St., Suite 306, Alexandria, VA 22314, tel. 703-548-7790

People with AIDS Coalition, 50 W. 17th St., 8th floor, New York, NY 10010, tel. 800-828-3280

People with AIDS Health Group, 150 W. 26th St., Suite 201, New York, NY 10001, tel. 212-255-0520

South Asian AIDS Action, P.O. Box 1326, Stuyvesant Station, New York, NY 10009, tel. 212-475-6486

Women and AIDS Resource Network (WARN), 30 Third Ave., Suite 212, Brooklyn, NY 11217, tel. 718-596-6007

Women at Risk, 252 Seventh Ave., 11th Fl., New York, NY 10001, tel. 212-255-5477

Women in Crisis, 360 W. 125th St., Suite 11, New York, NY 10027, tel. 212-316-5200

# ❖ Chapter 14

# Substance Abuse Issues

ANN B. WILLIAMS
PATRICK G. O'CONNOR

In many parts of the world, including North America and parts of Europe, a major risk behavior associated with the acquisition of HIV infection among women is injection drug use. The growth of the HIV epidemic among women has highlighted the serious and complex issues raised by women's substance abuse and requires that clinicians caring for women with HIV infection be well informed about the dynamics of substance abuse in women and about current treatment approaches.

In addition, the substance abuse activities of a sexual partner are a significant influence in the lives of the majority of North American women with HIV. This is true for two reasons. First, most women who use drugs have a male sexual partner who also uses drugs, and drug-using women are more likely than drug-using men to have drug-using partners. Second, in areas of the world in which injection drug use plays a large role in HIV transmission, heterosexual transmission from drug-using men to their non-drug-using female sexual partners is driving a rapid growth of the epidemic among women. Indeed, as of March 1993, 80% of the cumulative reported cases of AIDS in U.S. women were attributed to injection drug use, either to the woman's own drug injection or to heterosexual transmission from a male partner who injected drugs (Centers for Disease Control and Prevention [CDC], 1993b).

An additional important feature of the epidemic is the close relationship between substance abuse, specifically injection drug use, and pediatric AIDS. The overwhelming majority of children under 13 reported with AIDS in the United States are the children of men or women who inject drugs. Thus, substance abuse plays a major role in the epidemic of HIV/AIDS among U.S. women and children, and the dynamics of addictive disease and its treatment are a major influence on the experience of living with HIV/AIDS for these individuals and their families.

Discussion of the relationship between HIV/AIDS and substance abuse most often focuses on the use of heroin and cocaine. Although these drugs are not the most frequently abused drugs in the United States, they are the ones most often taken by injection. In addition, noninjection cocaine use, specifically the use of crack cocaine, is thought to play a large part in the growth of the HIV epidemic among poor, urban women through its association with exposure to multiple sexual partners in the exchange of sex for drugs or money (Chaisson et al., 1991). Noninjection cocaine use is also associated with the increased incidence of other sexually transmitted diseases that are responsible for significant morbidity among women, including syphilis (Greenberg, Singh, Htoo, & Schultz, 1991) and genital ulcer disease (Chirgwin, DeHovitz, Dillon, & McCormack, 1991).

Thus, it is essential that clinicians who care for women with HIV infection have an understanding of substance abuse patterns and addictive disease that is both intellectually sophisticated and emotionally compassionate. The issues of substance abuse are so intimately connected to the HIV/AIDS epidemic among North American women that they are addressed throughout this volume. In this chapter, we discuss a primary care approach to understanding, identifying, and treating addictive disease, with a specific focus on the features of this problem that are uniquely experienced by women.

## ❖ Addictive Disease: A Primary Care Approach

To diagnose and manage addictive disorders effectively in their patients, primary care providers need to be familiar with the basic concepts and principles associated with substance use and addictive diseases. The fundamental concepts of addictive disease are similar in both women and men.

### Definitions

For the primary provider, *substance abuse* might best be thought of as a chronic disease. As with other chronic diseases, substance abuse is characterized by (1) a long time frame, (2) a natural history that includes exacerbations ("relapse") and remission ("clean" and "sober" periods), and (3) varying responsiveness to treatment. Thus, substance abuse may, in part, be viewed in a manner similar to other chronic diseases, such as diabetes and chronic obstructive pulmonary disease. In substance abuse, "cure" is not necessarily considered as an objective; rather, the overall goal is to care for patients by helping them attain a drug-free state ("abstinence") and maintain this state for as long as possible. Other, more specific, concepts differentiate substance abuse disorders from common chronic diseases.

*Substance dependence* is diagnosed in DSM-III-R (1987)[1] when a minimum of three of the nine symptoms of dependence have been present for at least 1 month. Dependence symptoms include a progressive but unintentional increase in the amount of substance use over time, unsuccessful

---

[1] *The Diagnostic and Statistical Manual of Mental Disorders,* 3rd Ed. revised (DSM-III-R), and its future version (DSM-IV) categorize substance use disorders for all "psychoactive" substances (American Psychiatric Association, 1987).

efforts to cut down, a great deal of time invested in substance use activities, frequent intoxication or withdrawal symptoms, interference with work and family life, continued use despite the presence of persistent medical or psychosocial complications, the presence of tolerance (need for increased amounts to achieve intoxication), the presence of characteristic withdrawal symptoms, and the use of substance to relieve withdrawal symptoms. (The term *substance abuse* refers to harmful use without dependence.)

## Substances of Abuse

A number of substances have been identified as having abuse potential. These include both licit substances, such as alcohol and tobacco, and illicit substances, such as heroin and cocaine. A variety of classification schemes have been developed to describe substances of abuse. Major categories of substances, with routes of administration and common street names, are outlined in Table 14–1. Sedative-hypnotic drugs commonly include alcohol and prescription drugs, such as benzodiazepines and barbiturates. In this as in other categories, prescription drugs can be obtained both legally and illegally. Each of the major sedative-hypnotic drugs has similar patterns of intoxication and withdrawal. Intoxication is generally characterized by initial euphoria followed by decreased consciousness and, in severe cases, coma and death. Withdrawal from alcohol and other sedative-hypnotic medications is typically characterized by a state of excitation that can include hypertension, tachycardia, agitation, and hallucination.

The opioid drugs fall into three categories: naturally occurring, semi-synthetic, and synthetic (Jaffe & Martin, 1990). Naturally occurring opioids are derived from the poppy plant and are exemplified by morphine. Heroin (diacetylmorphine) was manufactured by the Bayer Company in 1898 as a potentially "nonaddictive" semisynthetic opioid for cough suppression. More recently, a variety of synthetic opioids, such as fentanyl, have been synthesized for use as analgesics and anesthetics. These synthetic opioids are often much more potent than street heroin, resulting in a higher risk of death from overdose. Opioids bind primarily to the $\mu$ receptor in the central nervous system to exert their effects. The withdrawal syndrome associated with opioids is similar to sedative-hypnotic withdrawal and includes hypertension, tachycardia, and agitation. Hallucinations and seizures, however, are typically not features of the opioid withdrawal syndrome.

Cocaine is perhaps the most notorious of the stimulant class of medications. Derived from the coca leaf, cocaine use has been described over many years. In the 1800s, cocaine was found in beverages such as Coca-Cola. The use of cocaine in this manner was banned by the Harrison Narcotic Act of 1914, although it remains available for pharmaceutical purposes. A variety of cocaine "epidemics" have been described since the late 1800s. The most recent epidemic in the 1980s was documented in greater detail than the others. Cocaine's clinical effects are based in part on the blockade of the

TABLE 14–1  Major Substances of Abuse

| Substance | Route of Administration | Slang/Street Name |
|---|---|---|
| *Sedative Hypnotics* | | |
| Alcohol | By mouth | Booze, brew |
| Benzodiazepines | By mouth | Tranks, valium |
| Barbiturates | By mouth parenteral | Barbs, downers |
| *Opioids* | | |
| Natural (e.g., morphine) | By mouth parenteral Inhalation (snorting) Smoking | Morph |
| Semisynthetic (e.g., heroin) | Same as natural opioids | Dope, jive, junk |
| Synthetic (e.g., fentanyl) | Parenteral | P-dope |
| *Stimulants* | | |
| Cocaine | Inhalation (snorting) Parenteral Smoking | Coke, snow Crack, hubba |
| Amphetamines | By mouth Parenteral | Dex, meth, speed Crystal, black beauties |
| *Cannabinoids* | | |
| Marijuana | By mouth Smoking | Weed, grass |
| Hashish | Same as marijuana | Hash |
| *Hallucinogens* | | |
| Lysergic acid diethylamide (LSD) | By mouth | Acid |
| Methylene dioxy-amphetamine (MDA) | By mouth | Ecstasy |
| *Inhalants* | | |
| Solvents | Inhalation | |
| Adhesives | Inhalation | |
| Tobacco | Inhalation | |

presynaptic reuptake of dopamine and norepinephrine (Gawin & Ellinwood, 1988). The excess of neurotransmitters that results produces a variety of physiologic effects, including tachycardia, hypertension, and vasoconstriction. The high, or euphoria, associated with cocaine is often described as intense and is associated with enhanced self-image and awareness of one's surroundings. Cocaine withdrawal, unlike withdrawal from sedatives or opioids, has been more difficult to characterize. Although no discrete physiologic phenomena characterize cocaine withdrawal, patients frequently present with a variety of psychological symptoms, including profound fatigue, depression, and anhedonia (Gawin & Kleber, 1986; Satel et al., 1991).

Powdered cocaine, when mixed with baking soda and water and heated, forms small pieces known as "rocks" of crack cocaine. These small pellets, which sell for between $5 and $10 each, are smoked to produce a rapid euphoria. Smoking delivers large quantities of cocaine to the vascular bed of the lung. The relatively low-cost, rapid intoxication and the powerful subsequent craving have combined to create a severe public health problem among women in many urban communities.

Other stimulants that have been known for their abuse potential are the amphetamines. The physiologic and behavioral effects of these substances are similar to those seen with cocaine. Intoxication with both amphetamines and cocaine can present with severe physiologic hyperactivity and psychological symptoms, including psychosis. Cocaine intoxication has also been associated with discrete medical complications, including cardiac and brain ischemia and infarction (O'Connor, Chang, & Shi, 1992).

Tetrahydrocannabinol (THC) is the active ingredient in marijuana. Marijuana is a preparation of the *Cannabis sativa* plant that consists of dried, crushed leaves. It is the resin of this plant that contains THC. A higher grade formulation of this resin is obtained to produce hashish. THC-containing substances can be smoked and consumed orally. The sought-after effects of marijuana and related substances include euphoria, enhanced self-esteem, and excitement (Jaffe, 1990). The effect of smoked cannabis lasts from 2 to 4 hours, while the effects of ingested cannabis can last up to 12 hours. Mild withdrawal symptoms have been described, including anxiety and insomnia. The harmful effects of marijuana use have been less clearly documented than those of other substances. Although psychological symptoms such as psychosis have been described, they seem to be uncommon. There is evidence to suggest that marijuana may exacerbate existing psychiatric problems (Thacore & Shukla, 1976). Studies have documented that THC may have some effects on reproductive hormones like testosterone (Smith & Ash, 1987). However, the long-term significance of these effects is unclear.

Hallucinogens represent another major category of substances of abuse. Major drugs that fall into this category include lysergic acid diethylamide (LSD), methylene dioxyamphetamine (MDA), and phencyclidine (PCP). LSD achieved notoriety in the mid-1960s. The hallucinogens result in a complex of symptoms that includes perceptual disturbances, both visual and auditory. In addition, users describe a variety of mood disturbances as well as depersonalization. Hallucinogens exert their effects through alterations in the secretion and actions of neurotransmitters like serotonin. The serotonin receptor 5-HT$_2$ is thought to be particularly important in mediating the effects of hallucinogens (Glennon, Tateler, & McKenney, 1984). Intoxication from hallucinogens can include acute anxiety, paranoia, and delirium.

Inhalant abuse is particularly common among younger individuals who may have limited access to other euphoriants. A variety of substances are commonly abused as inhalants, including solvents such as paint thinners and gasoline, aerosol sprays, and adhesives. The active ingredients in these products include toluene, acetone, methanol, and propane. Euphoria and headache are the major symptoms of intoxication. A variety of significant medical complications have been described in this population, including central nervous system, pulmonary, and psychiatric diseases (Sharp & Rosenburg, 1992).

## Screening and Diagnosis

Substance use disorders are highly prevalent in primary care populations; estimates range as high as 20% in the case of alcohol (Cleary, Miller, & Bush, 1988). Given this high prevalence, all patients seen in primary care settings should be carefully screened for substance use. Certain social or medical "red flags" should raise the provider's suspicion that a substance use disorder may be present. For example, patients who present with psychiatric or psychological symptoms like anxiety or depression may be more likely to have an underlying substance use disorder than patients without these symptoms. Among women, higher rates of suicide and attempted suicide have been related to psychotropic drug use (Fidell, 1981). Social dysfunction, such as repeated unemployment, divorce, or legal problems, may also be suggestive of substance use. Episodes of domestic violence, battering, or sexual abuse may reflect active substance use in the family.

Specific medical complaints may also give an important clue to substance abuse in patients. For example, alcoholic patients may present with hypertension, dyspepsia or peptic ulcer disease, acute hepatitis, or symptoms of peripheral neurologic disease. Common symptoms associated with cocaine use include palpitations, headache, or a recent history of cardiac or neurologic ischemia. Injection drug users may present with a specific set of problems relating directly to the fact that they use needles, including HIV infection, hepatitis, and soft tissue infection. Among women, recurrent gynecologic problems, sexually transmitted diseases, and menstrual irregularities, although not diagnostic of substance abuse, suggest the need for further evaluation. Thus, when any of these or other red flags are present, the primary care provider needs to be especially careful to obtain a detailed substance use history.

From a primary care perspective, women who use drugs are often elusive and difficult to identify. In the hospital, women at risk are found particularly in the emergency room, the pediatric and gynecology services, and on the inpatient units. Women conceal their drug use from health care professionals out of fear of rejection and in reaction to previous difficult encounters with the health care system. In turn, providers may be reluctant to confront women when substance abuse is suspected. Women who avoid care for themselves will often bring their children for care, and it may be useful to take advantage of this by providing care for mothers and children in one clinical setting. However, it is important to realize that women's concerns for their children, feelings of guilt, and fears about loss of custody may influence the nature of their relationship with providers.

## Substance Use History

Important components of the substance use history include the types of substances used, frequency of use, duration of use, route of administration, presence of complications, and prior treatment history. Clinicians must be aware that polysubstance use is common. For example, individuals who use cocaine frequently use alcohol or other sedatives to medicate some of the side effects of cocaine. Prior treatment history is particularly important if a thoughtful referral to treatment is to be made. Once a trusting patient-provider relationship has been established, periodic reassessment of substance use may yield information that was previously withheld.

## Discussing the Diagnosis

Even after the primary care provider has collected sufficient information to make the diagnosis of a substance use disorder, denial frequently interferes with the ability of patients to understand and accept this information. It is important that clinicians consider this issue and discuss the diagnosis with patients in a nonjudgmental and empathetic fashion. It is useful to educate patients carefully about the diagnosis of substance use disorder so that they can understand how their own symptoms or problems fit into this definition. It may not be unusual for patients to require several visits before they can fully accept this information. In addition, some patients may acknowledge their problem but be unwilling or unable to change their behavior.

## Initiating Treatment for Substance Abuse

Once the patient has accepted the diagnosis, the primary care provider needs to consider carefully how to initiate treatment in patients. The two phases of substance abuse treatment are detoxification and maintenance of abstinence. Goals for treatment must be discussed explicitly and in the context of the patient's life experience. Goals must also be realistic and must take into account the fact that a remission can be difficult to achieve and that relapse in substance use disorders is common. Successful drug treatment is best achieved with a multidisciplinary team approach that includes primary care providers, drug-treatment providers, and representatives from social work, nursing, and other providers. Many patients, perhaps the majority, will benefit from additional community-based specialty services for substance abuse treatment. Thus, it is imperative that the primary care provider has a thorough knowledge of local resources and an effective working relationship with drug-treatment providers. These are important not only in referral for treatment, but also in helping to monitor patients who are enrolled in substance abuse treatment.

**Detoxification**   Patients who are more severely dependent on substances may require supervised detoxification. The determination as to whether detoxification should take place on an outpatient or inpatient setting depends on such topics as prior treatment experience, level of dependence, likelihood of complications of withdrawal, presence of medical and psychiatric comorbidity, and the availability of social support, such as a place to live and someone to stay with during detoxification. It is imperative that the detoxification plan include clear follow-up contingencies to enroll patients in ongoing treatment for the maintenance of abstinence.

The goal for detoxification is to bring patients safely from a drug-using to a drug-free state. Commonly used therapies are designed to prevent complications of withdrawal, such as seizures, and the return to drug use. In many cases, detoxification is based on cross-tolerance; the substance of abuse is gradually withdrawn, and a pharmacologically similar substance is substituted and then slowly tapered. Examples of this approach include benzodiazepines for alcohol withdrawal and methadone for heroin withdrawal. Other therapies have been designed to provide partial relief of important symptoms, such as clonidine for heroin withdrawal and tricyclic antidepressants for cocaine withdrawal (Kosten, 1992).

**Pharmacologic Strategies for Maintaining Abstinence**   In addition to treating the withdrawal, pharmacological strategies have also been developed to promote the maintenance of abstinence for specific substances. Among the most well-known strategies for long-term treatment of heroin addiction is methadone maintenance. Methadone, which is a long-acting (greater than 24 hours), orally effective opioid, when substituted for heroin, effectively blocks heroin craving and withdrawal. Developed by Dole and Nyswander in the 1960s, methadone maintenance has come to be viewed as an effective, although controversial, treatment modality for heroin addiction (Dole & Nyswander, 1965). Its effectiveness has been demonstrated in a variety of studies of heroin addicts. Outcomes such as heroin use, injection drug use, legal problems, and other aspects of social functioning have been shown to be positively treated with methadone. The controversy around methadone maintenance often centers on the issue of substitute addiction. In addition, methadone maintenance may be required for many years to maintain some patients in a drug-free state.

The short-term goals for methadone maintenance are to help patients stop using injection drugs and cease addiction-supporting behaviors like theft and prostitution. Once patients have been stabilized, the process of improving their social and medical status begins. The long-term goals of methadone maintenance are a return to effective social functioning and, if possible, eventual methadone detoxification. Earlier in the course of treatment, patients are typically seen daily in the program where the methadone is dispensed. Other treatment modalities that are given along with methadone maintenance include counseling, vocational rehabilitation, and medical care.

An alternative approach to methadone maintenance can be the use of naltrexone, a long-acting, orally effective opioid antagonist (Jaffe & Martin, 1990). Naltrexone works by blocking the opioid receptors so that patients who use opioids are less likely to experience euphoria and thus are presumably less motivated to use drugs. Although effective in highly motivated patients, such as professionals whose jobs depend on the maintenance of abstinence, naltrexone is generally considered to be less effective in "street addicts" with less to lose. Naltrexone is typically administered in doses of 100 mg on Mondays and Wednesdays and 150 mg on Fridays. As with methadone maintenance, counseling and other activities are provided. The primary side effects of chronic naltrexone maintenance may include mild anorexia and nausea. In addition, naltrexone is potentially hepatotoxic; serum transaminase elevations have been noted and should be monitored with chronic therapy.

As noted earlier, unlike pharmacotherapy for opioid addiction, the search for pharmacotherapies for cocaine addition has been less fruitful. A variety of agents have been studied, including antidepressants and dopaminergic drugs. Antidepressants are believed to be useful in reducing cocaine craving. The substances studied include desipramine, imipramine, and lithium. Similarly, dopaminergic agents like bromocriptine have in some studies shown beneficial effects in terms of craving and cocaine use. Although the results of these studies have been promising, they have suffered from methodological difficulties, including low treatment samples and lack of long-term follow-up (Kosten, 1992). Buprenorphine has been studied as an alternative to methadone in opioid-addicted patients who are also using cocaine, with promising early results. Thus, although a variety of substances have been evaluated, none has been widely accepted for widespread use.

### Nonpharmacologic Strategies for Maintaining Abstinence

In addition to the pharmacotherapies evaluated earlier, a variety of nonpharmacologic strategies have been employed with some success in promoting the maintenance of abstinence from substance use. Specific modalities have included self-help groups, such as the 12-step programs of Alcoholics Anonymous and Narcotics Anonymous, as well as more formal substance abuse treatment program strategies, such as individual, group, and family therapy and behavioral interventions. These modalities are designed to help individuals identify high-risk situations and develop coping strategies to avoid relapse.

Generally speaking, successful substance abuse treatment may involve the use of multiple treatment modalities, including pharmacologic and nonpharmacologic interventions. For the primary care provider, brief intervention strategies used in the office setting represent an initial step in engaging patients in drug treatment. Often, providers can combine office-based management with the prescription of self-help meetings for individuals interested in this approach. Clearly, however, the primary care provider must be knowledgeable about local drug treatment programs, both outpatient and inpatient, for individuals in need of more intensive therapies.

In some situations, patients may benefit from referral to long-term residential treatment as part of a therapeutic community. However, the majority of these programs are not designed to meet the special needs of women.

### Anticipating Relapse

The primary care provider must consider the fact that relapse is part of the natural history of addictive disorders. Individuals may be at highest risk for relapse early in abstinence. Commonly, patients may complain of increased anxiety or depression prior to a relapse. It is the role of the primary care provider to be sensitive to the possibility of relapse and responsive to patients' needs so that relapse can be prevented, or should it occur, be kept as brief as possible.

## ❖ Addictive Disease: Special Issues for Women

### Physiologic Impact

Physiologic differences in addiction between men and women are poorly understood; very little basic or clinical research has been conducted on sex differences in the pharmacokinetics and pharmacodynamics of commonly abused drugs. Experience suggests that such gender-associated differences, if they exist, have little immediate impact and that differences in the natural history of drug dependence and treatment outcomes are the result of social context, access to care, and particular treatment modalities.

The most common gender-specific physiological effect of substance abuse among women is menstrual dysfunction. This may be the result of a stressful and disorganized life-style featuring lack of sleep, inadequate nutrition, and weight loss associated with active heroin and cocaine use or the direct result of opioid drug use. Amenorrhea is a well-known effect of narcotic agents (Santen, Sofsky, Bilic, & Lippert, 1975), often making its first appearance when women begin methadone maintenance therapy. The steady plasma levels of methadone achieved by regular daily dosing can induce amenorrhea even in women who do not experience this effect while using heroin, most likely because the total amount of opioid in heroin purchased on the street is low. Tolerance to the hypothalamic effects of methadone occurs during chronic methadone maintenance therapy, and the majority of women experience the return of menses after 12 to 18 months of therapy (Kreek, 1983). As a result of irregular menses, women may believe they are infertile, fail to use contraceptives, and fail to identify early pregnancy.

## Psychosocial Issues

Women who use drugs suffer more discrimination, stigma, and guilt than men who use drugs. The patterns, experience, and implications of drug use are different for men and women as a result of the culture and society in which they live and in which personality is formed. Recognition of the fundamental part that gender plays in personality development and role relationships is a prerequisite to understanding the dynamics of drug use in women. To a large extent, gender defines individual identity, the structure of an individual's life cycle, the nature of her life experience, and the opportunities and resources available to her. Some of these parameters, such as childbearing, are biologically determined, whereas others, such as economic independence and resources, are culturally determined, but all work to shape the patterns of women's drug use.

Men and women, particularly in economically impoverished and politically marginalized groups, live in a world that is often segregated by gender and in which there are very different expectations about appropriate behavior and roles for men and women. In this context, the stigma associated with drug use also differs for men and women. Drug abuse is viewed negatively for both, but for women, drug use, especially injection drug use, is considered directly antagonistic to the natural, "feminine" self. Men's drug use, although not approved behavior, is not "unmanly." A woman with a drug abuse problem, when identified, may be described as "sicker" than her male counterpart. In addition to the drug problem, she has an additional gender-related personality problem because she has a "male" disease. Attitudes, even among health care professionals and drug abuse program staff, are more negative toward women than men with addictive disease.

The differences in the patterns of drug use among men and women in our society are a reflection of social context. Women are more likely than men to use and become dependent on legal drugs, such as over-the-counter appetite suppressants or prescription antidepressants and psychotropics (Fidell, 1981). Historically, as long as a drug such as heroin was legal, it was a "woman's drug." Before the Harrison Narcotic Act of 1914, two times as many women as men were dependent on narcotics. This dependence among largely middle-class women was seen as unfortunate but neither unfeminine nor criminal. When the use of the drug became illegal and moved underground, it became associated with male criminality, and women who continued to use the drug acquired the stigma associated with criminal and lower-class behavior (Sutker, 1981). Heroin and cocaine were both originally marketed in the United States as patent medicines and followed the same route to the underground world of drug traffickers and crime.

Men and women who use dependence-inducing drugs derive essentially the same reinforcing effects from initial drug use: feelings of pleasure and relief from anxiety. However, for women, powerful life events that may trigger an initiation or return to drug use are often related to sex role and sexuality. Such self-reported events include childbirth and postpartum depression, abortion, miscarriage, divorce, a child leaving home, the death of a family member, infertility, hysterectomy, menstrual difficulties, and menopause. These crises all relate to aspects of the specifically female role in society, with an emphasis on childbearing and mothering.

Addicted women have lower self-esteem and higher levels of anxiety and depression than do addicted men or nonaddicted women from a similar socioeconomic background (Colten, 1979). In spite of the fact that they are survivors and fiercely protective of their children, they are often not assertive in their personal relationships and have little sense of control over their lives. They often mirror the negative attitudes of society, believing themselves unworthy of respect or care. Their value systems are frequently quite traditional and conservative, that is, they hold traditional beliefs about sex role behaviors and see themselves as personal failures when they are unable to maintain these standards.

Women who use drugs have fewer social networks and receive less support from male partners than men who use drugs or nonaddicted women from similar backgrounds (Tucker, 1979). They are likely to have few close relationships; their strongest relationship is often with their mothers, who are particularly likely to maintain the connection when there are young children requiring care. Addicted women have fewer psychological and practical resources and skills for coping with the problems of daily life than do their male counterparts or other women.

If they have a male spouse, he is also likely to use drugs and provide little in the way of support. Relationships are often dominated by the need to acquire drugs; drugs, particularly opiates, replace sex. The majority of women who inject illicit drugs are introduced to drug use by a male companion, and many remain dependent on men for a supply of drugs (Gomberg, 1981). However, often women will take on primary responsibility for securing money to purchase drugs for both partners through prostitution or shoplifting, activities that are seen as "easier" than the burglaries or more violent crimes men may perform for the same purpose. Their role as primary providers of drug money, however, does not bring concomitant power in the relationship.

Women who use drugs face very hard times on the street; they must take daily risks to survive and to support their addiction. They are frequently in physically vulnerable situations and, of course, risk death with each injection. In addition, in many cases they have been rejected by their families and isolated in their communities. Sexual relationships may have been abusive and exploitative. Drug dependence represents an extreme loss of autonomy and control; drug-dependent women occupy one of the most powerless rungs of society. It is not surprising that their lives are often shaped by violence, sexual assault, and prostitution. Moreover, it is remarkable the extent to which women in this situation are able to create a meaningful life for themselves and their children.

## Mothering

In the United States, the majority of women who use drugs are women of childbearing age. Many drug-dependent women have limited options as a result of poverty and inadequate schooling, and they may not see much potential for their own economic or social betterment. Motherhood is a role that is open to them and that is socially valued in both their immediate community and in the larger society. Children are a major source of strength to women; they offer the potential for love given and received and sometimes for the restoration of family ties severed during years of drug use. Concern for the well-being of a child can provide the strongest motivation for changing drug use patterns or for ceasing to use drugs altogether. A woman who takes good care of her children, in spite of drug use, is respected among her peers.

However, the reality of mothering may conflict with the demands of drug dependence. The need to acquire large amounts of money for drugs can lead to illegal activities, which carry the risk of arrest and imprisonment. Small children may be placed in physically dangerous situations in which drugs are traded and used or may be left at home with inadequate supervision. Pride in mothering skills is severely undermined by guilt when addiction impairs the ability to care successfully for a child. If women do lose custody of their children, it is devastating, especially when the children are placed with strangers as a result of protective services intervention. Women, recognizing the negative effect of their drug use but unable to stop, will frequently voluntarily send their children to live with extended family members, often an older female relative.

For many women who use heroin or cocaine, pregnancies are not planned. The drugs themselves and the chaotic life-style associated with their use disrupt the menstrual cycle, causing long periods of amenorrhea that lead women to believe they are infertile. Even women who do not want children often fail to use effective contraception. Also, as a result of irregular menstrual cycles, women may not realize they are pregnant until late in the pregnancy, forestalling access to early prenatal care or abortion services.

The obstetric and neonatal complications and problems associated with substance abuse in pregnancy are the result of either the direct effects of the drugs or the indirect effects of the life-style associated with drug use. Women who are actively injecting heroin or cocaine are at risk for inadequate weight gain, placental abruptio, and premature labor. Their infants may be premature, small for gestational age, and opiate dependent (Keith et al., 1989; Lewis & Watters, 1989). However, a clear and consistent description of the consequences of prenatal drug exposure has been extremely difficult to achieve for several reasons. First, the use of more than one drug is common; for example, cocaine is often used in conjunction with heroin, benzodiazepines, or alcohol. Second, drug use patterns are embedded in a dynamic social context and may change rapidly. Third, it is extremely difficult to establish accurately the composition of illicit drugs as well as the dose, duration, and timing of prenatal exposure. Fourth, the neurodevelopmental and behavioral abnormalities postulated to result from prenatal drug exposure are difficult to measure, may take years to develop, and are confounded by social variables like class, education, and family function. All these factors complicate attempts to conduct both prospective and retrospective studies of the effects of maternal drug use.

In spite of these research difficulties, it is clear that prenatal drug exposure has negative consequences for the infant. The infants of women who are dependent on opiates will also be opiate dependent and will require observation and possibly pharmacologic treatment for neonatal abstinence syndrome. Neonatal abstinence syndrome has been well described, and treatment regimens are established (Finnegan, 1979); however, even after successful drug withdrawal, these infants may be unusually irritable and difficult to feed and to mother. Infants exposed to cocaine also demonstrate increased irritability, tremors, and diarrhea and are difficult to feed and console (Fulroth, Phillips, & Durand, 1989; Oro & Dixon, 1987). A number of congenital malformations, including eye, cardiac, and genitourinary defects, have also been suspected but not established (Bingol, Fuch, Diaz, Stone, & Gromish, 1987; Chasnoff, Chisum, & Kaplan, 1988; Little, Snell, Klein, & Gilstrap, 1988; Zuckerman et al., 1989).

From a primary care perspective, the first goal must be to establish a positive relationship with the mother and engage her in prenatal care. Comprehensive prenatal care includes careful evaluation of the extent of substance use and the initiation of appropriate treatment. For women with a primary opiate dependence, appropriate treatment is most often stabilization on methadone maintenance therapy. It is believed that the advantages of ending the cycle of maternal drug craving, injection, intoxication, and withdrawal outweigh the disadvantages associated with neonatal opiate dependence. In addition, mothers-to-be can benefit from the social and psychological support services of a methadone maintenance program.

As discussed earlier, treatment modalities for cocaine addiction are much less well developed than those for opiate dependence. Pharmacologic therapies have not been studied in pregnancy and cannot be recommended; therefore, the emphasis is on behavioral and psychological approaches. The lack of successful, standardized treatment strategies for pregnant cocaine addicts is a significant problem as the cocaine epidemic grows.

The primary problem facing pregnant drug users and the clinicians who care for them is access to drug abuse treatment. Physicians and nurses in maternal and child health services are often overwhelmed and frustrated by the myriad of physical and psychosocial problems associated with maternal substance abuse. They desperately need the support of substance abuse specialists in a multidisciplinary team. However, many drug-treatment programs, especially residential programs (also overwhelmed and underfunded), have been reluctant to admit women during pregnancy. In spite of the development of a few specialized programs to address the needs of pregnant women as demonstration or research projects, in most parts of the country such services continue to be scarce.

## ❖ Medical Problems Associated with Addiction

Among both men and women who use drugs, especially injection drugs, a variety of health problems are common. These include conditions precipitated directly by drugs, such as heroin-associated nephropathy, cocaine-induced cardiac arrhythmias and arrest, and seizures from stimulant overdose, and conditions associated with drug administration. The latter fall into two groups: problems related to the trauma of drug administration and infectious disease complications. Traumatic complications are sclerosed or collapsed peripheral veins, sterile abscesses from drug infiltration, pneumothorax from needle puncture suffered in an attempt to inject into a jugular vein, and necrosis and perforation of the nasal septum as a result of the vasoconstrictive effect of cocaine inhalation.

HIV is only the most recently recognized infectious disease complication of substance abuse. Other bacterial and viral infections frequently encountered in drug users are bacteremia and endocarditis, bronchitis and pneumonia, hepatitis, abscesses, cellulitis, osteomyelitis, pyelonephritis, and spinal abscesses. Infections are most often due to common community-acquired organisms, but the possibility of infection with unusual agents must always be considered in the context of drug injection. Sexually transmitted diseases and pelvic inflammatory disease are of particular concern among women because of their long-term effects on health and childbearing.

## ❖ Addictive Disease: Interaction with HIV

The infectious disease complications of injection drug use, which were well known prior to the HIV/AIDS epidemic, are clearly more frequent among HIV-infected drug users. Bacterial infections, especially pneumonia, occur earlier in the course of HIV infection when the immune system is still relatively intact and may be considered a sentinel event. Tuberculosis disease, primarily reactivation of old infection, has been shown to occur more frequently among HIV-infected drug users than among noninfected drug users in methadone treatment (Selwyn et al., 1992).

It has not been shown that continued substance abuse accelerates the progression of HIV infection, although clearly, active drug injectors continue to be exposed to a wide range of pathogens, including additional strains of HIV. More significantly, active substance abusers are less likely to seek health care or to be compliant with treatment for medical problems. Health-seeking behavior may be erratic and crisis-oriented.

In addition, active drug use can complicate the presentation of a variety of clinical syndromes, making the differential diagnosis very difficult. Constitutional symptoms, such as weight loss, anorexia, myalgias, and diarrhea, may represent either the effects of drugs like cocaine, heroin, or alcohol or may be HIV-related. Similarly, the central-nervous-system effects of drug intoxication may be difficult to differentiate from HIV-related neurologic disease without repeated extensive evaluations.

Self-medication, pain management, and drug interactions are important considerations in the pharmacologic management of women with HIV disease. Women who use drugs are accustomed to self-prescribing and may attempt to treat soft tissue infections, vaginitis, urinary tract infections, and even HIV exposures with antibiotics and other medications acquired from friends. Women will often share medications with others who appear to have similar symptoms, especially male partners who may have more limited access to clinical services and medications through entitlement programs. It is important to ask very specifically and carefully about these possibilities because women may not see them as relevant to their care and may otherwise fail to mention them.

Pain management for HIV-infected women is a challenging problem; the complexities of the problem are exacerbated by active substance use and by the attitudes of health professionals toward former users. Although concern about drug-seeking behavior is appropriate, it is necessary to start from the premise that the primary goal is pain relief. Women who are opiate dependent, whether on illicit drugs or methadone maintenance therapy, have developed tolerance to these drugs and generally need larger doses of standard analgesic medications as a result. Based on previous experiences, many women expect to be undermedicated and approach potentially painful procedures with great anxiety. They may self-medicate before coming to the hospital with opiates, benzodiazepines, or other drugs obtained on the street.

Because both patients and providers approach the problem of acute and chronic pain management with preconceived attitudes based partly on personal belief systems and partly on previous experiences, it is important that the plan for addressing pain be openly discussed, thoroughly understood, and mutually agreed on. Women should feel that their pain is taken seriously and should know what they can expect from the provider in terms of medication dose and renewal.

A variety of interactions between drugs prescribed for management of HIV-related problems and methadone or other drugs have been described. Some interactions with methadone were well known before the onset of the HIV/AIDS epidemic and have achieved greater significance in this context. Rifampin has long been known to precipitate an opiate withdrawal syndrome in patients on methadone maintenance through the increased hepatic metabolism of methadone (Kreek, Garfield, & Cutjahr, 1976). It is important to preempt this response by increasing the daily methadone dose gradually but concurrently with initiation of rifampin; the eventual result may be as much as a 50% increase in the methadone. Failure to make this adjustment often leads to lack of compliance with the rifampin regimen. Rifabutin is another drug, related to rifampin, that is commonly used to treat mycobacterium avium complex (MAC) and that has recently been recommended as MAC prophylaxis therapy for individuals with late-stage HIV infection (CDC, 1993a). It is not known whether rifabutin increases methadone metabolism, but the possibility should be kept in mind. Phenytoin, commonly used to prevent or control seizures, is known to enhance methadone metabolism and precipitate a mild narcotic abstinence syndrome 2 to 4 days after beginning treatment (Tong, Pond, & Kreek, 1981). The reaction is milder than that associated with rifampin and can be managed with observation and appropriate increases in methadone dosage.

Pharmacokinetic studies have found no changes in methadone metabolism associated with zidovudine, although many patients believe that an interaction exists. It is important to include this information in the patient education given at the time of initiation of zidovudine therapy. Otherwise, women may attribute the early side effects of zidovudine, such as headache, nausea, and insomnia, to methadone withdrawal and stop taking the zidovudine. It is worth noting that some studies have documented reduced clearance and increased plasma levels of zidovudine in patients concurrently taking opioids, although the clinical implications of this finding are unclear (Schwartz et al., 1991).

## ❖ Substance Abuse Treatment Needs

Although women constitute a significant proportion of the clients in drug abuse treatment, research, outreach, and treatment programs have been designed for men and based on a paradigm in which addictive disease is seen as a male problem. Fewer women than men enter treatment, the retention rate is lower for women, and the treatment staff, particularly the ex-addict role models, are likely to be male. It is not surprising that substance abuse treatment programs, many of which center around a "therapeutic community," mirror many negative societal attitudes toward female addicts. Women are described as manipulative, emotional, difficult to treat, and sicker than men. Successful rehabilitation for women is more likely to be defined in terms of sex-role behaviors, relationships, and mothering than by completion of education or acquisition of employment.

Effective substance abuse treatment for women must respond to two categories of needs: practical and psychological. The most significant practical issue facing a woman considering entering treatment for drug dependence is how the treatment plan will accommodate her responsibilities as a mother. Women cannot engage in therapy without reassurance that their children are safe and that they will be able to maintain contact. In practice, this means that many women are excluded from a major treatment modality: long-term residential treatment. Within day treatment programs, inadequate or nonexistent child-care services deter many women from participation or make their participation a difficult and demeaning experience.

Traditionally, a major therapeutic approach in substance abuse treatment has focused on acceptance of individual responsibility for behavior and its consequences. Often, the technique used is one of group therapy in which addicts are confronted by their peers with the negative impact of their behavior on others. Because women begin drug abuse treatment carrying a heavy burden of guilt and with very low self-esteem, this approach is not appropriate for them and may even contribute to psychological distress.

Treatment programs for women should be designed to address the negative impact of substance abuse on women's self-esteem and should work to increase self-esteem and self-confidence by supporting women in the areas in which they feel positive about themselves. Paradoxically, women often feel the most guilt and the most pride in their activities as mothers, and thus an emphasis on mothering is appropriate. However, it is important to avoid a judgmental atmosphere that contributes to women's feelings of guilt about the impact of their substance abuse on their children because the vast majority of women begin treatment with an already overwhelming sense of guilt.

Supporting women in their efforts to be good mothers means helping women acquire the skills they need to provide and care for themselves and their children economically. Women who have little power to negotiate daily life in terms of rent, food, or clothing will find it difficult to feel good about themselves as parents. Failing to address, or at least articulate, these issues in treatment communicates to women that these social problems are their individual responsibility and perpetuates feelings of inadequacy and guilt.

## ❖ Provider Issues

Women who use injection drugs present a tremendous challenge to clinical care providers. The challenge reflects both the complex nature of the illness and the complex attitudes and beliefs of society toward drugs. To be effective, it is necessary to be aware of the dynamics of both aspects of the challenge. Health care professionals are committed to helping patients and are frustrated and puzzled by self-destructive behaviors, such as those associated with substance abuse. In their turn, women who use drugs are often mistrustful, angry, and scared. They have had tumultuous relationships with a variety of institutions in the past and have come into the clinic or the hospital ready to defend themselves. There they encounter professionals who often see them as noncompliant, manipulative, and unlikely to change. Clearly this is a prescription for a difficult relationship.

It is usually, though not always, possible to change this scenario with a carefully straightforward and honest approach. Remembering that women who have had negative experiences in the past are extremely sensitive to nuances and nonverbal behavior, it is important to convey genuine concern and a nonjudgmental attitude. Concern and acceptance do not imply condoning drug use or allowing unacceptable behavior, such as threats. A clear, structured, and consistent approach is most effective and will usually be appreciated by women, even though they may test the extent of the commitment to their care by challenging the boundaries of the relationship. Daily lives shaped by the dynamics of poverty and drug use are often chaotic and fragmented; in this context, clear expectations and limitations can be a relief and are often welcome.

Some specific aspects of this approach might include ensuring that women are cared for by one or two consistent primary care clinicians, establishing times and routes of availability for clinicians, discussing medication and prescription policies ahead of time and then adhering to those policies, and communicating frequently with other members of the health care team. When working with an angry or difficult woman, it is useful to try to hear the anxiety and guilt that is driving the anger. Until her real fears are addressed, her care will continue to be frustrating, incomplete, and less than effective.

Finally, because addiction is a chronic, relapsing disease, the effectiveness of professional interventions cannot be judged solely by abstention from drug use. Rather, effective primary care interventions are those that encourage women to care for themselves, facilitate appropriate treatment, contribute to an improved quality of life, and promote growth in self-esteem based on mutual respect.

## ❖ Summary

The growth of the HIV epidemic among women highlights the serious and complex issues raised by women's substance abuse and requires that clinicians caring for women with HIV infection be well informed about the dynamics of substance abuse in women and about current treatment approaches. Substance abuse is best thought of as a chronic, long-term disease, with periods of exacerbation and remission.

Substance use disorders are highly prevalent in primary care populations, and all women being followed for HIV disease should be carefully screened for substance use. In the context of the HIV epidemic, the use of heroin and cocaine is particularly relevant because these drugs are most often used through injection. Treatment modalities for heroin abuse are more fully defined than those for cocaine use. The two phases of substance abuse treatment are detoxification and maintenance of abstinence. Successful drug treatment is best achieved with a multidisciplinary team approach that includes primary care providers, drug-treatment providers, and representatives from social work, nursing, and other related areas.

Physiological differences in addiction between men and women are poorly understood, but experience suggests that such gender-associated differences have little immediate impact and that differences in the natural history of drug dependence and treatment outcomes are the result of social context, access to care, and particular treatment modalities. However, the social and psychological impact of substance abuse is more destructive to women's identity and self-esteem. HIV-infected women with a past or current history of substance use carry multiple burdens of responsibility and guilt.

For many women, children are a source of great strength; concern for children offers powerful motivation for ending drug use. However, the reality of mothering can conflict with the demands of drug dependence, creating additional stress. The obstetric and neonatal complications associated with substance use in pregnancy are the result of both the direct effects of the drugs and the indirect effects of the life-style associated with drug use. The primary problem facing pregnant drug users and the clinicians who care for them is a lack of substance abuse programs designed for women and their children.

HIV disease is the most recent in a large number of health problems associated with drug use in both men and women. Injection drug use in particular places women at risk for traumatic and infectious disease complications as well as for conditions precipitated by the drugs themselves. Active drug use complicates the presentation of many clinical syndromes and makes management of HIV very difficult. In working with patients who are abusing drugs, it is important to be concerned, but not judgmental, and to set clear, consistent limits. With patience and persistence, it is possible to establish a relationship of mutual respect; the rewards for doing so are great.

# References

American Psychiatric Association. (1987). *Diagnostic and statistical manual of mental disorders* (3rd ed., rev.). Washington, DC: American Psychiatric Association.

Bingol, N., Fuch, M., Diaz, V., Stone, R. K., & Gromish, D. S. (1987). Teratogenicity of cocaine in humans. *Journal of Pediatrics, 110*(1), 94–96.

Centers for Disease Control and Prevention. (1993a). Recommendations on prophylaxis and therapy for disseminated mycobacterium avium complex for adults and adolescents infected with human immunodeficiency virus. *Morbidity and Mortality Weekly Reports, 42*(RR-9), 17–19.

Centers for Disease Control and Prevention. (1993b). *HIV/AIDS Surveillance Report, 5,* 10.

Chaisson, M. A., Stoneburner, R. L., Hildebrandt, D. S., Ewing, W. E., Telzak, E. E., & Jaffe, H. W. (1991). Heterosexual transmission of HIV-1 associated with the use of smokable freebase cocaine (crack). *AIDS, 5,* 1121–1126.

Chasnoff, I. J., Chisum, G. M., & Kaplan, W. E. (1988). Maternal cocaine use and genitourinary tract malformations. *Teratology, 37*(3), 201–204.

Chirgwin, K., DeHovitz, J. A., Dillon, S., & McCormack, W. M. (1991). HIV infection, genital ulcer disease, and crack cocaine use among patients attending a clinic for sexually transmitted diseases. *American Journal of Public Health, 81*(12), 1576–1579.

Cleary, P. D., Miller, M., Bush, B. T., Warburg, M. M., Delbanco, T. L., & Aronson, M. D. (1988). Prevalence and recognition of alcohol abuse in a primary care population. *American Journal of Medicine, 85*(4), 466–471.

Colten, M. E. (1979). A descriptive and comparative analysis of self-perceptions and attitudes of heroin-addicted women. In *Addicted women: Family dynamics, self-perceptions and support systems* (DHEW publication no. [ADM] 80-762). Rockville, MD: National Institute on Drug Abuse.

Dole, V. P., & Nyswander, M. E. (1965). A medical treatment for diacetylmorphine (heroin) addiction. *Journal of the American Medical Association, 193*(8), 646–650.

Fidell, L. S. (1981). Sex differences in psychotropic drug use. *Professional Psychology, 12,* 156–162.

Finnegan, L. P. (1979). *Drug dependence in pregnancy: Clinical management of mother and child.* Rockville, MD: National Institute on Drug Abuse.

Fulroth, R., Phillips, B., & Druand, D. J. (1989). Perinatal outcome of infants exposed to cocaine and/or heroin in utero. *American Journal of Diseases in Children, 143*(8), 905–910.

Gawin, F. H., & Ellinwood, E. H. (1988). Cocaine and other stimulants. *New England Journal of Medicine, 318*(18), 1173–1182.

Gawin, F. H., & Kleber, H. D. (1986). Abstinence symptomatology and psychiatric diagnosis in cocaine abusers. *Archives of General Psychiatry, 43*(2), 107–113.

Glennon, R. A., Tateler, M., & McKenney, J. D. (1984). Evidence for 5-HT2 involvement in the mechanism of action of halucinogenic agents. *Life Sciences, 35,* 2505–2511.

Gomberg, E. S. (1981). Women, sex roles and alcohol problems. *Professional Psychology, 12*(1), 146–153.

Greenberg, M. S. Z., Singh, T., Htoo, M., & Schultz, S. (1991). The association between congenital syphilis and cocaine/crack use in New York City: A case control study. *American Journal of Public Health, 81*(10), 1316–1318.

Jaffe, J. H. (1990). Drug addiction and drug abuse. In A. G. Gilman, T. W. Rall, A. S. Nies, & P. Taylor (Eds.), *Goodman and Gilman's: The pharmacologic basis of therapeutics* (pp. 522–573). New York: McGraw-Hill.

Jaffe, J. H., & Martin, W. R. (1990). Opioid analgesics and antagonists. In A. G. Gilman, T. W. Rall, A. S. Nies, & P. Taylor (Eds.), *Goodman and Gilman's: The pharmacologic basis of therapeutics* (pp. 485–521). New York: McGraw-Hill.

Keith, L., MacGregor, S., Friedell, S., Rosner, M., Chasnoff, I. J., & Sciarra, J. J. (1989). Substance abuse in pregnant women: Recent experience at the perinatal center for chemical dependence of Northwestern Memorial Hospital. *Obstetrics and Gynecology, 73*(5), 715–720.

Kosten, T. R. (1992). Pharmacotherapies. In T. R. Kosten & H. D. Kleber (Eds.), *Clinician's guide to cocaine addiction: Theory, research and treatment* (pp. 273–289). New York: Guilford Press.

Kreek, M. J. (1983). Health consequences associated with the use of methadone. In J. R. Cooper, F. Altman, & B. S. Brown (Eds.), *Research on the treatment of narcotic addiction* (pp. 456-490). Rockville, MD: National Institute on Drug Abuse.

Kreek, M. J., Garfield, J. W., & Cutjahr, C. L. (1976). Rifampin-induced methadone withdrawal. *New England Journal of Medicine, 294*(20), 1104.

Lewis, D. K., & Watters, J. K. (1989). Human immunodeficiency virus seroprevalence in female intravenous drug users: The puzzle of black women's risk. *Social Sciences and Medicine, 29*(9), 1071–1076.

Little, B. B., Snell, L. M., Klein, V. R., & Gilstrap, L. C., III. (1988). Cocaine abuse during pregnancy: Maternal and fetal implications. *Obstetrics and Gynecology, 73*(2), 157–160.

O'Connor, P. G., Chang, J., & Shi, J. (1992). Medical complications of cocaine use. In T. R. Kosten & H. D. Kleber (Eds.), *Clinician's guide to cocaine addiction: Theory, research and treatment* (pp. 241–272). New York: Guilford Press.

Oro, A. S., & Dixon, S. D. (1987). Perinatal cocaine and methamphetamine exposure: Maternal and neonatal correlates. *Journal of Pediatrics, 111*(4), 571–578.

Santen, R. J., Sofsky, J., Bilic, N., & Lippert, R. (1975). Mechanism of action of narcotics in the production of menstrual dysfunction in women. *Fertility and Sterility, 26*(6), 538–548.

Satel, S. L, Price, L. H., Palumbo, J. N., McDougle, C. J., Krystal, J. H., Gawin, F., Charney, D. S., Heninger, G. R., & Kleber, H. D. (1991). Clinical phenomenology and neurobiology of cocaine abstinence: Prospective inpatient study. *American Journal of Psychiatry, 148*(12), 1712–1716.

Schwartz, E. L., Brechbuhl, A. B., Kahl, P., Miller, M. A., Selwyn, P. A., & Friedland, G. H. (1991). Pharmacokinetic interactions of zidovudine and methadone in intravenous drug-using patients with HIV infection. *Journal of Acquired Immune Deficiency Syndromes, 5*(6), 619–626.

Selwyn, P. A., Sckell, B. M., Alcabes, P., Friedland, G., Klein, R. S., & Schoenbaum, E. E. (1992). High risk of active tuberculosis in HIV infected drug users with cutaneous anergy. *Journal of the American Medical Association, 268*(4), 504–509.

Sharp, C. W., & Rosenburg, M. L. (1992). Volatile substances. In J. H. Lowinson, P. Ruiz, R. B. Millman, & J. G. Langrod (Eds.), *Substance abuse: A comprehensive textbook* (pp. 303–327). Baltimore: Williams and Wilkins.

Smith, C. G., & Asch, R. H. (1987). Drug abuse and reproduction. *Fertility and Sterility, 48*(3), 355–373.

Sutker, P. B. (1981). Drug dependent women: An overview of the literature. In G. M. Beschner, B. G. Reed, & J. Mondanero (Eds.), *Treatment services for drug dependent women* (pp. 25–51). Rockville, MD: National Institute on Drug Abuse.

Thacore, V. R., & Shukla, S. R. P. (1976). Cannabis psychosis and paranoid schizophrenia. *Archives of General Psychiatry, 33*(3), 383–386.

Tong, T. G., Pond, S. M., Kreek, M. J., Jeffery, N. F., & Benowitz, N. L. (1981). Phenytoin induced methadone withdrawal. *Annals of Internal Medicine, 94*(3), 349–351.

Tucker, M. B. (1979). A descriptive and comparative analysis of the social support structure of heroin-addicted women. In *Addicted women: Family dynamics, self-perceptions and support systems.* (DHEW publication no. [ADM] 80-762). Rockville, MD: National Institute on Drug Abuse.

Zuckerman, B. S., Frank, D. A., Hingson, R., Amaro, H., Levenson, S. M., Kayne, H., Parker, S., Vinci, R., Aboagye, K., Fried, L. E., Cabral, H., Timperi, R., & Bauchner, H. (1989). Effect of maternal marijuana and cocaine use on fetal growth. *New England Journal of Medicine, 320*(12), 762–768.

# ❖ Chapter 15

# Lesbians and HIV

MICHELE RUSSELL

The lesbian community responded to the first wave of the AIDS epidemic in gay men and the second wave in women and children with an outpouring of volunteer efforts. However, there has been only limited research on the risks, prevalence, and prevention of HIV in lesbians. This chapter examines some of the issues surrounding HIV infection among lesbians.

Lesbians are women whose primary emotional, psychological, social, and sexual interests are directed toward other women. Falco (1991) estimates that there are 11 million lesbians in the United States, members of all social and economic classes, educational levels, and religious, racial, and ethnic groups. The exact numbers are difficult to ascertain because many women are private about their sexual lives or do not identify as lesbian. Women may choose not to self-identify as lesbian for many reasons, including family, cultural, or societal bias, religious prohibitions, and internalized homophobia. Although a woman may not identify herself as a lesbian, she may be in a long-term monogamous relationship with another woman. Self-identified lesbians may also be sexually active with men for reasons ranging from sexual attraction to a need for money (Cochran & Mays, 1988; Young, 1992).

## ❖ HIV Risks among Lesbians

Injection drug use (IDU) has been identified by the Centers for Disease Control and Prevention (CDC) as the primary risk factor for lesbians diagnosed with AIDS. The very low incidence of AIDS among lesbians reported by the CDC (Chu, Birchler, Fleming, & Berkelman, 1990) may relate to the CDC's hierarchical classification of risk factors. For women, this classification system lists IDU first, then recipients of contaminated blood, heterosexual exposure, and finally, no identified risk. Because the CDC definition of a lesbian is a woman who has had sex exclusively with women, a single heterosexual contact on the part of a woman with HIV infection who identifies as lesbian, results in the woman being classified as bisexual and her transmission risk as heterosexual. Reports of woman-to-woman transmission have not been proved because the majority of lesbians with HIV infection have had coexisting behaviors of drug use or heterosexual contact (Marmor et al., 1986; Monzon & Capellan, 1987; Perry, Jacobsberg, &

Fogel, 1989). Although the results suggest that the confounding drug and heterosexual behaviors are responsible for the HIV transmission, more research is indicated before lesbian sexual transmission of HIV can be definitively ruled out.

Some research has been done on HIV incidence among lesbian injection drug users. Young and colleagues (1992) found that lesbian drug users were more likely to share syringes and to exchange sex for money or drugs than nonlesbian drug users. Lesbian injection drug users are often secretive about their drug use when among non drug-using lesbians (Denenberg, 1991b) because sex with men, IDU, prostitution, and HIV diagnoses are not readily accepted within the lesbian community. Therefore, lesbian drug users are often secretive about their drug use and their HIV status when among non-IDU lesbians (Denenberg, 1991a). For example, at a support group for lesbians with HIV infection at New York Hospital, the eight participants voiced feelings of fear of isolation from both lesbians and the larger society. The major issues for these women were difficulties in disclosing their HIV diagnosis, lack of pertinent information, societal bias, and social and familial rejection as a result of the combined drug use history and lesbianism. The primary themes were concerns of stigma, loss of control and powerlessness, anger, deterioration, and sex and safer sex. One woman lamented her status, "First we're black, then female, then gay, and now HIV positive." The women in this support group were poor or working-class, minority women, and their CDC-identified risk factors were heterosexual transmission or IDU.

This group felt that traditional HIV/AIDS support groups had not met their needs because these groups targeted gay men, injection drug users, and heterosexual women. "I joined a lesbian support group thinking, 'Great! I'm gonna meet some women.' One day the topic of HIV came up. None of the women were positive. They made comments like, 'Could you imagine if you met a woman who was HIV positive? I couldn't. I wouldn't touch her.' They went on and on. I sat there alone and afraid. I couldn't say anything."

One bisexual woman with a history of IDU reported that she shared needles with her husband until his death from AIDS in 1989. At that time, she learned she was HIV positive and entered Narcotics Anonymous. Although she was able to share her diagnosis in the 12-step program and in a women's HIV support group, she felt the part of her that was attracted to women was neglected and was uncomfortable discussing her sexual relationships with women in either of the two groups.

## ❖ Lesbians and Health Care

When lesbians seek heath care, they frequently will not divulge their sexual identity to their health care providers for fear of discrimination or negative reactions (Cochran & Mays, 1988; Smith et al., 1985; Stevens & Hall, 1988). In one study, 96% of lesbian respondents agreed with the statement, "You'd get poorer care if they knew you were lesbian" (Selvin, 1993).

When working with women, including those who have HIV infection, providers should not assume heterosexuality unless a woman specifically states this. Services for all women, indicating that the service is "lesbian friendly," should include the following:

❖ Information about safer sex for all sexual practices, allowing patients to make the appropriate choices
❖ Lesbian sensitivity training for all staff
❖ Substance abuse training for all staff
❖ Environment conducive to the confidential exchange of information
❖ Literature specific to lesbians for women in waiting rooms
❖ Lesbian HIV support groups
❖ Advocacy for increased research on the sexual habits of women who have sex with women

## ❖ Lesbians, Sex, and Safer Sex

The myth exists that lesbians are at low risk for HIV infection and that a study of woman-to-woman transmission is unnecessary because "lesbians don't have much sex" (Solomon, 1992). The low incidence of sexually transmitted disease among lesbians fuels the denial of risk among lesbians who feel protected from exposure to all sexually transmitted diseases, including HIV. Many lesbians feel that by avoiding women who are acknowledged bisexuals, sex workers, or drug users, they do not have to practice safer sex. In a study of self-identified lesbians in New York City, few of the women used safer sex methods identified with oral-vaginal sex. Many of them felt that they were at no risk of HIV because they had known their lovers for years, were monogamous, did not use drugs, or had not had recent sex with a man (Russell, 1992). The necessity to practice safer sex is a widely debated topic within the lesbian community. Its practice remains a personal decision because information about woman-to-woman transmission is limited and there is no evidence that female barriers are effective (Camlin, 1992).

For primary care providers, it is important to teach safer sex practices to all women, including lesbians. Transmission of HIV occurs with the exchange of blood and vaginal secretions during sexual activity, and this exchange occurs during both heterosexual and lesbian sex. Figure 15–1 describes lesbian sexual activities that may be high risk for HIV transmission. These should be discussed during sexual history taking. General guidelines include instructions to avoid sharing body fluids and to use barriers designed for women's sexual activities, such as dental dams, latex barriers, or latex or plastic squares. These barriers should be used only once, never shared, and never transferred from the vagina to the anal area. Sex toys should be cleaned after each use and used only with a condom or finger cot. Condoms should be replaced when switching sex toys between the anus and the vagina. Water-based lubricants, such as K-Y, should be used.

**High-Risk Sexual Activities**

- Oral-genital/anal sex without barrier protection
- Sharing uncovered or unclean sex toys (e.g., dildos)
- Placing uncovered fingers in the vagina or anus
- Sucking on breasts that are lactating or have galactorrhea, ulcerations, or skin breaks
- Kissing with open sores or blisters on lips or mouth
- Sadomasochistic sex that draws blood
- Sexual activity during menses without protection
- Activities that involve the exchange or intake of body fluids

**Lower Risk Sexual Activities**

- Kissing without open sores or blisters on lips or mouth
- Mutual masturbation with finger cots or latex gloves
- Sucking nonlactating breasts
- Oral-genital/anal sex with barrier protection

**Low-Risk Sexual Activities**

- Cuddling, fondling, hugging, stroking
- Sharing fantasies
- Watching erotic videos
- Self-masturbation

FIGURE 15–1    Lesbian sexual practices and risks.

## ❖ Summary

The majority of lesbians diagnosed with HIV/AIDS have risk factors of IDU and heterosexual transmission. Women who have sex with women are often "invisible" within the community; they will not always define themselves as lesbians, and they may not disclose homosexual or high-risk behaviors to health care providers. The regular practice of safer sex is not universally accepted among lesbians. It is important for health care providers to give as much health and sexual information as possible to all women, allowing them to make educated choices.

## ❖ References

Camlin, C. (1992, Summer). Dams be dammed! *Out Weekly*, 43.

Chu, S. Y., Buehler, J. W., Fleming, P. L., & Berkelman, R. L. (1990). Epidemiology of reported cases of AIDS in lesbians, United States 1980–89. *American Journal of Public Health, 80*(11), 1380–1381.

Cochran, S. D., & Mays, V. M. (1988). Disclosure of sexual preference to physicians by black lesbian and bisexual women. *Western Journal of Medicine, 149,* 616–619.

Denenberg, R. (1991a). A decade of denial: Lesbians and AIDS. *Off Our Backs,* 21–42.

Denenberg, R. (1991b). We shoot drugs and we are your sisters. *Outlook,* 30–36.

Falco, K. L. (1991). *Psychotherapy with lesbian clients: Theory into practice.* New York: Brunner Mazel.

Marmor, M., Weiss, L. R., Lyden, M., Weiss, S. H., Saxinger, W. C., Spira, T. J., & Feorino, P. M. (1986). Possible female-to-female transmission of human immunodeficiency virus. *Annals of Internal Medicine, 105*(6), 969.

Monzon, O. T., & Capellan, J. M. B. (1987). Female-to-female transmission of HIV. *Lancet, 2,* 40–41.

Perry, S., Jacobsberg, L., & Fogel, K. (1989). Orogenital transmission of human immunodeficiency virus (HIV). *Annals of Internal Medicine, 111*(11), 951–952.

Russell, M. (1992, July). *The perception of risk for HIV infection among lesbians in New York City.* Paper presented at the Eighth International Conference on AIDS, Amsterdam. (Abstract No. PoD5217)

Selvin, B. W. (1993, March 2). Doors opening for gay health care. *New York Newsday,* p. 68.

Smith, E. M., Johnson, S. R., & Guenther, S. M. (1985). Health care attitudes and experiences during gynecological care among lesbians and bisexuals. *American Journal of Public Health, 75*(9), 1085–1087.

Solomon, N. (1992, Spring). Risky business: Should lesbians practice safer sex? *Outlook,* 47–52.

Stevens, P. E., & Hall, J. M. (1988). Stigma, health beliefs and experiences with health care in lesbian women. *Image: Journal of Nursing Scholarship, 20,* 69–73.

Young, R., Weissman, G., & Cohen, J. (1992). Assessing risk in the absence of information: HIV risk among women injection-drug users who have sex with women. *AIDS and Public Policy Journal, 7*(3), 175–183.

# ❖ Chapter 16

# Ethical, Legal, and Policy Considerations

ELIZABETH B. COOPER

KATHLEEN POWDERLY

The HIV epidemic has raised profound ethical dilemmas for health care workers and for society in general. The HIV epidemic renewed the perceived conflict between public health priorities and individual civil liberties once seen with tuberculosis and venereal diseases. The demographics of those with HIV disease intensified the emotional component of the current debate. Initially, AIDS was identified primarily in gay men and intravenous drug users. When HIV was found to be transmitted through sex and drug use, societal stigmatization was intensified.

As the epidemic progressed, the face of HIV/AIDS changed dramatically. Most new cases were found in injection drug users, their sexual partners, and their children. Increasingly, newly infected individuals were poor, people of color, women of childbearing years, and children. The mobilization of resources that had been achieved by the largely middle-class gay community was much more difficult to achieve as HIV moved into highly marginalized communities (National Academy of Sciences, 1993). Although the increasing visibility of young children with HIV had the beneficial impact of mobilizing new resources for these children, this mobilization was often accompanied by characterizations of women with AIDS as evil vectors of the disease and of children as the innocent victims. This false paradigm continues to be the foundation for much of the ethical, legal, and public debate on issues about women and children with AIDS.

## ❖ Confidentiality

Confidentiality is an important ethical issue for all health care professionals. One only needs to sit in a hospital cafeteria to know that this principle is often violated by health care professionals. Although morally wrong and possibly illegal, hospital gossip occurs; yet, conversation about a patient's broken leg may not be as harmful a breach of confidentiality as when the diagnosis is HIV.

Although U.S. society has traditionally afforded a great deal of privacy to individual medical records and medical information, the government is

245

allowed to collect otherwise private information in certain situations. For example, state and local health departments maintain lists of people with illnesses like tuberculosis and syphilis for reasons that include surveillance, treatment (or cure), and control. AIDS is somewhat different from these conditions because it is still incurable as well as highly stigmatizing.

Persistent dangers of discrimination against people with HIV disease serve to emphasize the importance of maintaining HIV-related confidentiality. Recognizing that HIV-related information is extremely sensitive, many states have passed laws specifically protecting its confidentiality (California Insurance Information and Privacy Act, 1985; Massachusetts General Law, 1986; New York Public Health Law, 1985; New York Public Health Law, 1986). Such statutes frequently provide civil penalties or other deterrents to disclosure by health care personnel, government employees, or other individuals who come into contact with information that identifies another as having HIV disease. Unfortunately, some states have used AIDS surveillance data for nonsurveillance uses. For example, the state of Illinois passed legislation that would permit the state's health officer to notify all patients when a health care worker has AIDS and all health care providers when a patient has AIDS. Thankfully, this legislation has been neither funded nor aggressively enforced. Yet every state collects the names of individuals diagnosed with AIDS, encodes them, and transfers them without identifiers to the Centers for Disease Control and Prevention (CDC). The names of individuals who have tested positive for HIV antibodies are collected by about 26, mostly low-seroprevalence, states.

## ❖ Mandatory Testing

Since the discovery of tests to determine seropositivity, there have been demands for mandatory testing, most frequently for prostitutes, sexual offenders, pregnant women, and newborns (Simonds, Oxtoby, Caldwell, Gwinn, & Rogers, 1993; Task Force on Pediatric AIDS, 1992). Less common, but still heard, are calls for routine testing of all hospital patients, health care workers, emergency workers, and homosexual males.

If demands for mandatory testing for HIV antibodies were heeded, virtually every person in America would be tested. However, learning everyone's serostatus through mandatory testing programs would be neither cost-effective nor productive. First, HIV/AIDS remains a highly stigmatizing condition. People with HIV/AIDS continue to suffer from discrimination in housing, employment, insurance, access to health care, and interpersonal activities. If knowledge of one's serostatus were the quid pro quo for participating in a health service or program, many individuals might work hard to avoid needing or using that service. For example, a hospital requirement of HIV antibody testing of all newborns without parental consent might trigger an increase in the number of at-home births.

Second, pretest and posttest counseling must be offered with HIV-antibody screening to provide emotional support and education about the test, about HIV/AIDS, and about resources for HIV health care. The time and energy spent on counseling and education might not be possible in a large-scale mandatory screening program.

Moreover, extensive experience throughout the 11 years of the AIDS epidemic has shown that mandatory testing programs only serve to discourage people from seeking HIV-related care and general health care. Mandatory testing programs of pregnant or parturient women, or their newborns, will rightly be viewed as selective and repressive by women and will therefore be counterproductive to the goal of increasing the use of health care services for women and their children.[1]

The law is quite clear that a woman may choose to continue or to abort a pregnancy through the first trimester and, in certain circumstances, later in a pregnancy (*Roe v. Wade*, 1973; *Webster v. Reproductive Health Services*, 1989). This right to choose applies regardless of the woman's serostatus. Attendant on this right to choose is the obligation of health care providers or counselors to provide all seropositive women of childbearing age with the facts about vertical transmission of HIV in a noncoercive manner.

Legislative interference in women's reproductive decision making includes attempts to mandate the HIV antibody testing of pregnant women or their newborns. For example, in 1993, the New York State Legislature narrowly voted to table a bill that would reveal the participants in the state's newborn seroprevalence study. Although these attempts generally are well intentioned, they reflect a failure to understand the nature of HIV and to comprehend the decisions that women with HIV disease must make.

Reproductive freedom is based on an understanding of the transmission of HIV. Newborn infants acquire their mother's antibodies passively through the placenta and may carry them for as long as 18 months. Newborn testing may or may not reveal which infants are infected; it does, however, tell us which mothers are infected. In fact, the rate of maternal-child HIV transmission is approximately 25%. The mandated, unblinded testing of newborn infants is, in effect, the testing of mothers without their consent. Although the rationale for testing newborns is that they can be provided with better care, increased surveillance and meticulous well-baby care ought to be provided to all infants (Arras, 1990).

In such a mandatory testing program, the state interposes itself between the mother and her child with the message that the state is a better caretaker

---

[1]Perhaps the most egregious example of the dangers that could attend a mandatory testing program is the case of C.M., an HIV-positive woman living in a southern state. When C.M. received a positive pregnancy test from her local health clinic, a warrant was issued for her arrest. To the state, and a judge, the pregnancy provided evidence that C.M. was not complying with public health directives to use condoms and to disclose that she had an infectious illness to her sex partners. She served approximately 1 year in jail prior to her negotiated transfer to a drug treatment facility.

than the mother. This mode of state intervention sets the stage for broader intrusions of government into the lives of women and their children. Concern over such intrusions—particularly the removal of children to foster care—historically has worked to discourage women from accessing services that might otherwise be beneficial to them or their families.

In addition, because testing newborns reveals the serostatus of their mothers, mandatory HIV screening programs would remove the right of informed consent selectively from childbearing women. Health care for HIV infected mothers is not necessarily an outcome of mandatory testing. Obtaining information about the infants' mothers without their consent and then not offering women with HIV infection care and services is morally reprehensible. Mandatory, unblinded perinatal HIV testing will be legally contested as a violation of laws that require proper counseling and specific, written, informed consent prior to testing. It may even be challenged as being a violation of women's constitutional rights.

The priority should be to get appropriate health care for both HIV-infected child and parent. Experience has shown that when offers of HIV testing are linked to the actual provision of services, individuals consent to being tested. This is as true for pregnant and delivering women as it is for all others. Providers working in high-prevalence areas have found that when health care services are truly available, patients understand the importance of HIV testing and accept this testing for themselves and their children.

It would be a mistake to institute any program that creates additional disincentives to accessing prenatal and postnatal health care. Those who will lose the most in this case are those on whose behalf the advocates of mandatory testing profess to wish to protect: the children. As a society, we cannot afford to make this mistake.[2]

Concern about the potential for intrusion continues to deter people from seeking HIV testing and care. Moreover, in the interest of promoting voluntary access to testing, creating incentives for obtaining HIV-related care, and reducing the incidence of discrimination, people with HIV/AIDS and their advocates continue to ask for confidentiality protection and to fight against mandatory HIV testing (Krasinski et al., 1988; Landesman, Minkoff, Holman, McCalla, & Sijin, 1987; Minkoff & Landesman, 1988; Minkoff, Holman, Beller, Fishbone, Landesman, & Delke, 1988; Nolan, 1990).

## ❖ Contact Tracing and Notification

Publicly sponsored programs for contact tracing or partner notification of HIV-infected persons would also impinge on the critical principles of consent and confidentiality. These programs, when mandated, are counterproductive because they create a disincentive to early testing and

---

[2] In fact, two prestigious medical organizations, the American Academy of Pediatrics and the National Academy of Science's Institute of Medicine, have taken positions against mandatory perinatal testing.

treatment. Such programs are extraordinarily labor intensive and expensive; public funds might well be spent more effectively on more successful prevention programs. Partner-notification programs seriously impinge on an individual's privacy without satisfying the state's interest in preventing the spread of HIV or getting people into care. Furthermore, these types of programs implicitly lend themselves to breaches in confidentiality, thereby subjecting the index patient to even greater risks of discrimination and stigmatization.

Voluntary partner-notification programs may work, allowing the seropositive individual to notify contacts herself or to obtain the assistance of others, usually a state-funded counselor, to notify her sex or needle-sharing partners that she is HIV positive and to encourage them to be tested and seek appropriate follow-up care and services. By respecting the autonomy, privacy, and confidentiality of people with HIV/AIDS, this type of program is far more effective than others because there is no disincentive to voluntary testing, it is far more economical to administer, and civil liberties are not violated.

## ❖ Disclosure

Health care workers are sometimes concerned regarding their personal obligation to disclose or withhold HIV-related information concerning a patient to those who might have intimate contact with her. In 1976, in *Tarasoff v. The Regents of the University of California*, the Supreme Court of California held that a psychotherapist could be held liable for failing to warn an intended victim that his patient presents a serious danger of violence. The court's holding was particularly noteworthy because, while recognizing the duty of a health professional to maintain the confidentiality of an individual in treatment, it drew a limit to the bounds of that protection. The court clearly stated, however, that any decision to disclose highly confidential medical information must not be lightly undertaken and further must require a highly individualized assessment of the nature of the risk and the likelihood that a negative outcome will occur. Numerous other states have adopted the essence of the *Tarasoff* court's holding.

The application of *Tarasoff*, however, is difficult. The risk of danger must be imminent, and the nature of the danger must be serious. Mere suspicion that an HIV-positive client is engaging in unprotected sex or needle sharing would not be likely to provide a sufficient basis for a health care provider to inform the patient's suspected sex or needle-sharing partners. In addition, many state statutes explicitly protect the confidentiality of HIV-related information, including the identity of those either known or believed to be HIV positive. Finally, the health professional must bear in mind the impact of such a disclosure on the individual who is warned as well as on the patient.

Therefore, the health care provider who believes that a client is putting others at risk faces quite a dilemma. If there is reason to believe that an HIV-positive patient is putting others at risk, the provider would do well to seek legal advice, the advice of those to whom he or she reports, and even the advice of the revelant professional organization. This approach is likely to protect best the provider's patients, their partners, and the health professional.[3]

## ❖ Justice: Access to Health Care

The ethical principle of justice requires that people be treated with equity; that is, people in like situations should be treated the same. Yet for many women who are HIV infected, access to even routine medical and dental care is limited. Although women may struggle to gain access to health care for their children, they may neglect themselves. In addition, they may be dealing with family violence or their own substance abuse or that of their partners. In the daily struggles of many women's lives, obtaining health care is often secondary to satisfying the more immediate needs of food, shelter, or child care. Some women may not have the time or the resources necessary to seek health care. Others fear coming to hospitals and clinics lest their substance abuse or immigrant documentation be discovered. Finally, many women may generally harbor mistrust of health care providers or instituitions based on past experience of themselves or others, or based on more systemic abuses, such as the Tuskegee experiements.

Even when health care is a woman's priority, gaining access is often problematic. Day clinics with no child-care facilities may not be accessible to a working woman or to one with small children. Obtaining fragmented services requires many visits and long waits. In some facilities, HIV-infected women may not be treated with dignity. Other facilities attend to the woman's children, but neglect her health problems. Great perseverance and a measure of luck may be needed to get comprehensive services for the patient and her children, and still, access may be elusive.

Many women, rich and poor alike, receive their primary health care as gynecologic care services related to the prevention or facilitation of pregnancy or childbearing. Women are not likely to see an internist unless referred by a gynecologist for a specific problem. Gynecologic practitioners must be trained to detect signs of HIV infection, to discuss them with their patients, and to grasp opportunities for HIV prevention, early diagnosis, and treatment.

### Allocation of Resources

In January 1993, almost 12 years after the first woman was diagnosed with AIDS, the CDC amended the case surveillance definition of AIDS to include one gynecologic condition: invasive cervical cancer. For

[3] NYS Public Health Law Act 27-F §2782 specifically provides specific conditions under which a physician may disclose HIV-related information.

years, women with HIV and their health care providers had been telling the agency that because women's bodies differ from men's, HIV disease in women would present with gynecologic manifestations. Convincing the CDC to modify both the HIV classification system and the case surveillance definition was an arduous task. Prior revisions to the CDC case definition had been largely based on anecdotal case reports of white males. Scientific studies of HIV disease in women proved to be particularly difficult to establish. Virtually no money had been provided to study the natural history of HIV disease in women, and study sites had not been required to conduct gynecologic exams. Even the CDC's own sentinel site study of the natural history of HIV disease did not require the involvement of gynecologic personnel.

Ignoring the gynecologic manifestations of HIV disease has resulted in real harm to women. Health care providers have not been adequately educated to recognize signs of HIV infection in women. Gynecologic clinics and providers have missed opportunities for earlier diagnosis, and HIV clinics have sometimes disregarded the specific needs of women.

The omission of women from the AIDS surveillance definition also contributed to the invisibility of women with AIDS. Because many state and federal agencies based their allocation of benefits on the AIDS case surveillance definition, women were disproportionately excluded from benefits that were available to people with CDC-defined AIDS. Moreover, AIDS research dollars have not been used to identify ways to treat opportunistic infections unique to women.

The combined effect of the foregoing has been a perpetuation of the myth that women do not get AIDS, a failure to recognize HIV-related symptoms in women, and a delay in the diagnosis and treatment of women with HIV disease (CDC, 1989; Minkoff & Moreno, 1990).

## Clinical Drug Trials

Until recently, women with HIV have not received due attention in HIV research. Few federally sponsored clinical drug trials have examined the course of HIV disease or its manifestations specific to women. Because the "ideal" research subjects have been white, middle-class males, little is known about drug action in women and people of color (Dresser, 1992; Minkoff, Moreno, & Powderly, 1992).

Women are underrepresented in HIV research for numerous reasons. The use of male physiology as the presumed norm in an effort to obtain "clean data" specifically excludes women from clinical drug trials. Researchers have not recognized the importance of comparing data on both genders. Fear of teratogenicity has often been cited as the basis for either excluding women from drug trials or requiring proof of their sterilization prior to participation.

Clinical trials must be conducted with caution, and subjects must be protected from research risks as much as possible. However, teratogenicity is not always a concern, and women can be provided with the option of accepting the risk following full counseling and the opportunity to provide informed, written consent.[4] The Federal Drug Administration (FDA) has published draft guidelines designed to correct current government-sanctioned biases that exclude women from drug trials; yet, some remain concerned that the proposed modifications do not go far enough to facilitate women's involvement in clinical trials.[5]

Even if nominally given the opportunity to enroll in clinical drug trials, women often encounter other obstacles related to the cultural and racial biases of health care providers. Many women of color do not trust the health care system in general and are particularly concerned about participating in an experimental program. Low-income women often obtain their health care, if at all, from clinics and from emergency rooms where it may be difficult to provide the information, counseling, and support that could encourage participation in clinical trials. Poor subjects have been perceived to be non compliant or unable to understand adequately the informal consent procedure due to poor education. Finally, without financial or institutional assistance with child-care arrangements and transportation, many women cannot logistically participate in clinical trials that require frequent visits to the test site.

These inequities in access to clinical trials of HIV treatment raise serious ethical and legal issues. Previously, the regulation of clinical research has been directed toward the protection of human subjects from research risks. Access to clinical trials has never been viewed as a right. In the HIV epidemic, however, some of this has changed. Perhaps because there is little recognized therapy for HIV infection, experimental drugs and clinical trials are often perceived as treatment. As such, affected persons seek increased access to clinical trials. Yet, availability of "new treatments" must be balanced with protection from undue burden or risk.

However, women should not be denied access to clinical trials simply because of their reproductive capacity. Some of the drugs being tested may indeed be teratogenic, and potential research subjects must be informed of the known or possible teratogenic effects of these drugs. The possibility of unforeseeable consequences to a fetus should be discussed as part of the

[4] Providing a woman with full disclosure concerning a drug's expected effects, and the opportunity for waiving claims related thereto, would be consistent with existing legal principles (*International Union, UAW v. Johnson Controls*, 1991). Title VII of the Civil Rights Act precludes an employer from excluding women as a class from certain positions based on potential future harm to a fetus, especially when the positions in question also potentially could cause harm to a fetus through the male reproductive process.

[5] The existing FDA guideline calls for the exclusion of women of childbearing years from Phase I and early Phase II clinical trials. Although this guideline contained an exception for women with life-threatening illnesses, including HIV disease, investigators persist in relying on the FDA guideline to exclude women with HIV disease from otherwise appropriate clinical trials. One woman was told that she could not participate in such a trial even though she had had a hysterectomy.

informed consent. Women should be allowed to participate in clinical trials with fully informed consent. Both women and men in clinical drug trials should be advised to use contraceptives to avoid possible damage by the drug to female and male gametes as well as to fetuses (Minkoff, Moreno, & Powderly, 1992). Some would question the right of a pregnant woman to participate in a trial that might harm her fetus. When the clinical trial deals with drugs for end-stage disease, the right of a woman to participate becomes even more compelling. Ironically, earlier inclusion of women in clinical trials on ZDV (ACTG trail 076) might have made the information about the effect of ZDV on reducing perinatal transmission available well before 1994.

Government and private researchers must reform their guidelines and actions to provide women with full access to clinical drug trials. Health care providers must work with women to provide as much information as is available about the trials, to assuage fears when appropriate, and to respond to concerns openly and honestly. After all, it is only following a thorough informed-consent process that anyone, male or female, should participate in a clinical trial. At the same time, trials must be conducted in facilities in and near the areas in which women live; moreover, they must be financed so that the trials contain mechanisms that support women's participation.

## ❖ Special Issues for Children with HIV Disease

Whether the child is infected or the child of an affected mother, there are significant ethical and policy concerns for the professional caregiver. Access to treatment and clinical trials is influenced by society's protective position regarding children.

### Access to Treatment

Children with HIV disease face some of the same problems as their mothers. They are often poor and may have little access to preventive health care or proper diagnosis. In this respect, they differ little from their HIV-negative peers. For a child with HIV disease, however, early diagnosis and treatment may make a dramatic difference. In addition, HIV seropositivity may greatly exacerbate the plight of a child who already suffers the ills of the urban poor.

### Clinical Trials: Access Versus Altruism

What access should children have to clinical trials? Children may be quite vulnerable. Because they are unable to make decisions for themselves, children need strong advocates. Most parents try to do what is best for their children and to protect them from harm. Yet, because of the nature of HIV disease, an infected child's parents may not be capable of making such decisions, may be absent, or may have died.

Because children are vulnerable, society sometimes steps in to protect them, for example, removing children from abusive parents. In the area of human subjects research, children have also been afforded special protections. Therapies are generally not tried on children until they are proved to be effective on adults (Levine, 1986). On the one hand, this protects children from unnecessary burdens and harms. On the other hand, the oncology experience teaches us that therapies that fail in adults sometimes work with children. Thus, by designing clinical trials for children with HIV disease that include only therapies proved effective in adults, we may be bypassing and denying children access to something that would provide benefit to them.

## Access for Older Children

Parents have traditionally been the health care decision makers for their children who are under the age of 18. The informed consent for treatment of children is the responsibility of their parents. Often, children have been totally excluded from the process of informed consent. Some pediatricians and other pediatric health care providers have argued, however, that although parents may have the legal authority and responsibility to make decisions for their children, the children should at least be given the opportunity to assent (Leikon, 1983). They should be informed to their developmental level of understanding of decisions being made and should be given the opportunity to assent to them. Experience with chronically ill children indicates that they are often quite savvy about their health care and treatment decisions. They may be able to understand the relative benefits and burdens of a particular individual therapy quite well. They should be included in the process.

## HIV Orphans

Approximately one in four of the children born to HIV-infected women will be infected themselves. Those who are uninfected are not unaffected, however. It has been estimated that by the year 2000, approximately 100,000 children will be orphaned by HIV disease (Michaels & Levine, 1992). As many of the children who are infected will die from their disease, the majority of these orphans are not themselves infected. There are clear consequences and burdens for them, however. Older children may be left to care for younger children. Siblings may be split up and placed in different foster homes. Although some mothers may be able to place their children in homes of their choosing before they die, others may not. In addition to the profound grief these children may experience, they may also face a stigma due to their mother's disease. Although projects like the Orphan Project are beginning to identify the possible impact of HIV disease on these children and on adolescents, there are other problems and dilemmas faced by this population that will only be identified over time (Michaels & Levine, 1992).

## ❖ Strategies for Coping

Professionals experiencing stress in their caregiving role may find support by participating in ethical rounds as well as a formal ethics committee that sets health care policy and assists with resolving ethical dilemmas.

### Ethics Rounds

One way of reducing the stress associated with caring for HIV-infected women and children is to discuss the ethical dilemmas that arise. These discussions best occur in an interdisciplinary setting. Ongoing ethics rounds allow for a strong focus on this particular set of issues. Ethics rounds and the services of a full-time clinical ethicist are available in some facilities. However, many facilities may not be able to accommodate ongoing ethics rounds from à logistic perspective. In addition, they may not have a clinical ethicist or someone trained to provide input from an ethical point of view. This does not mean that the issues identified in this chapter cannot be discussed as one aspect of clinical management in already established inter-disciplinary forums. Although the physiological parameters often focused on in these sessions may be vitally important, so too are the ethical parameters—for patients and providers. Discussing beliefs about maternal-fetal conflicts or confidentiality and contact notification may go a long way toward reducing underlying disagreements, emotional conflicts, and stress. Only by facilitating communication about these difficult ethical issues can we reduce the stress associated with them.

### Ethics Committees

The vast majority of American hospitals have institutional ethics committees. Some of these committees function at a high level; others do not function as well. Although ethics committees are not a perfect solution, they may be the best available resource for patients, families, or health care providers who face ethical dilemmas they are unable to resolve on their own. Ethics committees do not make decisions. Rather, they serve as an educational resource, help design hospital policies and guidelines, and facilitate communication. It is the latter function that is probably most important in relation to HIV-infected women and children. Ethical dilemmas often create an atmosphere charged with emotional tension. Hearing all sides of the issue often diffuses the tension and allows for better decision making. The impartiality of the ethics committee, as well as the specific expertise that may be available, may greatly facilitate this diffusion. In addition, if an issue is raised several times, the ethics committee may be able to formulate better policy to help decrease the ethical dilemmas and stress.

## ❖ Summary

The issues discussed in this chapter are what present the greatest challenges to primary care professionals caring for women and children with HIV infection. Providers from all disciplines must advocate for their access to health care, clinical trials, and related support services. Women must have the autonomy to identify services most helpful for themselves and their children and adequate supports to alleviate the stress of working through complex ethical and legal dilemmas.

## ❖ References

Arras, J. (1990). AIDS and reproductive decisions: Having children in fear and trembling. *Milbank Quarterly, 68*(3), 353–382.

California Insurance Information and Privacy Act. (1985). California Insurance Code, s791, et seq.

Centers for Disease Control. (1989). Guidelines for prophylaxis against Pneumocystis carinii pneumonia for persons infected with human immunodeficiency virus. *Morbidity and Mortality Weekly Report, 38*, S–5.

Dresser, R. (1992). Wanted: Single, white male for medical research. *Hastings Center Report, 22*(1), 25–29.

International Union, UAW v. Johnson Controls, 111 S. Ct. 1196 (1991).

Krasinski, K., Borkowsky, W., Bebenroth, D., & Moore T. (1988). Failure of voluntary testing for human immunodeficiency virus to identify infected parturient women in a high risk population. *New England Journal of Medicine, 318*(3), 185.

Landesman, S., Minkoff, H., Holman, S., McCalla, S., & Sijin, O. (1987). Serosurvey of human immunodeficiency virus infection in parturients. *Journal of the American Medical Association, 258*(19), 2701.

Leikin, S. L. (1983). Minor's assent or dissent to medical treatment. *Journal of Pediatrics 102*(2), 169–176

Levine, R. (1986). *Ethics and regulation of clinical research* (2nd ed.). New Haven, CT: Yale University Press.

Massachusetts General Law. (1986). Ch. 111, s70(f).

Michaels, D., & Levine, C. (1992). Estimates of the number of motherless youth orphaned by AIDS in the United States. *Journal of the American Medical Association, 268*(24), 3456–3461.

Minkoff, H., & Landesman, S. (1988). The case for routine prenatal HIV testing. *American Journal of Obstetrics and Gynecology, 159*(4), 793-796.

Minkoff, H., Holman S., Beller E., Fishbone, A., Landesman, S., & Delke, I. (1988). Routinely offered prenatal HIV testing [Letter to the Editor]. *New England Journal of Medicine, 319*(15), 1018.

Minkoff, H., & Moreno, J. (1990). Drug prophylaxis for immunodeficiency virus infected pregnant women: Ethical considerations. *American Journal of Obstetrics and Gynecology, 163*(4), 1111–1114.

Minkoff, H., Moreno, J., & Powderly, K. (1992). Fetal protection and women's access to clinical trials. *Journal of Women's Health,* 1(2), 137–140 National Academy of Sciences. (1993). *Social Implications of AIDS.* Washington, DC.: Author.

New York State Public Health Law. (1985). s2307.

New York State Public Health Law. (1986). s206(l)(j).

Nolan, K. (1990). Human immunodeficiency virus infection, women and pregnancy: Ethical issues. *Obstetrics and Gynecologic Clinics of North America, 17*(3), 651–668.

Roe v. Wade, 410 U.S. 113 (1973).

Simonds, R. J., Oxtoby, M. J., Caldwell, M. B., Gwinn, M. L., & Rogers, M. F. (1993). Pneumocystis carinii pneumonia among U.S. children with perinatally acquired HIV infection. *Journal of the American Medical Association, 270*(4), 470–473.

Tarasoff v. The Regents of the University of California, 131 Cal. 14 (1976).

Task Force on Pediatric AIDS. (1992). Perinatal human immunodeficiency virus (HIV) testing. *Pediatrics, 89,* 791–794.

Webster v. Reproductive Health Services, 492 U.S. 490 (1989).

# ❖ Chapter 17

# Legal Concerns of Women with HIV Infection

Lauren Shapiro

Health care professionals are uniquely able to assist their patients in identifying legal issues and providing necessary information about their legal rights. They can also help patients secure needed legal assistance; this role is especially important for practitioners caring for women with HIV disease. Common legal concerns of women with HIV infection that arise from the course of their disease include planning for possible death or incapacity, the guardianship of children, and health care decision making. The onset of HIV illness results in many changes in a woman's life, ranging from the loss of a job and hospitalization to deciding to stop using drugs. These changes raise many legal issues involving foster care, custody, housing, and entitlements.

This chapter discusses how health care professionals can help patients get legal advice or representation and how to overcome the barriers to providing this service in the health care setting. The chapter also provides the health care professional with a basic understanding of common legal issues that arise for women with HIV, such as advance medical directives, custody and guardianship, foster care, and entitlements. Although many of the issues addressed in this chapter also apply to men, their discussion is limited to the perspective of women.

## ❖ Helping Patients Obtain Legal Services

The shortage of time in busy, overcrowded clinics makes it difficult to deal with the patient's legal problems. Other barriers to referring women with HIV infection for legal help are the patient's denial about her illness, her fear of death, and the range of crises she faces in the present. In addition, health care professionals may find it difficult to raise these topics with patients because of their own discomfort with discussing incompetency and death. Even when both the provider and the patient are ready to discuss these difficult issues, there may be other practical obstacles to addressing the patient's legal needs, including lack of knowledge on the part of both the health care professional and the patient about legal issues and resources. The patient's feelings of disempowerment in the health care setting and her trepidation about the legal system also present barriers to getting legal help.

Although overcoming these barriers is challenging and requires reallocation of limited resources, legal referrals should be an essential component of providing comprehensive primary care. The health profession can take many concrete steps to overcome these barriers. Addressing the patient's legal concerns and planning issues will reduce stress and may have a direct impact on her health.

Two specific activities can be integrated into the health care setting to ensure that patients learn about their legal rights and have access to legal help. First, providers can display written information about legal rights and resources in the waiting room. Patients do not always know that they can benefit from legal help because they do not know they have a legal problem or that they have particular legal rights. For example, patients may not have thought about writing a will to name a guardian for their children or may not know that they can appoint a health care agent to make health care decisions for them when they are no longer able to do so. Having information available that describes these rights and options will make it more likely that patients will think about these issues and discuss them with the health care provider.[1]

Second, it is critical for health care professionals to develop linkages with legal groups for referrals. One of the best places to refer patients with HIV infection is to a legal services office that has an HIV project. Specialized HIV projects at legal organizations are becoming more common and are more likely to be accessible and sensitive to the needs of patients with HIV infection. However, legal services programs that do not have specialized HIV projects may also be able to assist patients with legal problems.

In addition to legal organizations, some community-based AIDS organizations have attorneys on staff or otherwise available to advise or represent individual clients. Local AIDS hotlines are frequently a good source for identifying legal resources.

---

[1]Finding written information on legal rights may be difficult. The American Bar Association AIDS Coordination Project has produced the *Directory of Legal Resources for People with AIDS*, which provides information on national, state, and local legal services and legal referral programs. This publication can be ordered by calling 201-331-2248. Try contacting legal groups and local AIDS community-based or advocacy organizations in your area to see what is available or what they are willing to produce. Health departments and "death and dying" organizations, such as the Hemlock Society and the Concern for Dying, should have written information on advance directives. *Facing the Future: A Legal Handbook for Parents with HIV Disease* (1991) discusses advance directives and guardianship issues. Although it is based on New York law, many of the principles discussed are relevant in other states, and it can serve as a useful outline of the issues. A copy of the book can be obtained by calling one of the groups that published it: South Brooklyn Legal Services, 718-237-5546, or Gay Men's Health Crisis (GMHC), 212-337-3504. These organizations are also producing a videotape that will address barriers and issues concerning planning for the future. GMHC also has other documents on legal issues. Finally, the ACLU AIDS project, 212-944-9800, has information on discrimination.

Local bar associations often have a volunteer lawyers' program or may provide referrals to lawyers or law firms for free legal help. Law firms can also be contacted directly. Many law firms, especially large ones, have *pro bono* projects that offer free legal representation. Before referring patients to an organization for legal help, the health professional should try to find out who the organization serves, what the eligibility criteria are, and what type of cases are handled. Health care providers may even find an organization that may be willing to start a project to work with their patients.

## ❖ Advance Medical Directives

The now-established movement in the United States for patient control over health care decisions and "dignity in dying" has resulted in the widespread use and acceptance of advance medical directives. These are documents that express an individual's wishes for the future in the event the individual becomes incompetent. Although the names and the terms of advance directives vary from state to state, they all perform the function of allowing patients to document their wishes about future health care decisions. Advance medical directives, including health care proxies (surrogates), living wills (medical directives), and do-not-resuscitate orders (DNRs), are discussed in this chapter.

The purpose of advance medical directives is to ensure that the patient's wishes are carried out in the event she loses her competency or becomes unable to communicate her wishes. Most states now have laws authorizing some form of advance directive. The U.S. Supreme Court has held that institutions must recognize the decisions of patients who have expressed their wishes concerning life-sustaining treatment in a clear and convincing manner (*Cruzan v. Director*, 1990).

Informed consent, the cornerstone of health care decision making, is usually defined by state law and generally means that a medical procedure or treatment cannot be performed or refused without the patient's permission. Patients also are entitled to sufficient information on which to make a decision. Advance directives ensure that the patient chooses the person who will make her medical decisions if she becomes incompetent and that this person knows what the patient's specific wishes are. Patients can write advance directives only while they are competent and capable of informed consent. When a patient becomes incompetent with no advance directive, health care decision making must be made by either a next of kin or a guardian, according to the laws of the state.

A new federal law, the Patient Self-Determination Act (1991), requires health care providers to play a critical role in ensuring that patients write advance medical directives. The law applies to health care institutions that accept Medicaid or Medicare, including hospitals, skilled nursing facilities, home health agencies, and hospice programs. The act requires these institutions to provide written information to all patients concerning their rights under the laws of that state to make decisions regarding medical care, including the right to accept or refuse treatment and the right to make advance directives. The act also requires providers to document in patient records if an advance directive has been executed and to educate staff members on issues concerning advance directives.

## Health Care Proxies

A health care proxy names an agent to act on the patient's behalf if she becomes unable to make medical decisions on her own behalf. Usually, a doctor must make the determination of whether a patient is competent. A health care proxy may go in and out of effect as the patient's competency changes. The purpose of a health care proxy is to carry out the wishes of the patient. In New York State, if the wishes regarding a specific treatment are not known, the proxy may act in the patient's "best interests."

## Living Wills

A living will expresses the patient's specific wishes regarding either the refusal or provision of medical treatment. It generally takes effect when the patient is terminally or irreversibly ill. A living will can include the naming of a health care agent, or it can be a separate document from a health care proxy.

## Do-Not-Resuscitate Orders

A DNR order instructs medical professionals not to attempt cardiopulmonary resuscitation (CPR) when a patient suffers cardiac or respiratory arrest. In a very few states, such as New York and Montana, DNRs must be honored outside of health care facilities, including patients who are seen at home.

## ❖ Options for the Care of Children

A primary concern of mothers with HIV infection is who will take care of their children if they are unable to do so, either temporarily while they are in the hospital or on a long-term or permanent basis. Child-care issues may arouse feelings of guilt, denial, or despair in mothers. Guardianship issues also raise deep feelings of sadness and powerlessness in practitioners, making discussions with patients about these issues extremely painful and difficult. This section addresses how to deal with these difficult planning issues and discusses the specific legal options that are available to HIV-infected women.

## Planning Issues

Because the consequences of the failure to plan for children can be far-reaching, it is essential for women to make guardianship (custody) decisions as early as possible. Although failure to plan does not necessarily mean the children will be placed in foster care if someone steps in when the mother dies, there may be other harmful effects. Family members may feud about who should care for the children, or no one may be available to care for them. A child may need consents for medical treatment, and stability of finances and schooling after the death of a parent is certainly desirable.

Putting the mother's wishes in writing while she is competent is critical because she is then able to decide the best interests of her children. She is probably the best judge of the children's relationships with potential care-givers and the ability of these adults to meet the children's needs.

Each practitioner must find the best way of raising these issues with patients. For patients who are not ready to appoint a guardian in writing, decision making can be discussed at different times. Of course, the length of time each woman can wait to take action depends on how ill she is. If possible, providers can begin by giving patients written information about their options and by discussing those options. Some patients may wish to speak with peers who have already done guardianship planning. Providers can also suggest that patients speak with a lawyer to get more information and, if possible, can offer to call the attorney for them while they are in the office. Another option is to invite a lawyer to speak to a group of patients to provide general information about guardianship options.

Concern for early planning must be balanced with a mother's readiness to confront these issues. Some mothers are not psychologically prepared to deal with these issues, and facing them prematurely can be traumatic. An effective explanation of guardianship issues is that planning is not an act of defeat, but rather one of patients' taking control over their and their children's lives; although it may be very painful for a mother to discuss, the concern about her children is probably looming, and not making these arrangements ultimately feels worse than taking care of them. One HIV-infected woman reported that she "needed to accept her death and write her will so she could move on and live again."

Addressing guardianship issues with mothers is further complicated when they have not told family members about their illness, when they are dealing with more pressing concerns like physical abuse or homelessness, or when their living situations are in flux. Health care professionals can make legal and counseling referrals to address these other problems, which will help to achieve the stability that may be necessary to deal with more painful planning issues.

The mother should discuss her long-term planning decisions with each of the people involved, including the children if they are old enough to understand. This discussion is frequently avoided because of the fear and discomfort it raises; however, not discussing the plan can lead to an unworkable situation. Some women may not be ready to put their wishes in writing, but discussing guardianship plans and going to see an attorney are the first steps of the planning process.

## Legal Options for Child Care

There are a number of basic legal principles that practitioners should know in advising their patients and that parents should know for appropriate planning. Each person's situation is different, and optimally, patients should always consult with a lawyer to determine what options are best for them.

### Executing a Will or Deed of Guardianship

After the mother decides who she wants to care for her children, the decision should be put in writing. This can be done in the form of a will, which should be executed by a lawyer, or in a less formal document, such as a deed of guardianship.[2] These informal forms should be available at health clinics so that a patient can begin by putting her wishes in writing. If a patient is critically ill and hospitalized, her wishes should also be in writing in case there is not enough time to get an attorney to the hospital to execute a will. Where possible, the guardianship choice should be written in a will because it is a more formal document and thus better evidence in the event of a dispute.[3]

Although it is essential for mothers to execute wills or deeds of guardianship naming a guardian, only a court can appoint the guardian or custodian of a child. Although a mother puts her wishes in writing, she cannot be assured that the person named as guardian will actually be appointed by the court. In some cases, the woman may want to go to court as soon as possible to have someone appointed as guardian. An appointed guardian is responsible for making decisions concerning the child's medical, educational, and emotional needs. Transferring these rights is not the same as giving up parental rights.

Where both parents are deceased, the court is supposed to consider the "best interests" of the child in determining guardianship. Certainly, an executed will is a factor to be considered in this analysis. There are strong legal arguments that the mother's wishes should be presumed to be in the best interests of the child, absent evidence of harm to the child. In practice, the court determines this by looking at the ability of the person named to care for the child and the ability of any other parties who are seeking custody. In the event there is a dispute over the custody of the child, the importance of a

[2]The name of this document may vary from state to state. The document names a guardian and should be recorded in court. It can be done without an attorney.

[3]A will also serves the additional purpose of distributing property. Even though the parent may not have a lot of money, she may come into property unexpectedly or may have personal items she wants to distribute.

written will cannot be stressed enough. When the dispute is between two relatives, such as paternal and maternal grandmothers, the designation of a guardian in a will can make all the difference in the outcome of the case.

**Father's Rights** The biological father has a greater right to custody of his children than anyone else whom the mother has named in a will, unless the father is unfit or has abandoned the children. Most states follow the principle that a natural parent has the right to custody of the children except in "extraordinary circumstances." Thus, the father of the children has both the right to seek custody and the right to object to the mother's appointment of a custodian or guardian.

**Standby Guardianship and Co-Guardianship** In New York, the first Standby Guardianship Law, enacted in 1992, resolves the dilemma of guardianship planning for women who are terminally ill.[4] Under the law, parents who are likely to die or become incapacitated within two years can ask the court to appoint a standby guardian. The guardianship does not go into effect until the parent dies, becomes incapacitated, or consents for the guardianship to begin.

Even in states that do not yet have a standby guardianship law, it is possible to ask the court to appoint a guardian, which would only take effect on the death or incapacity of the parent. Another more likely possibility is to have the future caretaker named co-guardian with the parent. Naming the future caretaker as the co-guardian with the parent would give both the parent and the guardian rights and responsibilities with respect to the children.

Two other, less common, planning options are foster care and adoption. Adoption is permanent, while guardianship or custody is less final. With adoption, the mother loses parental rights, and with foster care, the mother loses custodial rights. When children are placed in foster care, they are in the custody of the commissioner of the state department of social services, which ultimately makes all the decisions about the children's care.

## Voluntary Foster Care Placement

In the event they become permanently unable to care for their children, mothers with HIV can arrange to voluntarily place their children in foster care. In almost all states, foster care is not available as an option for future long-term planning, but only as an immediate, possibly temporary, measure. However, an innovative program in New York City, the Early Permanency Planning (EPP) project, allows parents to use the foster care system for long-term planning. Parents may apply if they have no one who

---

[4]As of the time of this writing, only Illinois and Florida have enacted similar standby guardianship laws. HIV advocates in numerous jurisdictions, including Pennsylvania, Connecticut, and Washington, DC, are trying to get similar laws passed. Most likely, over time, such laws will become common.

can care for their children or if they have a relative or friend who they want to be certified as the foster parent of the children.

Under the EPP project, a parent with a terminal illness may apply for the program within 6 months of when foster care is likely to be necessary. The parent then signs a voluntary placement agreement (a contract with the city agreeing to place the children in the city's custody), which does not go into effect unless the parent dies, is hospitalized, or is otherwise unable to care for the children. If the parent does not have a potential foster parent, the city will identify a family through a foster care agency. The parent and the children will then have an opportunity to meet the potential foster parents, and the children will have the chance to spend time with them, thus smoothing the transition for everyone involved. If the parent has an identified foster parent, then the case will be assigned to a foster care agency for investigation of this potential foster parent.

### Adoption

For children to be adopted, both natural parents must surrender their parental rights, usually in a formal proceeding.[5] When a parent surrenders parental rights, she no longer has any rights with respect to the children. Instead, the adoptive parent has all the rights and duties of the parent, including the obligation to support the children. Adopted children gain the right to inherit from the adoptive parents and receive their Social Security benefits, good reasons for the chosen caregiver to adopt the children rather than to be the custodian or guardian. Adoption proceedings can also be filed after the parent dies so that the parent's rights do not have to be terminated.

Adoption is a sound choice when the parent would like a spouse who is not the biological parent to become the caretaker so that the children's future is secure. For this to occur, the birth parent would have to either be deceased or surrender parental rights.

### Temporary Options
#### Temporary Care and Custody

A parent may have a short-term need to have someone else care for the children while she is hospitalized or sick. For the most part, this can be done informally. The parent can sign a statement, which should be notarized, called a temporary care and custody document or agreement. Although this document is not a legal one in most states, it should be sufficient to enable the temporary caretaker to make the necessary arrangements for the children's medical and educational needs.

---

[5]Parental rights can also be terminated by the state in certain situations, such as where the parent has permanently neglected or abandoned the children.

## Voluntary Foster Care Placement

Another temporary option is voluntary placement of the children in foster care with either a stranger, a relative, or a friend for a limited period of time, for example, until the mother comes out of the hospital. Although voluntarily placing children with a relative or friend can be complicated and is discouraged by most child-protection agencies, it may be facilitated by a lawyer. Rules vary from state to state governing how children are voluntarily placed in foster care and how they are removed. Anyone considering this option should consult a lawyer. Placing children in foster care is a dramatic measure. It means that the parent no longer has custody of her children and loses many rights. Because it may be difficult to get children back from foster care, parents should try to make informal arrangements if at all possible.

## Foster Care

As a consequence of physical illness, past drug use, emotional trauma, or a combination of these factors, women with HIV infection may have children who are in foster care. Although federal law requires states to have a plan for providing preventive services to parents to avoid removal of children from the home and to ensure reunification of parents with children who have been placed in foster care, the system rarely works to achieve these goals. Parents are not advised of their rights, they do not have access to advocacy services, and the system frequently humiliates them and discourages reunification with their children.

Women with HIV infection, even if asymptomatic, do not have the time to let the system work its course. Concerned about their remaining time with their children, women with HIV disease will and should want to resolve foster care issues as quickly as possible. The most important service a health care practitioner can provide is to encourage patients to speak to an attorney about their rights in the foster care system.

Children are in foster care (1) because they were voluntarily placed there by their mother or caretaker by signing an agreement for placement for an indefinite or specific period or (2) through a child-protection proceeding, which the state brings against the mother based on her alleged danger to the children. Legal issues concerning foster care arise primarily when a mother wants to fight the initial removal of her children from the home, get her children out of foster care, or increase visitation rights while they are in foster care. Laws and rules governing foster care vary greatly by state and depend on how the children entered the foster care system.

The health care practitioner can play an important role by encouraging patients to fight for their rights in the foster care system and to seek the assistance of an attorney, if possible. For example, the amount of visitation a parent has with the children in foster care is usually very limited without advocacy. Visits are usually at the agency for limited time periods, possibly supervised, and maybe only once every two weeks. This may be difficult for parents who are ill. Parents have the right to ask for more visits, for visits in their home, and for unsupervised or overnight visits. Visits should be arranged for children to see mothers who are hospitalized. Advocacy on behalf of the parent for expanded visitation can be significant. The parent can also go to court to seek expanded visitation.

The HIV status of the mother is frequently raised in foster care proceedings as a result of ignorance or discrimination on the part of the court, the agency, the foster parents, or the children's lawyer. These prejudices are often masked behind claims of the mother's failure to plan for the children's future or to get proper medical treatment. Courts, agencies, and attorneys commonly assert that because she is going to die anyway, the children should not be returned to their mother. The health care provider may need to provide medical documentation regarding the life expectancy of women with HIV disease in general and the specific condition of the mother.

The HIV status of the mother should not be relevant except to the extent that it affects her ability to care for the children. Legally, the burden of the state to prove that the mother is a danger to her children is greater than that of the other parent to show that it is not in the children's best interests to remain with the ill parent. Medical documentation should state that the mother is compliant with treatment, comes to appointments regularly, and is responsive and communicative. Documentation of the mother's symptoms and how they would affect her ability to care for the children may be needed. The type of documentation that is needed depends on the issues raised by the agency or the court. For this reason, communication between the mother's attorney and the health care provider is essential.

### ❖ Visitation and Custody Issues

Women with HIV infection may face child custody and visitation issues for many reasons, including the desire to reestablish contact with children on learning of one's HIV status, the occurrence of illnesses, discrimination by the other parent or by relatives, and the incidence of past or present drug use. Laws governing these areas differ greatly by state and can be very complicated. This section describes general legal issues to aid practitioners in both advising their patients and in providing necessary medical or psychological documentation.[6]

[6]For a more extensive legal discussion of these issues, see L. Cooper, HIV infected parents, in N. Hunter & W. B. Rubenstein (1992). AIDS agenda: Emerging issues in civil rights. (New York: New York Press); N. Mahon, Public hysteria, private conflict: Child custody and visitation disputes involving an HIV infected parent, 63 *New York University Law Review*, 1092 (1988); and *HIV and family law: A survey* (New York: Lambda Legal Defense and Education Fund, 1992). The latter can be obtained by calling Lambda at 212-995-8585.

## Visitation

The issue of a mother's visitation rights with her children arises when the mother has not had regular visitation with her children because of drug use or illness or because the custodian learns of the mother's HIV status and denies continued visitation out of fear or anger.

A noncustodial parent has an absolute right to visitation with her children unless "visitation would endanger seriously the child's physical, mental, moral, or emotional health" (Uniform Marriage and Divorce Act, 1979, §407[a]). It is fairly well accepted that a parent's HIV status alone does not endanger her children, and the HIV status should only be relevant if the custodian can prove that the parent is unable to care physically or emotionally for the children during visits (e.g., alcohol or drug use).

Noncustodial parents initially can try to obtain visitation by asking the custodian for it. If unsuccessful, intervention of another family member, a social worker, or an objective party, such as a priest, should be tried before going through court. If the parent does have to go to court, it will be helpful to show that the parent reasonably tried to resolve the conflict with the custodian. Since court proceedings are stressful for all concerned, parents should resort to suing the custodian in court only when the custodian either refuses visitation or does not agree to regular visitation.

## Custody

Custody issues most commonly arise for the mother with HIV infection either when she has custody and another parent or relative seeks to obtain custody on the basis of her illness or when she is seeking custody of her children who are currently under someone else's care.

A custody dispute between the children's two parents is determined by the court based on the "best interests" of the children. The best interests standard is discretionary, and decisions are based on the individual facts of the case. Some states require the court to apply specific factors in deciding the best interests of the children. The Uniform Marriage and Divorce Act (1979, §402), which many states have adopted or use as a model, identifies five factors: the wishes of the child's parent(s); the wishes of the child; the relationship between the child and the parent(s) or sibling(s); the child's adjustment to home, school, and community; and the mental and physical health of the parties.

Custody disputes between two parents that occur after one parent already has custody are governed by a different standard. Usually, the parent who is seeking to change the custody arrangement must prove that there have been "changed circumstances." For example, one parent may make a motion to modify a custody order naming the other parent on the ground that the other parent started using drugs. Drug use may be a legitimate basis for changing the order. However, courts have found that a parent's HIV status is not sufficient to change a custody order unless it affects the parent's ability to care for the children.

### Practitioner's Role in Custody and Visitation Cases

The health care practitioner can play a critical role in the patient's custody and visitation case by providing medical documentation, where possible, that the mother is regularly receiving medical treatment, that she is compliant with treatment, that her symptoms are controlled by medication, and that her reported symptoms and conditions should not interfere with her ability to care for the children. The health care practitioner can also aid the mother in obtaining services that will allow her to continue caring for the children, such as home care, child care, or psychological counseling. The provider should also refer the mother for planning legal issues because, at times, the issue of whether the mother has properly planned for the future of the children will come up in a custody case.

## ❖ Women and Entitlements

Entitlement to HIV-related or disability-based benefits depends on the symptoms or conditions of the applicant. Thus, the recognition of the conditions that are specific to women and children becomes crucial in the determination of who is entitled to recieve benefits. Until the expansion of the Centers for Disease Control and Prevention (CDC) definition of AIDS in January 1993 to include cervical cancer, pulmonary tuberculosis, recurrent bacterial pneumonia, and a T cell count of less than 200, many women and poor people were excluded from receiving benefits that required a CDC AIDS diagnosis.

### . Federal Disability Benefits

In the case of Supplemental Security Income (SSI) or Social Security Disability (SSD) benefits,[7] the applicant must prove that she has one or more of a specific set of conditions included in the Social Security Administration's (SSA) HIV-related listing. The SSA is the federal agency responsible for administering SSI and SSD benefits. The SSA relied heavily on the CDC definition of AIDS to determine disability until December 1991, when the SSA promulgated interim regulations that listed numerous conditions particular to women, such as cervical cancer and vaginal candidiasis.

---

[7]SSI benefits are available to disabled individuals with income and resources below a specified amount. The amount of the SSI benefits varies slightly from state to state. Disabled individuals are entitled to SSD benefits when they have worked and paid Social Security taxes (FICA) prior to the disability. The monthly amount they are entitled to depends on the level of taxes paid. The definition of disability is the same for both SSD and SSI.

In July 1993, the SSA listing was finalized with many changes that made it easier for claimants to get benefits. The SSA offers materials that explain which conditions and symptoms now qualify a patient for benefits.

### Practitioner's Role

As treatment providers, health care practitioners play an extremely important role in the patient's application for benefits. To help patients obtain these benefits, providers should be familiar with materials from the SSA that explain the qualifying illnesses and conditions. This knowledge will assist the practitioner in completing the reports requested by the SSA in the proper manner.

### ❖ Summary

The most common legal issues that women with HIV infection face are discussed in this chapter. These include strategies to access legal services and specifics about advanced medical directives including health-care proxies, living wills, and do-not-resuscitate orders. Guardianship and long-term planning for childcare, including temporary care, foster care, adoption, and custody, are considered in the overall context of the primary care needs of women and children with HIV infection. Providers can play an important role in assisting patients to meet their legal and advocacy needs through education, assessment, and active referrals.

### ❖ References

*Cruzan v. Director, Missouri Department of Health*, 110 S. Ct. 2841 (1990).
Uniform Marriage and Divorce Act §407(a), §402 1979.

# ❖ Chapter 18

# Prevention and Education

Kathleen M. Nokes

Marilyn I. Auerbach

Primary prevention consists of activities directed toward decreasing the probability of specific illness, such as HIV infection (Pender, 1987). Preventing HIV transmission through education and the modification of behaviors is the most hopeful approach to stopping the spread of HIV/AIDS (Albee, 1989). The focus of this chapter is on preventing the spread of HIV infection through education and the modification of sexual and drug use behaviors. The transmission of HIV from an infected woman during pregnancy to the fetus is addressed in chapter 6. The Centers for Disease Control and Prevention (CDC) report that as of March 1993, 289,320 people in the United States have been diagnosed with AIDS and 32,477 (11%) of them are female. HIV infection is the leading cause of death in nine cities in the United States for women between the ages of 25 and 44 (Selik, Chu, & Buehler, 1993). The behaviors associated with the spread of HIV infection, injection drug use and unprotected sex, have been well established. However, 8% of the women with AIDS in the United States do not know how they became infected.

Prevention strategies for women are complicated. Some women do not know that they are placing themselves at risk because they do not know that their sexual or drug-sharing partner is HIV infected. People are not always truthful about their sexual and drug use histories. In one study of college students, 20% of the men and 4% of the women reported that they would lie about having a positive HIV antibody test (Cochran & Mays, 1990). The proportion of AIDS cases in bisexual men (men who have sex with both men and women) increased slightly during the 1980s (Chu, Peterman, Doll, Buehler, & Curran, 1992). Bisexuality is also an issue for women. Women in a lesbian-identified bar in New York City reported their sexual preferences as exclusively lesbian (82%), bisexual (women who have sex with both men and women, 15%), or heterosexual (3%) (Russell, Alcober, & McKinley, 1992). It is also well established that women of color are overrepresented in the number of female AIDS cases in the United States.

## ❖ Sexual Behaviors Associated with HIV Infection

The vast majority of Americans are sexually active. In one sample of college students, 77% reported that they had had intercourse during the preceding 3-month period (Jemmott-Sweet & Jemmott, 1991).

Many adolescents have had at least one sexual experience by the age of 16 (Ehrhardt, 1992). Sexual practices that increase risk for HIV transmission include anal, oral, and vaginal exchange of body fluids with an HIV-infected person. Although receptive anal sex is usually associated with men having sex with men, it is not uncommon among heterosexuals. Eleven percent of the women in one study (Saracco et al., 1993) and 19% in another study (Jemmott-Sweet & Jemmott, 1991) reported having engaged in anal intercourse.

When one sexual partner is HIV infected, the rate of HIV transmission from men to women is much greater than from women to men. Twelve percent of the men and 20% of the women in one group became infected. Factors associated with the increased risk of transmission from women to men include advanced stage of HIV disease; sexual contacts during menses, anal sex, and advanced age of the female partner, perhaps because of the increased fragility of the genital mucosa in perimenopausal women (over 45 years old) (European Study Group on Heterosexual Transmission of HIV, 1992).

Condoms provide a physical barrier to prevent the exchange of body fluids (Rosenberg & Gollub, 1992). In settings of high HIV incidence or among couples in which one of the partners was infected, condom use provided up to a ninefold protection of the uninfected partner, and regular use seemed to improve effectiveness (Cates, Stewart, & Trussell, 1992). However, condoms are not used consistently. A telephone survey of sexually active residents in the District of Columbia found that 40% of the respondents reported always using condoms, whereas 34% reported never using condoms. Women who reported two or more partners were not significantly more likely to use condoms than were women with one sex partner (CDC, 1993). In a study of sexual practices and AIDS knowledge among female partners of HIV-infected hemophiliacs, 60% always used condoms, 13% did so most of the time, and the remaining 27% did so sometimes. In this study, condom use was not significantly related to either frequency of intercourse, the woman's knowledge of AIDS and AIDS-risk reduction, the HIV status of either partner, the extent of the woman's worry about contracting HIV, or her mood, age, or education (Mays, Elsesser, Schaefer, Handford, & Good, 1992). In the European study of monogamous female partners of HIV-infected men (Saracco et al., 1993), 56% reported always using condoms, 18% reported not always using condoms, and 25% said that they never used condoms. The yearly seroconversion rate of the female partner was 5.7% for couples who never used condoms, 9.7% for couples who reported condom use as "not always," and 1.1% for those who always used condoms (Saracco et al., 1993). The higher seroconversion rate for people reporting occasional condom use as compared to never using condoms is clinically important. The risk of HIV seroconversion during anal sex was also reduced significantly in women whose male partner always used condoms.

The reasons given for not using condoms include difficulty changing sexual behaviors, decreased pleasurable sensation with condom use, lack of availability, decreased spontaneity of the sexual act, and fear of being seen as promiscuous or infected with a sexually transmitted disease.

## ❖ Drug Use Behaviors Associated with HIV Infection

Injection drug use has also been established as a route of HIV transmission when equipment is shared with an infected person. Women (N = 330) were significantly more likely to share a syringe during their last injection as compared to a sample of male drug injectors in New York City (Sotheran, Wenston, Rockwell, DesJarlais, & Friedman, 1992). Women were more likely to inject in social contexts, often sharing equipment with their male sexual partner. Heterosexual partners entering a methadone maintenance program were also questioned about their needle-sharing behaviors, and these women also reported more needle sharing than their male sexual partners. The men reported injecting first and then giving the equipment to their female sexual partner. African-American couples in this study engaged in less risky needle-sharing behaviors than white couples, and injection cocaine use was associated with greater needle and sex risk (Wells et al., 1992).

Crack cocaine use is associated with several high-risk sexual behaviors including increased sexual activity; unprotected vaginal, anal, and oral intercourse; multiple sex partners; and trading sex for drugs (McCoy & Inciardi, 1993). Among female crack cocaine users engaging in streetwalking, those who performed primarily oral sex were more likely to be infected with HIV than those who performed primarily vaginal intercourse. This finding is associated with possible oral trauma secondary to the heat of the crack pipe causing a break in mucosal integrity (Weiner, Wallace, Steinberg, Hoffmann, & Fielding, 1992). Crack has been attractive to women in part because it is smoked rather than administered by injection (Jonsen & Stryker, 1993) and also because it is comparatively less expensive than cocaine or heroin. Crack use augmented the risk of HIV transmission through an increase in sexual drive and more sexual partners, and men on cocaine maintained erections longer, which may have contributed to increased vaginal dryness and subsequent irritation (Jonsen & Stryker, 1993).

## ❖ Assessing Need for Prevention Programs

Before any preventive intervention is planned, a needs assessment should be done to identify and measure gaps between the needs of a particular community and the resources available to meet them (Windsor, Baranowski, Clark, & Cutter, 1984). Needs are not discrete, easily identifiable entities but are diffuse and interrelated. Communities and their needs are dynamic and in a constant state of flux (Siegel, Attkisson, & Carson, 1978). The community needs assessment addresses the existence of health and social services, educational programs, personnel, and resources and the community's perception of their adequacy. This evaluation technique helps to ensure that program goals and planned activities are appropriate and feasible for that community (Figures 18–1 to 18–3).

When health care providers are conducting needs assessment or assisting community members in conducting needs assessment, reflection on how their values may be different from those of community members is essential

---

- To identify unmet needs
- To clarify the community's perception, attitudes, and beliefs about its problems
- To describe the community's perception of the need for new services
- To identify target or high-risk populations
- To identify existing services and their duplication
- To identify barriers to the use of available services
- To provide baseline information for evaluation
- To identify community or agency resources for prevention, including money, personnel, facilities, equipment, materials, time, and technical support
- To identify resources of the target populations, including the time and money to participate in programs and the kinds and level of skills that members have, such as literacy and social support systems

---

FIGURE 18–1 Purposes of needs assessments.

---

- When must the information be available for decision making?
- How can interest groups and community decision makers be involved in the needs assessment from the beginning?
- What is the purpose of the needs assessment?
- Are there existing data that are valid, reliable, and applicable to the assessment?
- Who will be responsible for the various tasks in the needs assessment?
- What are the anticipated barriers to conducting a useful needs assessment, and how can they be overcome?
- Who will pay for data collection and analysis?
- What are the limitations of the data to be collected?
- How will the data be integrated to set priorities and make decisions?
- What are the ethical issues involved in conducting the needs assessment (privacy, raising expectations, unexpected adverse outcomes), and how will they be dealt with? (Basch, 1987, p. 70)

---

FIGURE 18–2 Needs assessment content.

- Review population data reports from the Centers for Disease Control and Prevention, and from the state and city departments of health.
- Conduct a literature review.
- Review use records of local services, such as HIV testing and counseling services.
- Conduct a community survey by mail, by phone, or face to face.
- Interview key informants from the community and service providers.
- Conduct a community forum.
- Conduct a focus group.
- Observe or measure the needs of community members.

FIGURE 18–3  Methods of data collection.

for a successful participative approach. The resources to explore include the time, money, personnel, facilities, equipment, materials, and technical support that are available within an organization, a community, and the target population. Resources may include the time and money to participate in programs, the kinds and levels of skills that members have, including literacy and social support systems. Targeting populations of women can be cost-effective because the woman is often the educator of her children and the caregiver for other family members.

Perceived needs for an intervention should be assessed from three audiences: representatives and leaders from the target population, leaders from the community and local organizations, and staff members who are most likely to be responsible for program implementation. Data collection for a needs assessment should include sources that are quantitative (objective) and qualitative (subjective).

One way to assess the knowledge, attitudes, and beliefs of a specific target population about HIV disease, transmission, and prevention is to give the group a test that assesses their knowledge, attitudes, and beliefs about HIV disease. Many different instruments have been developed to achieve this goal. Because validity and reliability data is often not established, however, it is virtually impossible to compare findings.

The focus group is another technique that has been used to assess the opinion of a target population. Eight to 12 group members with a shared experience are asked a series of guided questions by a trained leader to assess their attitudes, beliefs, and feelings about a specific subject. An observer records the interactions of the group and often tape-records the session. Focus groups are used to (1) explore a topic, (2) understand why people hold the beliefs they do about topics or messages, (3) address misconceptions about subject areas, (4) critique materials such as pamphlets and public service announcements, and (5) probe and generate spontaneous ideas that can be used to help develop programs and materials.

Eight focus group discussions were held with both men and women in drug-treatment programs, a prison, and an outreach clinic to elicit their opinions about condom use (Kenen & Armstrong, 1992). Participants did not hold one universal opinion about condoms, but most of the people did not like to use them. Group members varied in their knowledge about the benefits of a condom, in how and when to put on a condom, in the associations they made between condom use and trust and commitment, in the type of partner and conditions under which they would use condoms, and in their willingness to consider condom use as an integral part of their lives. In general, women in this study seemed more willing to use condoms than their male partners. Focus groups can be used to assess the knowledge and attitudes of groups when the provider is uncertain about the knowledge needs of the group. Focus groups are particularly effective if the target group is not comfortable with written materials.

## *Choosing a Theoretical Framework*

In addition to the needs assessment, it is important to identify a theoretical framework that will provide direction for practice. Social learning theory is becoming a metaparadigm in the health education field because it synthesizes knowledge from diverse fields, integrates cognitive and behavioral perspectives, and retains learning concepts as a central core. According to social learning theory, behavior and environment are best studied as reciprocal systems, which means that the influence is bidirectional. The environment shapes, maintains, and constrains behavior, and people have an impact on their environments.

Jemmott-Sweet and Jemmott (1991) used the theory of reasoned action to study condom use among black women ($N = 103$). They found that women who expressed more favorable attitudes toward condoms and greater support for condom use among their significant support system reported stronger intentions to use condoms in the immediate future. This theory is based on the assumption that humans are reasonable and that they systematically process and use the information available to them before taking action (Fishbein & Middlestadt, 1989). It addresses the relationships between beliefs, attitudes, intentions, and behavior. Intentions are defined by the four elements of action, target, context, and time. To change behavior, a change must first occur in the cognitive structure that underlies that specific behavior. The behavior in question must be directly observable and under the individual's control. Putting on a condom would be an example of a directly observable behavior that is under a man's control.

The health belief model was developed in the 1950s by a group of social psychologists and currently includes all types of health-promoting behaviors. Williams (1991) used the health belief model and the concept of self-efficacy to develop an AIDS education program. She used a qualitative research design to elicit responses from women who either injected illegal drugs or were the sexual partners of men who injected illegal drugs. These women perceived AIDS as a very serious health threat and were aware of their personal vulnerability to that threat. These perceptions of personal vulnerability were compromised when the women recognized that it would interfere with their relationship with their significant other. The women perceived themselves as capable of taking actions in some situations, such as buying condoms, but not in others. They especially did not perceive themselves as capable in situations requiring actions that involved interacting with significant others, such as their regular sexual partner and their family members. According to the health belief model, an individual performs a health-promoting activity as a result of the interaction of four factors: (1) perceived susceptibility to harm, (2) perceived severity of the problem to be avoided, (3) perceived benefits, and (4) perceived barriers.

Self-efficacy theory, the confidence a person has about performing a particular activity, is an important prerequisite for behavior change. Behaviors result from an interaction of expectations about the outcomes that will result from the behavior and expectations about one's ability to engage in or carry out the behavior (Green & Kreuter, 1991). A consideration of the concepts included in the health belief/self-efficacy theory highlights the complexity of trying to achieve successful health-promotion programs.

One concept in the health belief model is the perception of personal susceptibility to harm. Women occasionally speak about engaging in repeated unprotected sexual behaviors with an infected man and yet remaining negative on HIV antibody testing for long periods of time. These women are often surprised when the third or fourth HIV antibody test result indicates that they have become infected. Some people think that they are invulnerable, or they claim that their chances of suffering negative events are smaller than the chances of their peers. People tend to choose salient high-risk individuals to represent the "average" when making comparative risk judgments. To illustrate, when people compare their number of sexual partners with someone like Magic Johnson, they often arrive at the conclusion that their sexual behaviors have been low risk—but low risk in comparison to Magic, not to Mother Teresa. Motivations associated with drug use and sexuality, including interpersonal pressures, may be more powerful than the desire to avoid risk. Hazard appraisal reflects many factors, and people often acquire their notion of a threat's seriousness from acquaintances or from the mass media. People who have engaged in risk-increasing behaviors for AIDS but who have not become infected are likely to conclude that they have no personal susceptibility to HIV infection.

Catania, Kegeles, and Coates (1990) used both the health belief and self-efficacy models and added concepts of emotional influences and interpersonal processes to develop the AIDS risk reduction model (ARRM). This model describes three stages: labeling, commitment, and enactment. Social networks and norms may be particularly powerful forces guiding the labeling of health problems. The second stage, commitment, is conceived as a decision-making stage. Movement from stage to stage is dependent on achieving the goals of the prior stages. Internal factors, such as emotions, and environmental factors, such as alcohol and drug use, play important roles in maintaining motivation for change over time. In the ARRM model, clients are at different stages with respect to HIV primary prevention behaviors. Some clients may never use condoms, some use condoms inconsistently, and others always use condoms. Selection of a prevention strategy must consider the stage of the targeted audience.

Schaalma, Kok, and Peters (1993) combined the theories of reasoned action and self-efficacy to survey students ($N = 1,018$) in Dutch secondary schools about their sexual intercourse experience and attitudes, perceived social influences, and self-efficacy assessments regarding using condoms to avoid HIV infection. They found that pupils with sexual intercourse experience were more likely than sexually inexperienced students to subscribe to the belief that condom use had negative consequences in terms of "an annoying interruption," "decreased pleasure," "a decreased sensitivity," and "expense" and that the use of condoms is unnecessary "when being careful" and "when knowing each other for a while." Sexually experienced students were also more likely to consider that bringing up the subject of condom use "reduces the joy of love-making." Boys were more likely than girls to identify both the disadvantages as well as the preventive advantages of condoms and condom use. Non-condom adopters were less likely to have used a condom at their first intercourse (40% versus 91%), and male non-condom adopters were more likely to have had intercourse at an early age. Non-condom adopters were more likely to be girls than boys (71% versus 53%). Self-efficacy was an important determinant of intended condom use. Although it is recognized that there could be significant differences between adolescents in the United States and those in the Netherlands, similar research has not proceeded in the United States as a result of a variety of political influences (Francis, 1992).

Criticism is growing that social-cognitive models are not inclusive enough to be used to predict the risk-reduction behaviors necessary to prevent HIV infection. One question is whether the health belief model is more successful in predicting the initiation or the maintenance of such risk-reduction behaviors as consistent condom use (Montgomery et al., 1989).

Differences in learning styles will affect the type of intervention chosen for a target audience. In addition, women also process cognitive information differently from men, shifting from one mode of knowing to another. Five categories of women's ways of knowing have been identified: (1) silence, in which women experience themselves as mindless, voiceless, and subject to the whims of external authority; (2) received knowledge, in which women conceive of themselves as capable of receiving and reproducing knowledge from some omniscient authority but not capable of creating knowledge on their own; (3) subjective knowledge, in which women see truth and knowledge as personal, private, and subjectively known or intuited; (4) procedural knowledge, in which women learn and apply objective procedures for obtaining and communicating knowledge; and (5) constructed knowledge, in which women view all knowledge as contextual, experience themselves as creators of knowledge, and value both subjective and objective strategies for knowing (Belenky, Clinchy, Goldberger, & Tarule, 1986). A needs assessment should determine not only the content to be taught, but also the preferential learning style of the targeted audience.

There is a movement toward models that stress sophisticated interactive skills and practice rather than cognition (Abraham & Sheeran, 1993). Tones (1993) calls this alternative model "radical." This radical challenge to cognitive theories of health behavior has generated two strategies, both of which aim to redistribute power and resources in pursuit of equity. The empowerment model is consistent with the radical imperative.

Richie (1992) developed an empowerment curriculum that was used with incarcerated women on Rikers Island. The curriculum consisted of five units: coping with life at Rikers Island, health and healthy behavior, drugs and drug use, sexuality and relationships, and self-esteem and decision making. Within each of the two-hour units, four steps were addressed: sharing individual experiences, discussing the common theme, applying the theme to risk reduction, and developing action plans.

Nurse-managed peer education and support groups for AIDS prevention have also been developed by McElmurry. Included in these programs is the recognition of women as key health promoters for families and communities, the interaction between health and social conditions, and the emphasis on self-care and community competency in maintaining basic health (Norr, McElmurry, Moeti, & Tiou, 1992). These programs, which have been implemented in Chicago, Illinois, and in Botswana, consist of peer education and support groups led by trained community women and coordinated by a nurse. This peer education model focuses specifically on supports, such as sharing personal experiences within a supportive group. These strategies are associated with lasting behavioral changes that promote health. The key components of the empowerment model are seeing the situation lived by the participants, judging the causes of the situation, and acting to change the situation. Empowerment is a process designed to help individuals understand the ways they have been made powerless in society and to support them in taking action on their own behalf. This model is based on the belief that individual health problems exist within a larger social context that must be considered in facilitating behavior change. The group process is especially suited to the application of this model.

A metaparadigm that combines many of the previously mentioned concepts is the precede-proceed model developed by Green and Kreuter (1991). There are nine phases in the model: five phases in the precede component and four in the proceed part (Figure 18–4). The precede-proceed framework takes into account the many components that shape the health status of a person or a community. It defines targets for intervention and identifies

## Phase 1: Social Diagnosis

The first phase addresses quality-of-life issues, which are the subjective problems and priorities of the individual or the community. A study of social and health problems is a practical way to assess quality of life.

## Phase 2: Epidemiological Diagnosis

Phase 2 explores the health of the individual or the community by looking at vital indicators like disability, disease, fertility, morbidity, and mortality. The health problems are ranked based on data, and the problem for educational intervention is selected.

## Phase 3: Behavioral and Environmental Diagnosis

The next phase addresses the behavioral and environmental indicators of health. These are the risk factors that the health education intervention is tailored to address, so they must be specifically identified and ranked. Environmental factors are external to an individual and often beyond personal control, so it is important to be aware of the links to personal behavior change.

## Phase 4: Educational and Organizational Diagnosis

Phase 4 delineates the predisposing, enabling, and reinforcing factors that facilitate or hinder the motivation for change. Factors that have direct impact on the target behavior and on the environment are sorted and prioritized.

## Phase 5: Administrative and Policy Diagnosis

This phase critically evaluates the capabilities and resources available for implementing a program. It includes budgets, resources, personnel, policies, linkages, and time constraints of the organizations that will be providing the educational intervention.

## Phase 6: Implementation

The plan is converted into health education interventions, policy, organization, and regulation.

## Phase 7: Process Evaluation

Process evaluation occurs first because this information is available first. The early observation of problems helps the educator to adjust materials, content, and presentations in a timely manner.

*continued*

**Phase 8: Impact Evaluation**

The eighth phase assesses the direct effect of the educational program, which includes changes in predisposing, enabling, and reinforcing factors or behavioral/environmental changes.

**Phase 9: Outcome Evaluation**

The final phase assesses the effect of the education program on long-term changes in quality of life, social indicators, or mortality, disease, or disability rates.

FIGURE 18–4    Phases of the preceed-proceed model.

objectives and criteria for evaluation. Many health care providers are particularly interested in phase 4, the educational and organizational diagnosis phase, which describes predisposing, enabling, and reinforcing factors. Predisposing factors are established personal or community traits that impact on behavior change, including knowledge, attitudes, beliefs, values, and perceptions. To support behavior changes successfully, certain services and supports—enabling factors—must exist. They include the availability and accessibility of health personnel and resources, established policies and laws that show a commitment to health, and personal ability to perform health skills. Reinforcing factors help maintain behavior change. Positive reinforcement and social support from health personnel, community leaders and policymakers, family, employers, teachers, peers, and coworkers make this possible. When these specific factors are understood, objectives, criteria, and evaluation mechanisms can be focused on the specific population that is to be educated (Green & Kreuter, 1991). This model has been validated and applied in many types of health education programs. By focusing on behavior and health outcomes, it is a practical approach to AIDS education programming.

Based on the precede-proceed model, Freudenberg (1989) developed sample activities and objectives for women in drug-treatment programs. The activities included support groups for women in drug treatment, training peer educators, needle and works cleaning demonstrations, and small-group discussions on AIDS and reproductive decisions. The learning objectives were to discuss alternative stress-reduction techniques, to identify sources of peer and social support for continued drug-free behavior, and to explain perinatal transmission of AIDS. Three possible behavioral objectives were identified: the use of condoms to prevent the exchange of semen and blood for women not involved in long-term monogamous relationships, the discontinuation of drug use, and, for women who continued to use injection drugs, the sterilization of needles or the participation in needle-exchange programs. The overall program objectives were a decrease in the incidence of new HIV infection among women enrolled in the program and a decrease in the number of enrollees who used injection drugs. The proceed phases would include implementing and evaluating the program.

## Types of Interventions

Once the theory has been chosen and the needs assessment completed, the health care provider should choose the type of intervention which will best achieve the identified goals. Cognitive and decision-making theories of health behavior suggest the lecture/discussion format, in which an identified expert conveys information about the topic. After a 12-minute audiovisual educational program on AIDS, low-income black and Latino women attending a Women, Infants, and Children program indicated significantly more positive attitudes about HIV/AIDS and greater intention to use safer sex strategies (Flaskerud & Nyamathi, 1990).

Audiovisual materials can be used to supplement and enhance content presentation. Printed handouts can reinforce the material and can be used by the participant after the teaching session has ended. D'Augelli and Kennedy (1989) critiqued two AIDS brochures and found that respondents reacted strongly to sexually explicit visual and written material and that much variability was found in the reactions of the college students. Examples of HIV prevention materials targeted to women, children, and adolescents can be obtained from ETR Associates, P.O. Box 1830, Santa Cruz, CA 95061-1830, tel. 800-321-4407, and from Sunburst Communications, 39 Washington Ave., P.O. Box 40, Pleasantville, NY 10570-0040, tel. 800-431-1934. Low-cost printed materials are also available from not-for-profit agencies, the National AIDS Clearinghouse, and state departments of health. Handouts should be chosen carefully to ensure that they meet the needs of the participants with respect to factors like language, racial and ethnic sensitivity, and literacy level.

About 5% of the U.S. adult population has extreme difficulty in reading, about one third have some reading problems, and many find reading to be an easily avoidable chore (Root, 1990). The characteristics of written materials for low-literacy readers include the following (Doak, Doak, & Root, 1985):

* Overall message that covers a few critical points
* Vivid but simple narrative style (third- to fifth-grade reading level)
* Conversational style
* Pages with ample white space
* Simple line drawings
* Short length
* Close match to logic, language, and experience of the intended audience

The more interactive theories focus as much on the teaching process as they do on the content to be learned. The New York State Department of Health (Thomas, 1993) developed a computer program called Condomsense using a CD-ROM format. This software was designed for use by young adults who are sexually active. The content focuses on the importance of using condoms to reduce the risk of HIV and other sexually transmitted diseases and offers ideas on negotiating with a sexual partner. The software is available without charge to educational or human service programs in New York State. Interactive theories indicate different interventions depending on where the client is in the behavior-change process (Valdiserri, West, Moore, Darrow, & Hinman, 1992). An HIV prevention delivery system that uses an interactive approach is characterized by increased emphasis on client assessment prior to service delivery, heterogeneous provider skills, specialized training needs for providers, and mechanisms to coordinate service delivery across sites and through time.

Schilling, El-Bassel, Schinke, Gordon, and Nichols (1991) compared HIV risky behaviors between two groups of women attending a large methadone maintenance program. The experimental group ($N = 48$) participated in five 2-hour sessions, conducted by experienced female drug counselors, which were intended to build skills. The control group ($N = 43$) participated in one session of AIDS information routinely provided by the clinic. There were significant differences between the two groups on several sexual outcome measures. Subjects in the experimental group reported that they initiated discussion more frequently and that they felt more comfortable talking about safer sex with their partner, using condoms during sexual intercourse, carrying condoms, and taking condoms from the clinic. They also perceived themselves as more able to reduce their exposure to AIDS, were more interested in learning about AIDS prevention, and were less likely to attribute AIDS to luck or other external factors. Follow-up data were collected from these women 15 months after the intervention (El-Bassel & Schilling, 1992). At this point, skills-building subjects did not appear to obtain or carry condoms more than did control participants and were more likely to attribute AIDS risk to luck. However, most of the posttest gains did not erode over time.

Probably the most extensively used prevention strategy is the one-to-one counseling that occurs in relation to testing for the HIV antibody. Almost 1.5 million HIV antibody tests were performed in publicly funded testing sites in 1990. It is estimated that between 12% and 30% of all HIV antibody tests are being performed on people who had been previously tested (Valdiserri, Jones, West, Campbell, & Thompson, 1993). All of these people have received individual teaching about HIV transmission and a risk assessment. It is unknown how many people have changed their behaviors as a result because many of these sites provide anonymous testing and therefore client data for follow-up is lacking.

## Tailoring the Prevention Strategy

Prevention strategies are most effective when they consider sociodemographic factors like ethnicity, age, gender, educational level, and culture. Many people believe that learning is facilitated when the information is taught by a person who is similar in sociodemographic factors to the target audience. The type of strategy used will be influenced by these sociodemographic issues. To illustrate, the exclusive use of printed materials with a low-literacy population not only might be ineffective, but might also be offensive to the audience. The language of the target audience must also be considered. Although a patient may be fluent in a second language, more intimate matters may be understood better when taught in the subject's primary language. However, language is greatly influenced by geography, and so the meaning of a word in one area may not be the same in a different area of the world. Flaskerud and Uman (1993) found that Hispanics with little education and low levels of acculturation into the dominant U.S. culture were not knowledgeable about HIV/AIDS and had many erroneous beliefs. As a result of these findings, Flaskerud and Uman argued that to consider all Hispanics as a single group may be "ineffective, irrelevant, and insulting" (p. 303).

The impact of social determinants (norms, roles, expectations, and relationships) on sexual risk-reduction behaviors must also be considered. McCoy and Inciardi (1993) drew from a sample of noninjecting female sexual partners of injection drug users and found that sexual risk behaviors were significantly related to crack cocaine use, dislike of condoms, discomfort with talking about condoms, increased number of sexual partners, and employment status. Personal attitude toward condoms was more important than the partner's attitude. The role of women in a specific target group will be shaped by cultural rules and standards. If the woman belongs to a cultural group that rewards submissiveness, an empowerment strategy that emphasizes assertive behaviors can be counterproductive. Instead, an intervention might target both the woman and her sexual partner and work within the values of the culture to promote healthy behaviors. To illustrate, meeting together with a couple and stressing the importance of condom use to safeguard the family may be better received than teaching the wife alone to refuse sex without a condom. Cultural factors can work to facilitate, rather than prevent, safer sex behaviors (Kline, Kline, & Oken, 1992).

Sexual orientation or preference must also be considered. If the woman is exclusively lesbian, it is essential that primary prevention strategies are targeted to address sexual practices between two women. Glove use, care of sex toys, dental dams, and sex during the menstrual period need special instruction. The Gay Men's Health Crisis (212-807-6655) has published a comprehensive pamphlet that provides clear directions related to HIV risk-reduction practices for lesbians.

## Evaluating the Prevention

Irrespective of the type of strategy used to promote HIV risk reduction, evaluation must occur. Evaluation refers to the process of determining the value of a program through a careful examination of its design and objectives, quality of implementation, and short- and long-term outcomes (Rugg, 1990). A complete evaluation plan consists of four elements: (1) formative evaluation conducted prior to project implementation (needs assessment); (2) routine process evaluation of a particular component of the project, such as a class or skills-building session; (3) outcome evaluation to determine the effects of the intervention on HIV incidence or prevalence, the incidence of other sexually transmitted diseases, behavioral outcomes like condom use or number of sexual partners, and changes in AIDS knowledge and attitudes; and (4) summative evaluation that reviews the entire project in terms of cost and accomplishments (AIDSTECH, 1992). A comprehensive evaluation plan is difficult to establish and implement but is the only true test of whether the intervention was helpful and whether it should be replicated on a larger scale or become part of an standardized intervention.

## *Primary Prevention for HIV-Infected Women*

Many of the strategies identified for uninfected persons hold true for women who are already infected. Their needs should be assessed and an intervention should be targeted to address those needs. However, there may be greater tension during sexual activity when the woman is HIV infected, especially if the male partner is uninfected. In this situation, safer sex strategies become even more important, and it is essential to ensure that the woman understands how she can protect herself and her sexual partner. The dynamics of condom use must be completely explored, condoms must be made readily available, and the woman should be encouraged to use contraceptive creams and foams or the female condom during sexual intercourse. The infected woman must also learn how to handle blood spills during everyday activities. She should be encouraged to keep chlorine bleach in the home. Special care should be taken to instruct the woman on how to dispose of her menstrual products and how to handle blood on her clothing. The instruction should be focused so that she understands what areas need special attention (blood, sexual fluids) and what areas do not require any adaptation (laundry, eating utensils, casual touching and hugging, to name a few).

## ❖ Summary

To prevent becoming infected with HIV, certain behaviors must be done consistently. It is not enough to use condoms with casual sexual partners and ignore them during sex with a steady partner. The steady partner could be infected and be unaware of it. Patients need clearer directions about the continuum of behaviors related to HIV transmission. It is not realistic to advise a person never to exchange sexual fluids, nor is it a good idea to stress asking partners about their sexual and drug use history because this history can be replete with gaps. The challenge of primary prevention is to develop clear directives about the continuum of risk behaviors, to instruct on how to engage in those behaviors with the maximum degree of effectiveness, and to develop reinforcement strategies that support the client in sustaining these healthy behaviors over time. Theory-based interventions will generate effective strategies as data are gathered in a variety of settings and with different populations. The challenges are great, but the cost of not trying is the continued spread of HIV and great suffering from AIDS.

## ❖ References

Abraham, C., & Sheeran, P. (1993). In search of a psychology of safer-sex promotion: Beyond beliefs and texts. *Health Education Research, 8*(2), 245–254.

AIDSTECH. (1992). *Tools for project evaluation: A guide for evaluating AIDS prevention interventions.* Durham, NC: Family Health International.

Albee, G. (1989). Primary prevention in public health: Problems and challenges of behavior change as prevention. In V. Mays, G. Albee, & S. Schneider (Eds.), *Primary prevention of AIDS* (pp. 17–22). London: Sage.

Basch, C. (1987). Assessing health education needs: A multidimensional-multimethod approach. In P. Lazes, L. Hollander Kaplan, & K. Gordons (Eds.), *Handbook of health education* (pp. 49–73). Baltimore: Aspen.

Belenky, M., Clinchy, B., Goldberger, N., & Tarule, J. (1986). *Women's ways of knowing.* New York: Basic Books.

Catania, J., Kegeles, S., & Coates, T. (1990). Towards an understanding of risk behavior: An AIDS risk reduction model (ARRM). *Health Education Quarterly, 17*(1), 53–72.

Cates, W., Stewart, F., & Trussell, J. (1992). Commentary: The quest for women's prophylactic methods—Hopes vs science. *American Journal of Public Health, 82*(11), 1479–1482.

Centers for Disease Control and Prevention. (1993). Sexual behavior and condom use—District of Columbia, January–February, 1992. *Morbidity and Mortality Weekly Report, 42* (20), 390–397.

Chu, S., Peterman, T., Doll, L., Buehler, J., & Curran, J. (1992). AIDS in bisexual men in the United States: Epidemiology and transmission to women. *American Journal of Public Health, 82*(2), 220–224.

Cochran, S., & Mays, V. (1990). Sex, lies and HIV. *New England Journal of Medicine, 322*(11), 774–775.

Doak, C. C., Doak, L. G., & Root, J. H. (1985). *Teaching patients with low literacy skills.* Philadelphia: Lippincott.

D'Augelli, A., & Kennedy, S. (1989). An evaluation of AIDS prevention brochures for university women and men. *AIDS Education and Prevention, 1*(2), 134–140.

Ehrhardt, A. (1992). Trends in sexual behavior and the HIV pandemic. *American Journal of Public Health, 82*(11), 1459–1461.

El-Bassel, N., & Schilling, R. (1992). 15-month followup of women methadone patients taught skills to reduce heterosexual HIV transmission. *Public Health Reports, 107*(5), 500–504.

European Study Group on Heterosexual Transmission of HIV. (1992). Comparison of female to male and male to female transmission of HIV in 563 stable couples. *British Medical Journal, 304,* 809–812.

Fishbein, M., & Middlestadt, S. (1989). Using the theory of reasoned action as a framework for understanding and changing AIDS-related behaviors. In V. Mays, G. Albee, & S. Schneider (Eds.), *Primary prevention of AIDS* (pp. 93–110). London: Sage.

Flaskerud, J., & Nyamathi, A. (1990). Effect of an AIDS education program on the knowledge, attitudes, and practices of low income Black and Latina women. *Journal of Community Health, 15*(6), 343–355.

Flaskerud, J., & Uman, G. (1993). Directions for AIDS education for Hispanic women based on analyses of survey findings. *Public Health Reports, 108*(3), 298–304.

Francis, D. (1992). Toward a comprehensive HIV prevention program for the CDC and the nation. *Journal of the American Medical Association, 268*(11), 1444–1447.

Freudenberg, N. (1989). *Preventing AIDS: A guide to effective education for the prevention of HIV infection.* Washington, DC: American Public Health Association.

Green, L., & Kreuter, M. (1991). *Health promotion planning: An educational and environmental approach.* Mountain View, CA: Mayfield.

Jemmott-Sweet, L., & Jemmott, J. (1991). Applying the theory of reasoned action to AIDS risk behavior: Condom use among black women. *Nursing Research, 40*(4), 228–234.

Jonsen, A., & Stryker, J. (Eds.). (1993). *The social impact of AIDS in the United States.* Washington, DC: National Academy Press.

Kenen, R., & Armstrong, K. (1992). The why, when and whether of condom use among female and male drug users. *Journal of Community Health, 17*(5), 303–317.

Kline, A., Kline, E., & Oken, E. (1992). Minority women and sexual choice in the age of AIDS. *Social Science Medicine, 34*(4), 447–457.

Mays, S., Elsesser, V., Schaefer, J., Handford, A., & Good, L. (1992). Sexual practices and AIDS knowledge among women partners of HIV-infected hemophiliacs. *Public Health Reports, 107*(5), 504–514.

McCoy, V., & Inciardi, J. (1993). Women and AIDS: Social determinants of sex related activities. *Women and Health, 20*(1), 69–85.

Montgomery, S., Joseph, J., Becker, M., Ostrow, D., Kessler, R., & Kirscht, J. (1989). The Health Belief Model in understanding compliance with preventive recommendations for AIDS: How useful? *AIDS Education and Prevention, 1*(4), 303–323.

Norr, K., McElmurry, B., Moeti, M., & Tiou, S. (1992). AIDS prevention for women: A community-based approach. *Nursing Outlook, 40*(6), 250–256.

Pender, N. (1987). *Health promotion in nursing practice.* Norwalk, CT: Appleton & Lange.

Richie, B. (1992). *The empowerment program: A curriculum for health education groups for women at Rikers Island.* New York: Hunter College Center on AIDS, Drugs, and Community Health.

Rosenberg, M., & Gollub, E. (1992). Methods women can use that may prevent sexually transmitted disease, including HIV [Commentary]. *American Journal of Public Health, 82*(11), 1473–1478.

Rugg, D. (1990). Evaluating AIDS prevention programs. *Focus: A Guide to AIDS Research and Counseling, 5*(3), 1–2.

Russell, M., Alcober, J., & McKinley, P. (1992, July). *The perception of risk for HIV infection among lesbians in New York City.* Paper presented at the Eighth International Conference on AIDS, Amsterdan, The Netherlands. (Abstract No. PoD 5217)

Saracco, A., Musicco, M., Nicolosi, A., Angarano, G., Arici, C., Gavazzeni, G., Costigliola, P., Gafa, S., Gervasoni, C., & Luzzati, R. (1993). Man-to woman sexual transmission of HIV: Longitudinal study of 343 steady partners of infected men. *Journal of Acquired Immune Deficiency Syndromes, 6*(5), 497–502.

Schaalma, H., Kok, G., & Peters, L. (1993). Determinants of consistent condom use by adolescents: The impact of experience of sexual intercourse. *Health Education Research, 8*(2), 255–269.

Schilling, R., El-Bassel, N., Schinke, S., Gordon, K., & Nichols, S. (1991). Building skills of recovering women drug users to reduce heterosexual AIDS transmission. *Public Health Reports, 106*(3), 297–303.

Selik, R., Chu, S., & Buehler, J. (1993). HIV infection as leading cause of death among young adults in US cities and states. *Journal of the American Medical Association, 269*(23), 2991–2994.

Siegel, L., Attkisson, C., & Carson, L. (1978). Need identification and program planning in a community context. In C. Attkisson (Ed.), *Evaluation of human service programs* (pp. 215–252). New York: Academic Press.

Sotheran, J., Wenston, J., Rockwell, R., DesJarlais, D., & Friedman, S. (1992). *Gender differences in the social context of syringe sharing among New York injecting drug users.* Paper presented at the International Conference on AIDS, Amsterdam, The Netherlands. (Abstract No. PoD 5093)

Thomas, R. (1993). *CondomSense.* (Available from New York State Department of Health, Bureau of Community Relations, Room 1084 Corning Tower, ESP, Albany, NY 12237.)

Tones, K. (1993). Radicalism and the ideology of health education [Editorial]. *Health Education Research, 8*(2), 147–150.

Valdiserri, R., Jones, S., West, G., Campbell, C., & Thompson, P. (1993). Where injecting drug users receive HIV counseling and testing. *Public Health Reports, 108*(3), 294–298.

Valdiserri, R., West, G., Moore, M., Darrow, W., & Hinman, A. (1992). Structuring HIV prevention service delivery systems on the basis of social science theory. *Journal of Community Health, 17*(5), 259–269.

Weiner, A., Wallace, J., Steinberg, A., Hoffmann, B., & Fielding, C. (1992, July). *Intravenous drug use, inconsistent condom use, and fellatio in relationship to crack smoking are risky behaviors for acquiring AIDS in streetwalkers.* Paper presented at the Eighth International Conference on AIDS, Amsterdam, The Netherlands. (Abstract No PoC 4560)

Wells, E., Clark, L., Calsyn, D., Saxon, A., Jackson, T., & Wrede, A. (1992, July). *HIV risk behaviors of heterosexual couples in methadone maintenance.* Paper presented at the Eighth International Conference on AIDS, Amsterdam, The Netherlands. (Abstract No. PoC 4656)

Williams, A. (1991). Women at risk: An AIDS educational needs assessment. *Image: Journal of Nursing Scholarship, 23*(4), 208–213.

Windsor, R., Baranowski, T., Clark, N., & Cutter, G. (1984). *Evaluation of health promotion and education programs.* Mountain View, CA: Mayfield.

## ❖ Chapter 19

# Caring for the Caregiver

JANICE BELL MEISENHELDER

Just as the person with AIDS is vulnerable to a host of physiological, social, and emotional affronts, the caregiver also may face numerous battles in the effort to remain effective in the delivery of care. This chapter addresses the emotional journey experienced by all health professionals—those new to AIDS care as well as those seasoned by experience. Self-care strategies may differ among caregivers, depending on the length of time they have been exposed to this unique pandemic. Although health care professionals are addressed here, the same needs and interventions apply to the patient's family and friends as they struggle to provide care for a loved one with HIV. The intent of this chapter is to give insight into the responses elicited by the disease, to identify the needs of caregiving colleagues and clients, and to suggest supportive interventions for all caregivers.

## ❖ Fear of Contagion—The Meanings of HIV

Many primary care providers feel afraid on their first encounter with patients with the HIV. Such fear may seem unacceptable to them as health care professionals, making a new situation somewhat harder to handle. Surveys of nurses, physicians, and mental health workers have identified fear of contagion as a significant factor in their lack of willingness to work with HIV-infected people (Bolon, Zimmerman, Rodriguez, & Patrone-Reese, 1989; Campbell, Maki, Willenbring, & Henry, 1991; Dow & Knox, 1991; Ficarrotto, Grade, & Zegans, 1991; Makadon & Phillips, 1989; Martindale & Barnett, 1992; Thurn, Campbell, & Henry, 1989; Wiley, Heath, Acklin, Earl, & Barnard, 1990). These studies report 20% to 50% of those sampled as having moderate or severe distress, concern, or desire to avoid people with HIV. Nurses have admitted to avoiding entering the room, touching, or speaking to a person with HIV when such avoidance was possible (Kelly, St. Lawerence, Hood, Smith, & Cook, 1988). Even providers specializing in HIV care experience an occasional, fleeting bout of anxiety over the risk of occupational exposure to infection. This discomfort is distressing to both the health care professional and the patient. People living with HIV often sense the caregiver's anxiety and feel rejected and outcast. Health care professionals try to hide their feelings, which are often expressed indirectly. Caregivers who are comfortable in HIV care would be naive to assume that all of their colleagues share their comfort. Likewise, those with discomfort and a

291

desire to avoid HIV care need reassurance that their reaction is understandable and not uncommon.

This fear of contagion is an anxiety response to the perceived threat of "catching" HIV. Although in reality, HIV is contracted only through very limited and specific situations, the perception of contagion is what leads to avoidance behaviors. Illnesses that have not yet been conquered by science trigger the greatest fear and may therefore be perceived as more contagious than evidence portrays (Sontag, 1977, 1988). The unknowns about HIV disease—its cure, the exact mechanism of transmission, the triggers of disease progression—heighten the perception that the virus is contagious and add to the fear of being out of control and more vulnerable. Cancer, with its unknown cause, sudden appearance of symptoms, and association with death, elicits a similar fear response.

AIDS is symbolically connected to three basic human fears: loss of control, resultant punishment, and death. The connection of sexual and drug-using behaviors with AIDS transmission arouses fear about the loss of personal control to sexual urges and illicit substances. Both drug-related and sexual HIV transmission carry social condemnation and elicit feelings of shame, disgrace, and ostracism. To deny our own vulnerability to death, we often further separate ourselves from terminal patients by finding a reason to blame the victim. This helps to explain the association of deadly diseases with punishment. This assumption of guilt unconsciously clings to all illness, but especially to diseases with devastating consequences; here illness takes on a judgmental meaning. AIDS represents a cultural finger pointed at a guilty party, punished for violation of social taboos (Sontag, 1977, 1988).

The judgment/punishment meaning of AIDS is compounded by its association with sexuality, which, along with death is a taboo subject in our culture. Open expressions of sexuality and homosexuality are viewed as distasteful or disgusting. This theoretical framework can explain fear of contagion with HIV and is supported by studies of nurses and physicians that have shown a relationship between fear of contagion and homophobia, a cultural distaste for homosexuality (Blumenfield, Smith, Milazzo, Seropian, & Wormser, 1987; Campbell et al., 1991; Kelly et al., 1988; Lester & Beard, 1988; Martindale & Barnett, 1992; Merrill, Laux, Wente, & Thornby, 1989; Mills, 1990; Reed, Wise, & Mann, 1984).

Thoughts of death are avoided in our culture, not only by seeking eternal life in medicine, but also by removing death from our consciousness. We no longer bury our loved ones in the community churchyard or lay the recently deceased in private homes. We section off death and hide it in hospitals, funeral homes, and cemeteries. Illness identified with death illicit the same reactions of avoidance and concealment.

Fear of contagion and the perception of AIDS as highly contagious are not a result of casual transmission, but rather of the social meanings of AIDS and the symbolic incorporation of the three powerful fears of loss of control, condemnation, and death. Encouragingly, educational and physical solutions exist to overcome the common but unfortunate reaction of fear. The educational solution to fear of contagion is to acknowledge one's feelings, understand their cultural origin, and ground oneself in the facts of science. The physical solution to fear of contagion is to strictly enforce universal precautions with the same adherence for all patients, regardless of diagnosis.

## ❖ The Educational Solution

Both misunderstanding and lack of sufficient knowledge add to the fear of HIV in our society. When HIV-experienced health care professionals feel fearful, they remind themselves of the facts:

- ❖ HIV is a blood-borne illness.
- ❖ HIV is not contagious via social contact.
- ❖ The occupational risk to health care workers has consistently been calculated at less than 0.5% (Bell, 1990; Fahey, Beekman, Wasserman, Fedio, & Henderson, 1990).

The first step in lowering discomfort is education. Studies have found less fear of contagion with higher educational levels and more accurate knowledge of HIV transmission (Dow & Knox 1991; Gallop et al., 1989; Valenti & Anarella, 1986). However, education alone is insufficient to deal with the powerful, symbolic meaning of HIV disease (Ficarrotto et al., 1991; Lester & Beard, 1988; Link, Feingold, Charap, Freeman, & Shelov, 1988; Martindale & Barnett, 1992). These symbolic effects disappear only as people begin to identify personally with those who are infected. As health care providers work more with people with HIV, they become more comfortable and less concerned with contagion (Strunin & Culbert, 1989; Dow & Knox, 1991; Smith, Godeau, & Katner, 1989; Taylor, Skinner, Eakin, Kelner, & Shapiro, 1989). This is a result of both the volume of exposure and the quality of the social contact (Anderson, Finn, Vojir, Lyne, & Johnson, 1990; Campbell et al., 1991; Lester & Beard, 1988; O'Donnell, O'Donnell, Pleck, Snarey, & Rose, 1987). As experience working with HIV-infected patients grows, identification with those affected becomes more powerful and symbolic connotations become less operational. Once AIDS has a "face" with whom we can identify and empathize, it is no longer a symbol but an undeserved tragedy of life. Once we see people with HIV as folks just like us, we perceive HIV more accurately as an indiscriminate virus causing intense and catastrophic human pain.

Health care professionals need an empathic understanding of the people to whom they give care, especially those from different cultures and lifestyles. Professional exposure is only one way to gain this understanding. For those who are fearful of HIV, volunteer work with an AIDS-prevention organization or other HIV-associated community activity provides a way to learn about and know those involved in the HIV community. These activities provide opportunities for emotional links with HIV-affected people and surround the individual with people who are not fearful of either HIV or the people infected with it. Creating a support network of nonfearful, nonanxious people is critical to remaining effective in providing care to those with AIDS. All educational sessions for health care workers should include an opportunity for people with HIV to share their experiences. Hearing the feelings of people with HIV disease, seeing their expressions, and feeling their pain can decrease the symbolism and replace fear with comfort and empathy (Meisenhelder & Rice, 1993).

As health care professionals, we need to acknowledge fear of contagion as a legitimate feeling and help decrease the anxiety associated with it by a firm embracing of the scientific realities of transmission and a courageous reaching out to patients with HIV infection.

## ❖ The Physical Solution

The only effective way to protect against workplace exposure to HIV is by using universal precautions—the same precautions with everyone. More than this is unnecessary, and less than this increases risk. Health providers must train themselves in the use of precautions until they are automatic. If necessary, an infection-control consultant can watch the professional's practice and provide feedback; failure to meet practice standards may be unconscious behavior. An estimated 50% of occupational exposures could have been prevented if the individuals had been using universal precautions.

For those new to AIDS care, an initial preoccupation with self-protection and the meticulous overuse of barrier precautions are classic manifestations of the fear of contagion. Although excessive fear is nonproductive, providers must focus on learning and implementing appropriate practices for physical self-protection at all times. An opposite reaction can occur with experienced AIDS providers who become careless about universal precautions. As patients with HIV become more like their acquaintances or friends, their perceived need to don gloves and mask sometimes decreases to a dangerous level. These providers need to focus on maintaining respect for the virus at all times. Health care professionals also put themselves at increased risk when they are certain that they can identify the patients who are HIV positive and therefore feel they know when to take "extra" precautions. When protection becomes inconsistent or careless, it is the unsuspected or unidentified client who is likely to cause an exposure.

## ❖ Cumulative Grief

Grief is the deep distress or sadness caused by the loss of someone or something dear to us. It is most intense immediately following the loss but may overwhelm us at unexpected moments. Grief comes in waves that force us to think of that which was lost, and it floods us with sadness.

Grieving is an automatic consequence of caring. It is a part of living. Every change in life is associated with some loss. Yet in our culture, openly expressing grief is taboo. Jacqueline Kennedy was acclaimed for her stoic ability to endure the shock and trauma of her husband's assassination without breaking down in public and without demonstrating grief. Because of our cultural discomfort with grief, it is often submerged inside and banished from consciousness. There, like other contained emotions, grief builds, seethes, and continues to cause misery.

A more useful and healthy way to handle grief is to acknowledge and express the loss. Because loss is a part of everyday living, grieving is like breathing, like letting out carbon dioxide to make room for oxygen. By letting out the pain, we make room for feelings of well-being. The comfort achieved by expressing grief and pain is an essential health-maintenance activity not only for those in AIDS care; it is critical for everyone.

The act of grieving honors that which was lost (Phillips, 1989), and grief enables us to remember the lost person. When we fight the instinct to remember, the images of the lost one haunt us during our daily activity, distracting us from work and play. When we acknowledge the loss and allow time to grieve, we find relief from the memories and can engage in life more freely. In this way, the Names Project, the sponsor of the AIDS Memorial Quilt, has served an invaluable service for all those who have contributed panels. The Names Project represents a national, voluntary effort to create a continuous memorial to those who died of AIDS. The Names Project facilitates grieving and provides a tangible outlet for feelings and a concrete expression of remembrance (Names Project, 23-62 Market St., San Francisco, CA 94107, tel. 415-882-5500).

For health professionals, the challenge is to allow for grieving, to give in to the memories, and to feel the pain in order to let it go. Structured opportunities to express grief are helpful for providers. One inpatient unit sends cards to the families, giving all caregivers an opportunity to write personal notes. Many attend funerals or wakes, which provide an opportunity for closure of the relationship. Support groups at the work site provide a wonderfully effective means for processing feelings in a shared environment. Many organizations sponsor spiritual healing services for those affected by HIV, offering comfort and hope in addition to support.

For some, grieving is a private activity. It may include planting a garden in memory of those for whom they have cared or keeping a journal, scrapbook, or photo album. It may be just setting aside time to reflect or meditate. The means of expression is not important, but taking the time to confront whatever emotions are brewing is important. Pain and grief must be allowed to escape constructively, providing the opportunity to renew and reenergize for the next day.

Some health care professionals protect themselves against experiencing grief by detaching from clients. This coping mechanism is helpful only to a point. To give effective care, attachment and detachment must be balanced so that caregivers can identify and empathize without feeling overwhelming personal loss with each death. Too much attachment cripples our effectiveness by the enormity of the emotions; too little leaves us uncaring and unresponsive. As health professionals, we need to strike the balance between meeting our responsibilities to our clients and to ourselves (Carmack, 1992).

Detachment may be a necessary coping strategy when we encounter clients who are too much like ourselves. Strong identification with a patient may make the caring too painful or too emotionally intense. This situation is intensified as more women and children with HIV infection are seen, giving their female providers personal distress and an increased awareness of their own vulnerability. Providers may find detachment the only way to continue to work with this population. Setting boundaries between the professional and personal areas of life is one way to separate the issues.

Finding a support group of peers who are confronting the same issues may be critical to working through the emotions sufficiently to remain effective in giving care. Often, such gender- and role-specific groups must be created from scratch, but sufficient perseverance and commitment make them worthwhile. Even a small support network that understands the clinical setting and identifies with our own concerns can be tremendously helpful. It is important for primary care providers to focus on the areas in which we can have a positive impact and to let go of those areas in which we have no control.

## ❖ Self-Care

One of the biggest problems in AIDS care is the feeling of frustration associated with our inability to conquer the disease. The more overwhelmed we feel by the tragedy of AIDS, the more compelled we are to work. For some of us, work becomes the means to run from the feelings inside us or to convince ourselves of our own irreplaceability. Work might also be a struggle to control that which we cannot control: illness, death, other people's behaviors. With mounting frustration, we hurl ourselves even more into our efforts, as if by working harder we could have more control. As primary care professionals, we often feel compelled to help others, even at the expense of ourselves. We need to resist this temptation. We cannot help anyone unless we first take care of ourselves. Burned-out health care professionals are ineffective and might do more harm than good.

Rather than trying to control the uncontrollable, we need to acknowledge our human limitations as well as our human potential and to set realistic objectives for our contributions. Then we must see that our contributions are dependent on our ability to keep ourselves healthy: emotionally, spiritually, and physically. Self-care must come before caring for others, for we must maintain our own stamina as well as be role models of self-care for others. All health-maintenance principles apply to health care professionals: Eat nutritiously, exercise regularly, sleep sufficiently, and laugh frequently. Taking time for self-care is not being selfish, but rather being wise and prudent.

For AIDS caregivers, the constant exposure to tragedy mandates a personal life-style that thrives on hope, optimism, and humor. The more we are confronted with life's pain in the workplace, the more we need levity and relief in our personal time. For this reason, we should choose comedies rather than dramas, swing in the playground or play softball rather than watch the news, read a humor magazine instead of a serious journal. The more deadly serious our lives are at work, the more lightheartedness we need in our time off to keep our balance and our perspective. We can cultivate recreational activities and habits that focus on creativity, life, hope, and laughter. We can read the newspaper comics before the headlines. For most of us, our commitment to the caring professions and to serving those in need is so intense that letting go of that seriousness, even in our personal lives, can be a struggle, but it is a necessary struggle. We must critically examine how we spend our time and must consciously construct a life that will sustain our hope and our health for years to come. This may mean working fewer hours. However, the significance of a lasting contribution may be greater than that of a brief, intense outpouring that results in burnout.

A major safeguard of mental health for primary care providers is a support network. The more relationships that offer such comfort, the greater the emotional margin of safety against life's traumas. The key to meeting our needs for social reinforcement is to find the right reference group. One effective strategy for creating a support network is through professional groups or subgroups of professional organizations. If it is important to feel empowered, a politically focused group may be appropriate. Spiritual groups may provide the peace needed to continue with work that can make us feel helpless and powerless. A combination of several of these possibilities may be best to provide reinforcement in different areas.

Health professionals should also seek out those who make up a critical reference group for them and should make this commitment a priority. A network of support improves the enjoyment and satisfaction of life and provides comfort when confronting pain. Connecting with others offers emotional protection from the perpetual losses experienced by AIDS caregivers. Family and friends are indispensable. Take the time to cultivate people with whom you can share, and maintain those relationships. Relationships require continuous investment; they rarely maintain themselves. Yet, the support of human understanding is immeasurable. All humans need affection, someone to hold us when we are in pain. Even a loyal pet can provide companionship. The context of the relationship is not important, but its existence is.

## ❖ Summary

For those providing AIDS care, the challenge is to take time to nurture and renew ourselves—physically, emotionally, and spiritually. Physically, we need to protect ourselves appropriately with the consistent use of universal precautions and stable eating, sleeping, and exercising habits.

Emotionally, we need to acknowledge and express the full gamut of our feelings, ground ourselves in scientific knowledge, and surround ourselves with optimism and new life by connecting with others. Spiritually, we need to focus on the eternal, the hope of life, trusting in that which is beyond our control in order to handle the frustration of our daily tasks. The better we care for ourselves, the more we will have to offer those to whom we give care—the women and children affected by HIV.

## ❖ References

Anderson, D. G., Finn, J., Vojir, C. P., Lyne, B., & Johnson, E. J. (1990). Caring for AIDS patients in rural settings: Nursing's challenge for the 1990's. *Sixth International Conference on AIDS: Final Program & Abstracts, 3*, 307.

Bell, D. (1990, June). *Occupational risk of HIV-infection in health care workers in the United States.* Paper presented at the Sixth International Conference on AIDS, San Francisco.

Blumenfield, M., Smith, P. J., Milazzo, J., Seropian, S., & Wormser, G. P. (1987). Survey of attitudes of nurses working with AIDS patients. *General Hospital Psychiatry, 9*, 58–63.

Bolon, T., Zimmerman, R., Rodriguez, M., & Petrone-Reese, J. (1989). HIV-related risk, worry and behavior changes among emergency medical workers: Personal and job-related factors. *Fifth International Conference on AIDS: Abstracts*, 724.

Campbell, S., Maki, M., Willenbring, K., & Henry, K. (1991). AIDS-related knowledge, attitudes, and behaviors among 629 registered nurses at a Minnesota hospital: A descriptive study. *Journal of the Association of Nurses in AIDS Care, 2*, 15–23.

Carmack, B. J. (1992). Balancing engagement/detachment in AIDS-related multiple losses. *Image, 24*(1), 9–14.

Dow, M. G., & Knox, M. D. (1991). Mental health and substance abuse staff HIV/AIDS knowledge and attitudes. *AIDS Care, 3*(1), 75–87.

Fahey, B. J., Beekman, S., Wasserman, B., Fedio, J., & Henderson, D. K. (1990). Assessment of risk for occupational HIV-1 infection in health care workers (HCW) and follow-up of HCW electing zidovudine (ZDV) chemoprophylaxis. *Sixth International Conference on AIDS: Final Program & Abstracts, 1*, 274.

Ficarrotto, T. J., Grade, M., & Zegans, L. S. (1991). Occupational and personal risk estimates for HIV contagion among incoming graduate nursing students. *Journal of the Association of Nurses in AIDS Care, 2*, 5–11.

Gallop, R., Taerk, G., Lancee, W. J., Coates, R., Fanning, M., & Keatings, M. (1989). Knowledge, attitude and concerns of hospital staff about AIDS. *Fifth International Conference on AIDS: Abstracts*, 720.

Kelly, J. A., St. Lawrence, J. S., Hood, H. V., Smith, S., & Cook, D. J. (1988). Nurses' attitudes towards AIDS. *Journal of Continuing Education in Nursing, 19*, 78–83.

Lester, L. B., & Beard, B. J. (1988). Nursing students' attitudes toward AIDS. *Journal of Nursing Education, 27*, 399–404.

Link, R. N., Feingold, A. R., Charap, M. H., Freeman, K., & Shelov, S. P. (1988). Concerns of medical and pediatric house officers about acquiring AIDS from their patients. *American Journal of Public Health, 78*, 455–459.

Makadon, H. J., & Phillips, R. S. (1989). Attitudes and practices of general internists regarding care of people with HIV infection. *Fifth International Conference on AIDS: Abstracts*, 724.

Martindale, L., & Barnett, C. (1992). Nursing faculty's knowledge and attitudes towards persons with AIDS. *Journal of the Association of Nurses in AIDS Care, 3*(2), 9–13.

Meisenhelder, J. B., & Rice, L. (1993, April). *Evaluating interventions for fear of contagion.* Poster presented at the annual Region V conference of Sigma Theta Tau, Boston.

Merrill, J. M., Laux, L., Wente, S., & Thornby, J. (1989). Improving the care of AIDS patients: Roles of provider gender and specificity of training. *Fifth International Conference on AIDS: Abstracts*, 697.

Mills, C. (1990). Interns' and residents' knowledge and attitudes concerning HIV infection. *Sixth International Conference on AIDS: Final Program & Abstracts, 3*, 306.

O'Donnell, L., O'Donnell, C. R., Pleck, J. H., Snarey, J., & Rose, R. M. (1987). Psychosocial responses of hospital workers to acquired immune deficiency syndrome (AIDS). *Journal of Applied Social Psychology, 17*, 269–285.

Phillips, J. (1989). Sustaining our hope. In J. B. Meisenhelder & C. L. Charite (Eds.), *Comfort in caring: Nursing the person with HIV infection* (pp. 31–38). Glenview, IL: Scott, Foresman/Little, Brown.

Reed, P., Wise, T. N., & Mann, L. S. (1984). Nurses' attitudes regarding acquired immunodeficiency syndrome (AIDS). *Nursing Forum, 21*, 153–156.

Smith, M. U., Godeau, R. E., & Katner, H. P. (1989). Knowledge and attitudes of rural Georgia physicians concerning AIDS. *Fifth International Conference on AIDS: Abstracts*, 720.

Sontag, S. (1977). *Illness as a metaphor.* New York: Farrar, Straus & Giroux.

Sontag, S. (1988). *AIDS and its metaphors.* New York: Farrar, Straus & Giroux.

Strunin, L., & Culbert, A. (1989). Medical students' knowledge and concerns about HIV infection. *Fifth International Conference on AIDS: Abstracts*, 722.

Taylor, K. M., Skinner, H. A., Eakin, J. M., Kelner, M. J., & Shapiro, M. (1989). Physicians' perception of personal risk from AIDS. *Fifth International Conference on AIDS: Abstracts*, 723.

Thurn, J. R., Campbell, S., & Henry, K. (1989). The impact of AIDS on acute care hospitals: A survey of infectious disease teaching hospitals in the United States. *Fifth International Conference on AIDS: Abstracts*, 697.

Valenti, W. M., & Anarella, J. P. (1986). Survey of hospital personnel on the understanding of the acquired immunodeficiency syndrome. *American Journal of Infection Control, 14*, 60–63.

Wiley, K., Heath, L., Acklin, M., Earl, A., & Barnard, B. (1990). Care of HIV infected patients: Nurses' concerns, opinions, and precautions. *Applied Nursing Research, 3*(1), 27–33.

# ❖ Index